THE BODY Soviet

THE BODY Soviet

Propaganda, Hygiene, and the Revolutionary State

Tricia Starks

THE UNIVERSITY OF WISCONSIN PRESS

This book was published with the support of the History Department, the Graduate School, and the Fulbright College of Arts and Sciences, all at the University of Arkansas.

The University of Wisconsin Press
1930 Monroe Street, 3rd Floor
Madison, Wisconsin 53711-2059

www.wisc.edu/wisconsinpress/

3 Henrietta Street
London WC2E 8LU, England

5 4 3 2 1

Printed in the United States of America

Library of Congress Cataloging-in-Publication Data
Starks, Tricia, 1969–
The body Soviet : propaganda, hygiene, and the revolutionary state / Tricia Starks.
p. cm.
Originally presented as the author's thesis (Ph. D.)—Ohio State University, 1999.
Includes bibliographical references and index.
ISBN 978-0-299-22960-3 (cloth : alk. paper)—ISBN 978-0-299-22964-1 (pbk. : alk. paper)
1. Soviets (People)—Health and hygiene. 2. Hygiene—Political aspects—Soviet Union. 3. Public health—Political aspects—Soviet Union. 4. Propaganda, Communist—Soviet Union. I. Title.
RA395.S65S72 2008
362.1089′917—dc22 2008011972

An earlier version of chapter 4 appeared as "A Revolutionary Home: Housekeeping and Social Duty in the 1920s," *Revolutionary Russia* 17, no. 1 (2004): 69–104; reprinted with the permission of Taylor and Francis Group (www.informaworld.com). An earlier version of chapter 5 appeared as "A Fertile Mother Russia: Pro-Natalist Propaganda in Revolutionary Russia," *The Journal of Family History* 28, no. 3 (2003): 411–42; reprinted with the permission of Sage Publications.

TO

my parents

CONTENTS

ILLUSTRATIONS

Figures

ACKNOWLEDGMENTS

Za vashe zdorov'e! ("To your health!") The toast that has launched a million celebratory gatherings in Russia—and dozens that I have had the great joy to attend personally—seems a fitting beginning to the most enjoyable part of any book—the moment when the author thanks all those who have helped to bring it into existence. I wish a hearty "To your health!" to all who helped me in the long journey from research to completion of the writing of this book, with all the twists and turns into archives, museums, parks, and pastry shops that the trip entailed.

Of course, the journey has been enjoyable but also expensive. The research for this work was funded by a Fulbright-Hays Dissertation Research Fellowship, the Kennan Center for Advanced Russian Studies at the Woodrow Wilson Center, and The Ohio State University Slavic Center. While in Russia I was assisted by affable, able scholars, including the knowledgeable and helpful Natalia Lvovna Pushkareva, who introduced me to others in Russia working on both Soviet history and gender studies. I also wish to thank the members of her family, who always made me feel at home at their kitchen table, feeding me and supporting me as I bumbled along. In addition to Russian scholars, I met with many generous women at archives and libraries. I am especially indebted to the perennially cheerful and interested Svetlana Nikolaevna Artamonova, of the Graphics Department of the Russian State Library, for her help in locating, reproducing, and interpreting the images used in this book.

On American shores, I wish to convey special thanks to Leila Rupp for her support and example, Eve Levin for her encouragement and spirit, and David Hoffmann for his suggestions and dry humor. While the zealous Allan K. Wildman did not get to see the completed dissertation, he guided me in my early years of graduate school and encouraged me in the project. I wrote many of the passages in this manuscript in dialogue with his memory. I could not have survived graduate school without my comrades-in-arms here and in Russia: Jen Anderson, Victor Boldeskul, Elizaveta Gorchakova, Paul Hibbeln, Pam Pennock, Aaron Retish, Bill Risch, Matt Romaniello, and Kurt (Koba) Schultz. They helped me to see the light at the end of the tunnel yet not miss the fun along the way. Aaron deserves a special award for suffering through multiple drafts of chapters, introductions, and grant proposals yet always giving good advice and asking provocative questions. Since leaving school, I have benefited from discussions with other scholars both abroad and at home. Greta Bucher, Michael David-Fox, Michelle DenBeste, Diane Koenker, Karen Petrone, A. K. Sokolov, and Kate Transchel all gave generously of their time, offering advice both academic and professional.

At the University of Arkansas I lucked into a group of fine scholars and great colleagues. David Chappell, Charles Robinson, Kathryn (M. D.) Sloan, and Beth (M. F.) Schweiger provided camaraderie and strength, while Evan Bukey, Lynda (P. G.) Coon, and Robert Finlay read early drafts of the manuscript and provided excellent comments from outside the field. Lynda challenged me to think in ways both broad and deep about gender, space, and cultural history. Anything remotely interesting that I might have to say I owe to her keen mind. Suzanne Maberry initially edited the manuscript with incredible attention to detail and left wry comments in the margins that provoked laughter to soothe the sting. I was fortunate to find Natalia Shchegoleva in the wilds of Arkansas to check the Russian throughout the manuscript. Anonymous readers for the University of Wisconsin Press further honed the analysis by pointing out flaws and omissions. Of course, whatever problems remain are purely a result of my own stubbornness in the face of strong argument and inexorable logic.

In the final stages of preparation, Larry Malley of the University of Arkansas Press showed the true spirit of academic support by providing advice and introductions. Revisions have been supported by funds from the University of Arkansas and Professor Jim Jones, who fully lived up to the title of Distinguished Professor of History by giving me—as well as all the junior faculty at the time—financial support and sage advice. Steve Salemson initially and Gwen Walker subsequently shepherded the manuscript through the University of Wisconsin Press. They were both attentive to my many questions as were Michel Hogue and Adam Mehring. Henry Krawitz's careful edit saved me from making many errors. The printing of color visuals was subvented by funds from the following agencies of the University of Arkansas: the Fulbright College of Arts and Sciences, the Graduate School, and the Department of History.

Finally, from start to finish, I have been aided by my family. I owe the greatest thanks to my mother and father, who always encouraged me to go, do, and try; to Mike Pierce, who helped me to keep going, do more, and try harder; and to Ben, who provided a respite from it all. I would not have finished without your love and unflagging support.

THE BODY *Soviet*

Introduction

In the midst of the devastating Russian civil war, V. I. Lenin turned his attention from the bourgeois parasite to another bloodsucker—the louse. "Either the lice will defeat socialism," he cautioned the 1919 All-Russia Congress of Soviets, "or socialism will defeat the lice."[1] Concern for health is not often associated with the years of revolution, but even in the thick of war Lenin's attention to hygiene made sense.[2] From 1919 through 1923 three quarters of the population suffered from starvation. As hunger weakened immune systems, waves of louse-born typhus, Spanish influenza, cholera, smallpox, and even plague coursed through Russia. Disease and famine killed as many as ten million Russians from 1914 to 1921 and left many times that number crippled or chronically ill.[3] The Bolsheviks inherited a sick population as well as an industrially defunct and militarily weak state. To restore Russian might and create a model state, Lenin saw the need for a more virile population, insisting "the fight for socialism is at the same time the fight for health."[4]

While historians are familiar with Lenin's battle cry against the louse, its relevance to political, cultural, and social issues has been lost.[5] Health was of immediate, vital importance to the new state for political stability, productive industry, and military manpower, but revolutionaries characterized health programs as necessary for more than mere survival. Caring for the population was a duty. Capitalism had stunted workers' lives and banished them to fetid basements. Revolutionaries pledged to provide the people with better living quarters, improved working conditions, and universal medical care. Reformers moved workers from overcrowded barracks into confiscated bourgeois housing. The government enacted protective legislation, and in 1918 the Narodnyi komissariat zdravookhraneniia (People's Commissariat of Public Health; hereafter Narkomzdrav) began a quest to protect the health and welfare of all citizens.[6]

Revolutionaries agitated for health as a matter of survival, duty, and political change. Narkomzdrav advocates worked alongside cultural and revolutionary theorists, who considered clean living part of their own utopian projects.[7] These professionals and supporters can collectively be termed "hygienists" for their unified support of habits for body, home, and life centered on order, rationality, and balance.[8] Just as many agendas included hygienic measures, not all hygiene recommendations can be ascribed to concerns about disease. Hygiene carries with it connotations far beyond health. The word "hygiene," rooted in the cult of the goddess Hygeia, retains much of the Greek emphasis upon balance and reason as the basis for personal and societal health.[9] As such, hygiene implies more than a condition of the body or environment and entails the creation of order and political systems. As did most medical authorities around the globe, Soviet activists included these classical concepts in their programs to cultivate the people and bring function to the state.

Hygienists' concerns, while seemingly cultural in form, were political in motivation. In their language, pamphlets, and programs, Soviet hygienists associated mental acuity, political orthodoxy, and modernity with lives lived according to the concepts of balance and reason. These presumed benefits from a regulated, hygienic lifestyle informed medical inquiry, education, and state programs. Soviet hygienists believed that ordered lives produced healthy bodies and politically enlightened, productive, and happy populations; strong bodies generated balanced minds that would, in turn, choose the most rational, equitable, and inevitable of political, social, and economic structures, namely, socialism. Furthermore, the cleansed body was not just a building block of the socialist utopia; it became the material manifestation of the revolution's success. Since the state, the nation, and the family would all "wither away," it was the population whose transformation would signal the success of revolution. Thus, the rationalized Soviet body was more essential to the socialist utopia than even the state; the creation of the body Soviet was the creation of the socialist utopia.

State-sponsored institutions and campaigns disseminated the message of hygiene in their quest to reform the population. Museums demonstrated the positive effects of fresh air, sunshine, and exercise. Actors staged show trials of people exhibiting "holdover" behaviors, such as the illiterate, the drunkard, the slob, the libertine, and the spitter.[10] Tuberculosis treatment centers and workers' vacation homes counseled hygienic behavior as the foundation of an entire "healthful" lifestyle, showing Russians how to eat, bathe, and decorate the house, as well as what kinds of activities could replace the usual boozing and romancing hygienists associated with worker leisure. Workers' clubs held lectures, screened films, and sponsored discussions on health themes, while workers' commissions organized weeklong campaigns to clean transit areas, barracks, and factories.[11]

Hygienists' plans were grand, and their dreams often exceeded their grasp. When lack of funding made it difficult for hygienists to counsel every citizen, cheap propaganda bridged the gap. Pamphlets and posters trumpeted a clean, ordered life, while brochures, magazine articles, leaflets, postcards, and newspapers also spread the word.[12] Contemporary observers and later historians have noted the ubiquity of Soviet propaganda and commented upon the massive amount of health messages in these posters, pamphlets, and newspapers. The numbers support their casual observations. Between January 1919 and June 1922, during a period of relative austerity, hygienists published over thirteen million pieces of public health literature and put out millions more pieces over the decade, with titles as diverse as *Tuberculosis and the Home, Strengthening the Will, Why Is Tobacco Dangerous?, To the Book or for a Beer?*, or *The Art of Dressing.*[13]

While hygienists provided a barrage of propaganda, health inspectors—medical professionals or citizen volunteers—served as the shock troops of sanitation. The government gave inspectors authority to examine living conditions, recommend changes, provide rewards, and relocate families. Inspectors patrolled factories, schools, buildings, and even individual apartments. Narkomzdrav permitted volunteers—whose sole qualification seems to have been a willingness to serve—to assist inspectors and, in severe cases, evict tenants.[14] These inspectors and volunteers proffered personal advice and left propaganda brochures in their wake.

The prevalence of propaganda and the companion surveillance institutions brought Soviet approaches to public health in line with other programs around the world. Soviet public health was built upon the German economic theory of cameralism, which emphasized controlling the population for economic and political stability, and expanded upon the examples of treatment and monitoring centers worldwide. But in Russia—and later in the Soviet Union—utopian ideas, political objectives, and a different interpretation of the divisions of public and private led to an application of health programs at a more invasive and pervasive level than elsewhere. Health activists, cultural revolutionaries, and major political figures treated issues of home, body, life, and leisure as public concerns essential to the Soviet project. Control became a central issue of public health and took on particular importance in the Soviet Union. Divisions of public/private and political/cultural are much more delineated in liberal states (albeit blurred, as Foucauldian scholars have noted), but the Soviets stretched these boundaries still further.[15] Soviet health programs were more thoroughly applied, more intense in their surveilling, and more radically conceived than anywhere else.[16] Though Narkomzdrav never managed to receive the budget or personnel necessary to completely implement universal health care and observation, the importance of hygiene decisions to citizenship and the success of the state resulted in a system of Soviet health care that was more expansive than that of any other contemporary state.

The program of public health did not spring fully formed from the pate of Lenin. There existed similarities of process and programs from across two divides—the geographic and the temporal. A long tradition of Western and Russian public health influenced the creation of Soviet programs. During the nineteenth century Russian public health physicians studied the connections between social conditions and disease and touted social change as a means to substantive progress in health. The Soviet use of health inspectors to control private lives mirrored programs in the United States, Britain, France, and Germany.[17] The similarity of Soviet programs makes the detailing of Soviet public health important for the history of global public health since it has been marginalized for too long. While the Soviets rejected capitalism, they adapted Western and prerevolutionary population control techniques—especially the surveillance state and the medicalized gaze—in their pursuit of socialist success.[18]

The tracking of the discourse of health—all manner of expression designed to coerce, edify, and transform the population into what political, scientific, and cultural experts deemed healthy citizens—does not reveal the condition of Soviet health. Its concrete impact on Soviet lives and identities is difficult to gauge.[19] The didactic messages do not mirror reality, nor does their ubiquity even indicate popular interest. Health statistics showed a rise in the population's health, but the numbers themselves are suspect and any improvement could have been due to better diets, cleaner cities, or more comprehensive water and sewage provisions. Within Narkomzdrav, budgetary and personnel problems left the countryside with insufficient care or a lack of materials for decades; low literacy and poor distribution lessened the impact of propaganda outside of the center. The state's lack of resources in the 1920s ensured that the battle for better health would be largely symbolic rather than coercive, but this should not be gauged as lack of importance. The influence of hygiene campaigns cannot be measured in terms of the piles of rubles spent or the number of institutions founded. As bureaucratic decisions and economic necessity led to the watering down of programs, hygienists waxed on about ideal programs, utopian societies, and perfected citizens, revealing new ideas of citizenship, state authority, and revolution alongside new techniques for control.

The fervor of reformers in defining and creating health programs was important in and of itself, revealing the anxiety of hygienists and leaders over the population's state of disorder.[20] The mere conception of these reforms reaffirmed the primacy of science, the necessity of rationalization, the need for order, and the centrality of hygienic control to revolutionary action. Whereas nation-states trust in a common, imagined past to provide community, the Soviets relied upon an idealized, imagined future. Ideas held strong currency in this world's construction—particularly concepts of cleanliness. Hygiene became part of an all-encompassing ideology of enlightened, Soviet behavior. Ideologies are more than beliefs or ideas. According to Dale B. Martin, they can become a "symbolic matrix that makes sense of and supports a particular exercise of power and the power structures that exist."[21] These ideologies created, tamed, and tempered the individual and the corporate body in the quest to create a political organism. Soviet definitions of dirt reinforced ethnic, class, and political prejudices.[22] Notions of hygiene, purity, and health involved more than just the care of the body; they informed the construction of Soviet institutions and identity.

The present study of Moscow highlights the ideal of health care, the aspirations of reformers, and the discourse of health surrounding the policy makers of the day as well as subsequent decades. Only major urban areas witnessed anything close to an ideal application of health programs, and Moscow's centrality to government, society, and culture created a vortex of need and attention. While it was hard to find medical care in the countryside, Moscow was blessed with an overabundance of medical professionals. Before and after the revolution, the majority of medical personnel and resources gravitated to Moscow. Although far from ideal circumstances reigned during the 1920s, Moscow was the best supplied of the major cities.[23]

Muscovite health was most vital since this environment influenced the decisions and rhetoric of Soviet governance and the creation of the state. Health problems in Moscow took on added urgency after the capital was moved from Petrograd to Moscow in 1918. In 1920 Lenin argued that Moscow had to be cleansed not just for the health of its inhabitants but for the health of the worldwide revolution: "We must do this so as to set an example to the whole country where this filth . . . is becoming more and more prevalent. We must set this example here, in Moscow."[24] Lenin's attention to the sanitation of Moscow materialized not just out of concern for stability but also based on his understanding of the symbolic significance of the capital. Moscow was a city of revolution, with monuments and celebrations that glorified its history, but it was also a living example of revolutionary change. Government officials and interested parties could not avoid seeing the problems at their doorsteps, and they could not hide them from visiting politicians and international workers' delegations. For these bureaucrats, revolutionaries, hygienists, workers, and interested foreign observers, the health of Moscow testified to the health of the revolution.

By examining the rich sources of health care propaganda, from posters and pamphlets to traveling museums and theater troops, and by scrutinizing the institutions that displayed, performed, and produced health care propaganda, this book places hygiene and the rhetoric of health at the heart of the revolutionary endeavor. Archival collections from health departments at city, regional, and state levels provided information on the activities of institutions, but collections of pamphlets, books, posters, and museum exhibits proved equally important for plotting the rhetoric of health. As a result of this novel source base, research from outside the archives and influences from beyond the field of history—including theoretical paradigms drawn from cultural studies, film theory, museum studies, and postmodern critiques of the Enlightenment—inform the present analysis. In order to make this work more useful for those interested in public health globally, comparative work and brief historical narratives have been provided where context seemed necessary. Finally, while this book highlights Narkomzdrav institutions—especially those in Moscow—it does not attempt to detail the full history of the commissariat. The investigation of propaganda and use of interdisciplinary techniques make this not an institutional history but rather a cultural investigation of the ideologies forged, transformed, and transmitted by health organizations and revolutionary activists, which in time flowed through all areas of the Soviet Union.

The book is comprised of six thematic sections, starting with the macrocosmic level of impersonal ideologies of the corporate body Soviet and moving to the microcosmic sphere of the individual Soviet body. Chapter 1, "Revolution: Destruction, Cleansing, and Creation," details the genesis of the Soviet preoccupation with hygiene in the language of revolution and the concerns of utopian tradition. The October Revolution provided both the opportunity and the impetus for reform, and in revolutionary rhetoric hygienic language framed political discussion. An overview of major themes of utopian literature illustrates how their glorification of science, medicine, communal ideals, and concern for individual behavior grounded the visions of hygienists and political figures. For hygienists dirt and disorder bred disease. They thus argued that if society were reorganized, the conditions for disease would disappear. Like the family and the state, the military and diplomacy, with the growth of socialism disease itself would wither and die. While Lenin and other revolutionaries imbued dirt with political significance, not all revolutionary groups looked upon untidiness with suspicion. The population resisted the imposed structures of the hygienists and seemingly regarded dirt according to their own biases. Some viewed pressed pants and well-maintained lodgings as bourgeois rather than revolutionary.

Chapter 2, "The State: Diagnosing, Monitoring, and Disciplining," links Soviet health care of the 1920s to worldwide trends toward pronatalism, surveillance, and public health. Hygienic concepts of order and rationality founded the ideology of revolution, and European and Russian institutional forms guided the imposition of these behaviors. Through institutions such as the dispensary and consultation, Narkomzdrav attempted to monitor and treat the population, but infighting by unions and other government agencies for scant material resources conspired to limit the reach of new programs. Narkomzdrav relied upon worker initiated programs alongside propaganda to implement and spread the call for preventative care. Although propaganda constituted the most prevalent form of health intervention in the lives of average citizens, it was subject to problems as well.

Chapter 3, "The City: Instruction, Regulation, and Isolation," addresses hygienists' attempts to control leisure in order to increase worker productivity and smooth the functioning of the state. Hygienists' diagnosis of the evils of modern life provided a conceptual basis for attacks upon dissolute living, slatternly appearance, and poor leisure habits. Within the city reformers hailed the activities of worker clubs, red corners (smaller versions of the club), night sanatoriums, and youth groups as healthful leisure activities that could counter the corrupting influences of the boulevards and beer halls. As a more drastic remedy, Narkomzdrav set up a system of Houses of Leisure and sanatoriums in the countryside to isolate workers periodically from pernicious, urban influences and to provide them with a regimen of healthful living, including cleanliness, physical activity, and correct nutrition, as well as less health-related skills such as etiquette and cultural appreciation. Resistance from the population limited the impact of these programs since popular views concerning leisure often differed from expert opinion.

Chapter 4, "The Home: Housekeeping, Social Duty, and Public Concern," includes recommendations for maintenance of a clean home that appeared in the Soviet press, posters, and pamphlets. While authorities emphasized the importance of maintaining the home for the health of society, this did not result in a glorification of household labor. Despite calls for the liberation of women, the dissolution of the family, and the creation of communal facilities to end the drudgery of housework, Soviet hygienists' programs for the upkeep of the home did not differ sharply from Western or prerevolutionary Russian ideas. Hygienists' recommendations for increased attention to domestic maintenance without the provision of laundry, child care, or other programs undermined Soviet promises to liberate women from the tyranny of the hearth. Exacerbating these contradictions, hygienists overlooked the lack of communal facilities and the impossibility of fulfilling these dictums given the crude domestic situation. Instead of liberating women from the home, hygienists increased the chores of women, more firmly connected housework to women's responsibility, and complicated domestic tasks.

Chapter 5, "The Family: Maternity, Birth, and Parenthood," investigates Narkomzdrav's Department for the Protection of Motherhood and Infancy (Otdel okhrany materinstva i mladenchestva) to offer a picture of the changing experience of parenthood in the 1920s. While campaigns for natal health elevated the importance of child care, the dependence upon doctors' advice devalued women's caregiving in favor of a new, rationalized, skilled type of motherhood in which anyone could become proficient if given professional instruction and supervision. Calls for higher birth rates and lower infant death rates motivated the professionalization of motherhood and placed Soviet natalism on the same trajectory as European and American movements."[25] Although hygienists vilified traditional caregivers and gave preference to a new, scientific, doctor-managed child care, the provision of new care facilities lagged.

Chapter 6, "The Body: Hygiene, Modernity, and Mentality," addresses recommendations for personal care. Drawing upon military and mechanical metaphors, health care authors attempted to order the worker's day and consequently the worker's body. Posters emphasized the impact of intimate decisions on the body politic and presented a healthy, Soviet lifestyle that encompassed not just work habits but leisure activities, health rituals, and techniques for maintaining the body. The state used the danger to the body politic to justify its intrusion into personal life. Gendered rhetoric framed hygienists' interpretations of the strengths, weaknesses, and dangers of male and female bodies. Worries about the potency of the Soviet state in the international arena weighed down discussions of gender and the mind/body connection and spurred attempts to strengthen the will, intellect, and leadership potential of male bodies.

The conclusion follows the path of the body Soviet after the closing of the 1920s. With Stalin's "Great Turn," the state committed itself to heavy industry and large-scale collectivization. Stalin answered the call to revolution differently than Narkomzdrav's early leaders. The purge of administrations of the late 1920s demonstrated the power of hygienic language but resulted in a turnover in personnel within Narkomzdrav. New leaders abandoned the quest for universal care, preferring worker-centered care in a state that declared the class war had been won.[26] In an ironic twist, the utopian dreamers were themselves "cleansed" when bureaucrats lacking medical training took over Narkomzdrav. While this may have ripped the heart out of Narkomzdrav, the institution—with its programs, propaganda, and promise—continued to lurch forward and extend its reach.

I Revolution

Destruction, Cleansing, and Creation

Though his doctors had ordered him to rest, the enfeebled V. I. Lenin would not allow the German socialist Klara Zetkin to end her visit in 1922 until he had read her a letter sent to him by a class of rural schoolchildren. He began, "Dear little grandfather Lenin, we want to tell you that we have become very good. We study diligently. We already read and write well. We make lots of pretty things. We wash ourselves carefully every morning and wash our hands every time we eat. We want to make our teacher happy. He does not love us when we are dirty." When he had finished, Lenin turned to Zetkin and remarked, "Do you see, dear Klara, we are making progress in every sphere, serious progress. We are learning culture, we wash ourselves—and every day too! The little children in the villages are already helping us to build up Soviet Russia. And then can we fear that we shall not triumph?" Zetkin left Lenin for the last time, his face beaming "his old, happy smile, which expressed such goodness and certainty of victory."[1]

Zetkin left us a curious image—the ruthless, battle-hardened Bolshevik enthusing over well-scrubbed schoolchildren. Still, Lenin's comments to Zetkin—that children studied "culture" by washing, that their actions were "building up" Russia, and that hygiene would lead to "triumph"—assigned great importance to individual behavior—especially hygiene. In Lenin's response to the schoolchildren's letter, he made hygiene a powerful weapon in the campaign to transform rural Russia. The peculiarity of the situation dissipates upon closer examination. Lenin and his fellow Bolsheviks depended on a rich tradition of utopian literature to plan their society of tomorrow. Utopian theorists constructed their immaculate realms of equality and brotherhood in pristine, gleaming settings and implicitly argued that if society were organized, the conditions of illness—and even disease itself—would disappear. Inspired by fictional utopias and concrete examples of rationalization from the West, the Soviets embraced purity of mind, body, and environment in their fight against capitalist disorder. The battle for people's hearts and minds began by lathering their children with soap and water.

In their quest for order, the Soviets defined and categorized the existing world by interpreting political orthodoxy and citizenship in terms of hygiene. The criteria of cleanliness appropriated by Lenin had been used for centuries to define desirable behaviors. As nineteenth-century scientific discourse penetrated bureaucratic institutions, the medicalized understanding of dirt and disease gained influence in the diagnosis of various behaviors; cultural concepts, in turn, influenced medical diagnoses. Science merged with prevailing assumptions about purity and propriety to create a vision of cultured life that included cleanliness, proper behavior, and politics all rolled into one big civilizing project. Steeped in this discourse, the Soviets associated cleanliness with desirable behavior and extended the metaphor of hygiene to domestic maintenance, political opinion, and leisure choices.

In the rhetoric of Lenin and political leaders, hygiene became a symbolic system and cleanliness developed into a political statement. In this schema, however, dirt was not always what it seemed. Anthropologist Mary Douglas argues that the fight to eradicate dirt is a battle of more than just hygienic proportions. Noting that the discomfort of civilization with dirt predated the revelations of nineteenth-century scientists like Joseph Lister, Douglas holds that dirt is not an absolute but "exists in the eye of the beholder." Rituals and efforts to cleanse a body, a home, or a society focus on dirt as a signifier of "disorder."[2] Because of its connection to order and disorder, dirt infiltrates discussions of behavior and becomes part of racial stereotypes, class commentaries, and sexual prejudices. In the West blacks, the lower class, and women were all associated with disorder and were consequently identified as "filth" in various modernizing contexts.[3] For the Soviets the creation of ordered, urban environments and hygienic, modulated citizens served as a critique of moribund, filthy capitalism and those recalcitrant peoples who resisted the revolution.[4]

Lenin's tale of purity and peasants concealed biases about the groups targeted for domestication. Workers, women, and the peasantry all worried authorities because of their perceived ignorance, intransigence, and general "disorder." The Bolsheviks took power with the avowed goal of creating a system for and of the dispossessed, but this pledge did not translate into an acceptance of the people as they were. They had to be bathed, groomed, and transformed or, as Leon Trotsky roared, be consigned "to the dust-bin of history!"[5] For many a total transformation proved difficult, for the dirt of the past clung more fiercely to their heels. Although dirt and disease lurked in the rhetoric surrounding the woman question, the Bolsheviks saw the peasantry as the most backward of citizens and therefore in greatest need of correction.

Hygienists repeatedly attempted to penetrate the countryside, an endeavor fraught with difficulty and resistance. While the hygienists, who marched forth certain of the natural appeal of their message, remained befuddled, not all people took to hygienic prescriptions and started scrubbing away. Living conditions and popular conceptions promised a different reception. One Soviet author's recounting of the story of Lenin, Zetkin, and the schoolchildren's pride had a comment appended indicating that the letter came from the *glukhoi* (deaf) countryside;[6] the term implied that the letter had emerged from an area so remote that it had heretofore been untouched by modern life. Distance and ignorance were not the only determinants of how the population received the message of hygiene. For many who heard the message, lack of basic services ensured that maintaining new standards of cleanliness for bedclothes and home was nearly impossible. For others it seemed unnecessary. Not everyone was convinced of the evils of dirt, and some even saw revolution in the presence of filth. Propaganda did not lull a quiescent audience seeking guidance, for questions of hygiene are always more than skin deep.

Only dreamers could hope to build a Marxist, industrial utopia upon the ruined Russia of 1917.[7] Russia entered the twentieth century too weak to battle with the forces of the modern age even as leaders pressed for conflict with the industrialized nations of Europe. Russian agriculture could barely feed the nation, and despite extraordinary growth in the 1890s, Russian industry still could not compete with the rest of Europe. Nicholas II, tsar of all the Russias, proved himself incapable of the vision required to keep up with the forces of change buffeting Russia. Clinging desperately to the privileges of autocracy, he resisted representative government, organization by civic groups, and programs to break down traditional barriers to land development. His intransigence alienated and splintered Russian society.[8]

Russia's entry into war exacerbated the weaknesses of tsarism and fractured the society upon which it rested. World War I, a war of attrition among industrialized nations, left Russia dependent on bad weather and poor roads to slow the enemy's headlong rush. Frontline forces, at times compelled to wage war without munitions, rebelled or deserted. Unable to arm its soldiers or feed its citizens, in February 1917 the autocracy was overcome by the pressures of war and unrest. An International Women's Day demonstration turned into a citywide strike in Petrograd and culminated in a massive upheaval that brought down the Romanov dynasty. A hasty coalition government prevented complete chaos, but it was challenged by a shadow government comprised of workers, peasants, and soldiers' soviets (assemblies). While the Provisional Government was recognized on the world stage, the Soviets wielded considerable power as well.[9]

The good will of the soldiers, workers, and peasants evaporated as war dragged on and elections to a constituent assembly were delayed. The exiled Vladimir Iliich Lenin capitalized on this discontent following his return to Russia in April 1917. Trained as a lawyer but with the mien of a revolutionary, he had been agitating for the Marxists since the late nineteenth century. The events of 1917 presented him with a great opportunity. Through fiery speeches that appealed to an increasingly radicalized population, Lenin elevated the Bolsheviks from a minor actor to the majority party by the fall of 1917. In October, Lenin and the Bolsheviks took Petrograd and Moscow from the Provisional Government with little effort.[10] Lenin installed a Bolshevik-led government and subsequently disbanded the Constituent Assembly in January of 1918, but power was not secure. Discontent with the Bolsheviks led to Civil War, and for the next several years, "Red" forces struggled for control against the disjointed "White" forces of liberals, monarchists, peasant supporters, World War I allies, and national minorities, until the Bolsheviks finally triumphed.[11]

The Bolsheviks in power proved far less assured than they had been while struggling for power. According to Marxist theory, the state would prove unnecessary following the revolution, and the government would wither away in favor of the diffused authority of worldwide communism. When revolution did not erupt in Germany, Britain, or the United States, the possibility of the state's disintegration seemed uncertain and the probability of a worldwide revolution remote. Not only did the external situation contradict the theoreticians' predictions, but the internal political structure did not develop according to Marxist dictates. Instead of a weakened state vanishing in the inexorable logic of the dialectic, the civil war had necessitated a strong, centralized state to supply the front lines. The Soviet government took shape in this environment, with centralization continuing to characterize its institutions as they matured.[12]

The war years created great internal disruptions, and droughts in 1920 and 1921 crippled agriculture. Industry was at a standstill. Urban populations fled to find food and work in the countryside; Moscow turned into a ghost town half its previous size.[13] Hunger, unemployment, and decay haunted the streets. Hard hit by food shortages and factory closures, Moscow entered the 1920s with production at 15 percent of prewar levels. In 1921 one traveler reported,

"The stranger in Moscow or Petrograd could not fail to see evidence of underfeeding wherever he went."[14] While the Bolsheviks made the revolution in the name of the workers, during the years of war, civil war, and domestic unrest, the working classes vanished and the cities were depopulated.

Uprisings underscored the distance between the ruling Bolsheviks and their subjects. Faced with a discontented and even riotous population, Lenin chose to change course rather than press forward. In March 1921 he inaugurated the New Economic Policy (NEP). In this temporary retreat from socialism, the government retained control of the "commanding heights" of industry and finance while permitting small-scale, capitalist enterprise. At the same time, the government extended a hand to the peasantry by moving away from forced requisitioning to a tax in kind that allowed the peasants to dispense surplus grain as they wished. The conciliatory policies of NEP enabled the Russian economy to rebuild itself and by the mid-1920s production rebounded.[15]

Despite economic recovery, NEP had immediate and disastrous effects on social welfare. For revolutionary activists any economic development under NEP was compromised by complicity with bourgeois capitalists and the consequent social problems brought on by massive unemployment and lack of funds for social programs.[16] Working women—considered too expensive, less skilled, and less serious by employers—were hard hit.[17] Women without means turned to prostitution—visible symbols along the boulevards that the Bolsheviks had failed to defeat the worst inequities of capitalism.[18] NEP's return to capitalism left many behind, while a conspicuous few benefited. Entrepreneurs came to Moscow to make fortunes, and enlivening the streets of the city, which doubled in size. Business picked up and more goods appeared in stores. Along the avenue the new policies meant a profusion of bourgeois pleasures to tempt these nouveau riche NEP men, businessmen who benefited from the new economics yet were far from loyal to the new political order.[19]

For the committed communist, capitalist consumption infected the heart of the socialist metropolis. Parisian-style boutiques sold the latest fripperies, including Coty face powder and exotic-sounding perfumes; chic cafés offered up expensive libations, accompanied by wild jazz and tango dancing. These were symptoms of decay to activists, and they blamed the prostitutes, the bootleggers, and the crime of the boulevards on the decadent appetites of the voracious NEP men. Propagandists and pamphlet writers argued that NEP fostered a hazardous urban environment oozing with noxious temptations. Fellow-traveling intellectuals—who even before the revolution had despised the rise of market capitalism and equated it with immorality—criticized the appetites of the urban dweller, who gorged on petty entertainments and consumer goods.[20]

Revolutionary activists mapped a city fraught with dangerous spaces where temptation lurked, such as boulevards, restaurants, and drinking halls. Because of biases about consumption and disgust with capitalism, these sites were simultaneously politically suspect and morally corrosive. While acknowledging the need for economic recovery, revolutionaries spurned the fruits of capitalism, which profaned the revolution and sullied the streets of the city.[21] Within this charged environment, individual behavior came under intense scrutiny. A proper Soviet citizen avoided the cafés, lived a simple life, and navigated the streets of the city carefully. To enjoy capitalist diversions was obviously taboo, but the proper way to handle other questions of daily life was not so clear. Debates over the creation of the new Soviet man and woman and their behavior, home, and family mushroomed. Popular interest spurred discussion still further.[22] In these uncertain times people hungered for answers to questions on communist deportment. How was a communist to live, to love, or to marry? Articles, pamphlets, posters, and plays addressed everything from diet to etiquette. Even though the new world was not yet upon them, Soviet citizens were obsessed with how they were supposed to live in the interim and what their lives would be like once it arrived. These esoteric discussions of cultural construction for an as yet uncompleted world assumed the same level of importance as decisions on the week's production drive.[23]

There were many depictions of the sublime future to provide inspiration. While Lenin and his fellow "scientists" chafed at being called utopians, this school of thought was highly important in the 1920s. From classical and European philosophers Soviet revolutionaries inherited a disgust for the visible symbols of oppression and poverty—overcrowding, disease, and filth—and became convinced that dirt and sickness were incompatible with the new state. Earlier utopists had cleansed their worlds for humanitarian, religious, and aesthetic reasons rather than for questions of health. Utopists included baths, clean clothes, and sweet-smelling surroundings in their fanciful agendas, but the ordering of the environment yielded political results as well as hygienic benefits, for these sanitized, sanctified spaces produced perfected, protected bodies impenetrable to disease.[24] Both Plato and Thomas More (1478–1535) had proposed rationalization of behavior, of services, and balance in all aspects of daily life as a remedy for illness.[25] While Classical and Renaissance governments did not dwell on hygiene, this indifference was not true of their utopists.[26] Such equations of cleanliness with political change were prevalent in Russia, too, and had appeared as early as the sixteenth century. Perhaps most notoriously, during the reign of Ivan IV (1533–84), his dreaded henchmen, the *oprichniki,* were said to ride around with not just horrific figures of dogs upon their saddles but also brooms, denoting their efforts to sweep clean the state.[27]

In response to the industrial revolution, European utopists tailored their worlds to address the more visible ills of capitalism and applied scientific principles to the problems of industrialization, in particular its detrimental effects upon workers.[28] The utopists who perhaps most influenced Friedrich Engels (1820–1895) and Karl Marx (1818–1883)—Henri Saint-Simon (1760–1825), Robert Owen (1771–1851), and Charles Fourier (1772–1837)—all attempted to apply scientific rules to the construction of society and preached the inevitability of change.[29] From them came some of Marxism's obsession with detail, liberation, and the plight of the working class.[30] Utopists influenced the templates of Marx and Engels and fueled the plans of other writers, artists, and architects.[31] In Russia designs for ideal homes, peoples, and societies spread well beyond the Marxists and found a ready audience.

This popular utopian literature was important in the construction of hygienic discourse in the 1920s. Ideas from utopian novels of the prerevolutionary period reemerged as planners discussed forms for the developing society. Three authors whose utopian visions remained influential in the 1920s were Nikolai Chernyshevskii (1828–1889), Edward Bellamy (1850–1898), and Alexander Bogdanov (1873–1928).[32] Each had his own vision of a world where the evils of capitalism were replaced by just and humane systems infused with socialist elements.

Chernyshevskii, the son of a priest, rose to prominence as a result of his contributions to the radical journal *The Contemporary* from 1853 to 1857. His criticism of the regime and serfdom led to his exile in Siberia. While in prison he wrote his seminal work *What Is to Be Done?* (1863). The book caused a sensation, affecting an entire generation of radicals.[33] In his philosophical tract-cum-novel Chernyshevskii portrayed the life of the agitator. Chernyshevskii's heroic revolutionary, Rakhmetov, impressed everyone with his natural strength, even earning the nickname *bogatyr,* after the burly heroes of Russian folklore. Rakhmetov was not content with his natural abilities. He followed strict dietary and health regimens to harden his body for revolution, going so far as to sleep on a bed of nails. Using his own body as a utopian space, he became a perfected model of hard work, determination, and patience. In effect, Rakhmetov's purified body provided an archetype—a key—for entrance into utopia. Acolytes, and future revolutionaries, learned to put their present lives on hold in order to triumph sometime in the future. Chernyshevskii's influence was widespread. Lenin counted *What Is to Be Done?* among his favorite books.[34]

For those perhaps less capable of the restraint exemplified by Rakhmetov, Chernyshevskii presented a softer approach to utopia in the person of his heroine, Vera Pavlovna. Chernyshevskii's vision of the future, related through Pavlovna's dreams, gave substance and direction to the plans of revolutionary reformers. Pavlovna saw a future world, framed in glass and steel, where communal institutions eased life. Her new world turned upon the transformation of prostitutes—women polluted by capitalism both physically and morally—into ideal citizens. Pavlovna liberated women from wage slavery through sewing cooperatives, infused them with a communal spirit, combated the problems of modern urban life, and permanently changed the individual's political outlook. Although Pavlovna may have been an inspiration to many, Elizabeth Wood convincingly argues that for Lenin it was the revolutionary Rakhmetov who mattered most. In his own "What Is to Be Done?" (1902) Lenin emphasized not change in women's status but the need for a professional, hardened revolutionary.[35]

While Chernyshevskii's novel held perhaps the greatest resonance for older revolutionaries, other works contributed to the utopian atmosphere. Edward Bellamy's *Looking Backward: 2000–1887* (1888), imported from America, enjoyed great popularity, going through multiple Russian translations before the revolution.[36] Bellamy's future world provided a detailed description of the organization and manners of a utopian society. Russian radicals embraced it even as Bellamy took communists, anarchists, and labor unions to task. In Bellamy's novel a man of the 1880s awakens in the year 2000 in the home of a doctor and his family, who then serve as his guides. The presence of a man of science added clinical precision to the account of Bellamy's utopia and gave the story of the transformation of life from the nineteenth to the twenty-first century the veneer of prescription rather than description. Bellamy sketched a world where centralized distribution networks, rationalization of consumption, and communalism ordered life and ensured a paradise for all. Bellamy's utopia reflected a strong relationship between personal attitudes—communalism and egalitarianism—and the perfect society. Like Chernyshevskii, he underscored the importance of individual action in the creation of a harmonious future.

Alexander Bogdanov's novel described not the future of Earth but a perfected society on Mars, whose recently observed "canals" had inspired much contemplation in the fin-de-siècle. Bogdanov's *Red Star* (1908) and *Engineer Menni* (1913) detailed the development and workings of an engineer-led Marxist civilization on Mars, where science had transformed life.[37] Bogdanov, a Bolshevik organizer and cultural theorist, believed that education could transform workers without being condescending or paternalistic. As an activist he encouraged workers to create their own culture as a pathway to a unique proletarian ideology that promoted cultural and political change. Even though he left the party before the revolution, Bogdanov inspired the movement for the glorification of proletarian culture known as Proletkul't (Proletarskie kul'turno-prosvetitel'skie organizatsii), which became a popular phenomenon, claiming approximately four hundred thousand members throughout the Soviet territories in its heyday in the early 1920s.[38]

Bogdanov's hero, Leonid, journeys from Earth to Mars to learn all about the Martians' perfected world. Bogdanov, a medical doctor by training, emphasized the importance of science in his novel, just as he did in his work with Proletkul't, where he encouraged the development of a proletarian science that would consolidate all areas of knowledge in one system that served the workers' interests.[39] In his novel he made the love interest a Martian doctor and had Leonid visit a hospital (although he pointed out that illness was rare on Mars because a perfected society created healthy citizens). To make the connection of politics and health more explicit, communalism literally coursed through the veins of the Martians since they regularly shared their blood in transfusions in order to prolong life. These transfusions united the social body in a physical embrace. Through the exchange of bodily fluids individuals joined together as one society; as a Martian doctor noted, "Our regular comradely exchanges of life extend beyond the ideological dimension into the physiological one." Bogdanov was so convinced of the power of transfusions to triumph over death that he set up an experimental clinic, where he died in 1928 as a result of the mingling of his healthy blood with that of a comrade who had both malaria and tuberculosis. The comrade survived.[40]

Like Bogdanov, the joining together of political consciousness and physical body proved the undoing of Leonid, the heroic, space-traveling revolutionary. On Mars Leonid grew ill because he lacked a worker's background and true communal spirit. His difficulties manifested themselves in nausea, hallucinations, headaches, and, ultimately, the profoundly antisocial act of murder. The Martian doctor treated Leonid for these psychologically induced illnesses with calming suggestions and soothing lights, implying that physical ailments, even for the transplanted earthling, were problems of consciousness.[41] Bogdanov's presentation of illness in utopia was somewhat unique. Many authors blamed illness upon the material conditions of capitalism, which forced workers into poor housing and unfavorable labor conditions. By extension, in their utopias illness vanished with the implementation of ideal environments. Bogdanov retained illness, including suicide, in his idealized world, perhaps hinting that the transformation of the psyche would be more difficult than economic change.

These were by no means the only utopian novels in circulation, but they were the most widely read. Aside from a strong attraction to medicine, these novels celebrated communal living, a concern for individual behavior, the conflation of private behavior with political/public issues, and a glorification of science, medicine, and mechanization.[42] Many of these ideas found resonance in the policies of the young state. Faith in the beneficial and transformative power of science underscored Bolshevik plans for the future as it had for earlier generations of Russian revolutionaries. The idea that science could be of tremendous benefit to humanity was at the core of the plans of Dmitrii Pisarev (1840–1868) and the nihilists of the 1860s. The nihilists considered all knowledge not applicable to the betterment of society as useless and focused upon the scientization of peasant life as a measure of a society's progress.[43] This faith in science and its companion, general education, to transform people and life inspired a variety of movements in the late nineteenth century promoting general literacy, scientific education, and university training.[44] The Soviets expressed their faith in science by pushing for stronger education and greater regimentation. Intricate studies, which included photographic series and statistical analyses, attempted to document proper work habits in order to replicate them and minimize industrial injury.[45] At the base of all of these studies was always a healthy body—the foundation of productivity and progress. In his investigation of the Bolshevik obsession with time, Stephen E. Hanson argues that the Soviets hoped to rationalize time so they could triumph over it, compress it, and jump forward through it.[46] Regimenting time and worker use of it could speed up the dialectical process and bring utopia that much closer. Because the stakes were so high, time studies minutely regulated workers; even their smallest actions could not be left to chance.

Contemporary examples proved the effectiveness of time-motion studies and rationalization. The American engineer Frederick Winslow Taylor (1856–1915), building upon earlier explorations in fatigue and body mechanics, became a worldwide force as his ideas spread to France, Germany, and Russia.[47] Taylorism, as well as the production techniques of Fordism, obsessed the industrial community. Lenin considered the application of a socialist version of Taylorism an ideal way of solving production problems.[48] The pursuit of Taylorism betrayed a fascination with the mechanization, rationalization, and acceleration of all aspects of life.[49] Institutions and clubs welcomed these hopes. By the mid-1920s over eight hundred cells and eight laboratories devoted their energies to applying Taylor's concept of scientific management, introduced to Russians as the Scientific Organization of Labor (Nauchnaia organizatsiia truda [NOT]), to all aspects of society.[50] NOT theorists applied their techniques not just to work but also to leisure. The detailed schedules of NOT for daily life included bathing, diet, and exercise recommendations intended to micromanage the worker's life outside the factory, a particular locus of concern.

Lenin and other leading Bolsheviks drew upon these models of rationalized life and the perfected, cleansed futures depicted in literature to order their own world, using the language of hygiene as a symbolic system to create and define the revolutionary state and citizen. Concern for ideological purity was intrinsic to the Bolshevik agenda, but the specific context of NEP made these questions more heated. NEP's introduction of capitalist contagion forced a confrontation and definition of the opposition.[51] Revolutionary rhetoric relied upon binaries of pure/polluted and healthy/diseased to frame ideological evaluations of the world.[52] Determinations of communist/capitalist and new/old were couched in the language of purification. Because communism was a perfected environment, hygienic metaphors resonated; metaphors of purity defined the ideal and delineated the past. The imposition of an order onto the existing world ensured that many practices would not fit, and the concept of utopian purity necessitated defining—and finding—dirt. Those things that defied communist order became pollutants. All choices became politicized, as did every speck of real or perceived dirt.[53]

Ordering and purifying the world was a difficult task during the NEP period, when impure economic relations continued to exist and were deemed necessary to prop up the state even as they were depicted as rot. NEP's depredations led to a glorification of the harsh Civil War years because they served as a simple contrast to the complicated present.[54] To organize the environment meant fighting the vestiges of capitalism and tsarism and redefining their presence as disorder and dirt. Interested in creating a new civilization, the Bolsheviks found in relics of the past the "danger and power" of the old, which imperiled the new.[55] For example, in a speech delivered in 1919 Lenin predicted that communism would make a "clean sweep of the landowners and capitalists."[56] The image of Lenin, the energetic janitor, appeared elsewhere. The popular Viktor Deni poster entitled "Comrade Lenin Sweeps Clean the Earth of the Unclean" (plate 1) linked the old order with filth. A comically oversized, broom-wielding Lenin energetically flicks a banker, priest, and king from the world. Lenin also attributed dirt to the fruits of capitalism when he described bourgeois exploiters as those who "wallow in filth and luxury."[57]

Lenin further utilized the accompanying dangers of filth as metaphors in attacks on the bourgeois, the kulak (rich peasant), and the priest, comparing them to diseases, parasites, or vermin.[58] Lenin often called for attacks on the "idlers and parasites that suck the blood of the working people."[59] In a lengthy tirade against "the rich, the rogues, the idlers and the rowdies" delivered in 1917, Lenin referred to them as "dregs of humanity . . . hopelessly decayed and atrophied limbs, this contagion, this plague, this ulcer that socialism has inherited from capitalism." He insisted that the people must take collective action "to *clean* the land of Russia of all vermin, of fleas—the rogues, of bugs—the rich."[60] During his speech he described the bourgeoisie variously as filth, rot, infection, vermin, and even crippled limbs, thereby connecting capitalism to dirt, disease, and degeneracy. Extending the metaphor of parasites and disease to his political opponents, in the article "The Itch" (1918) Lenin portrayed scabies as evidence of inchoate, unorthodox political thought. Here again Lenin presented cleansing as the solution: "Put yourself in a steam bath and get rid of the itch."[61]

Theoretically it was simple to spot the unclean. By comparing capitalist sympathies and unorthodox politics to dirt and disease, Lenin suggested the visibility of these dangers—that one could spot capitalists by outward appearance or behavioral cues. In their study of revolutionary rhetoric Orlando Figes and Boris Kolonitskii note that according to Russian revolutionary tradition the enemy had long been demonized as "dark" and "disgusting in every way—morally, aesthetically, hygienically—so that just to touch him was to invite mortal danger."[62] In the discourse of the 1920s, corpulence, suits, watch chains, and jeweled stick pins became the symptoms of the capitalist male. The capitalist female, dripping with furs and slathered with makeup, incarnated capitalism as the prostitute.[63] The clean escaped easy definition. A simple cleansing was not a cure-all, for the absence of dirt was often not enough. No one was pure. Those who professed the right politics were still suspect because of their origins.[64] Furthermore, in the complicated 1920s, foul capitalism remained and the regime found itself tainted by the exigencies of NEP and dependency upon bourgeois specialists. The dirty and clean lived side by side and contact with the contagion of capitalism could not be avoided.

Party operatives had to work with the unclean yet never be corrupted. The difficulty of negotiating this relationship spurred interest in party etiquette. Lenin provided a guide when he applied the metaphors of cleansing to the party faithful as well as the bourgeois holdovers. In a 1922 speech he referred to the survival of Oblomovism[65] at all levels, with "people sitting endlessly at meetings, setting up commissions and drawing up plans without end." Lenin concluded, "Oblomov still lives; and it will be necessary to give him a good washing and cleaning, a good rubbing and scouring to make a man of him."[66] Lenin implied not only that cleansing could take care of the remnants of the old order but also that party actives should worry about their own purity.

Even the outwardly politically conscious might harbor some remnants of the old order, which had to be scraped away. More than just a superficial problem, immersion in political effluvia compromised the vitality of a communist and resulted in political sickness. In 1924 the Central Control Commission of the party came up with a list of seven problems, evocatively termed "party illnesses," which they associated with the turbulent times: sexual, alcoholic, or personal excesses; marrying someone of the bourgeoisie; religious participation; capitalist acquisition; and factionalism.[67] Printer activists diagnosed improper leisure among workers as a "yellow infection."[68] Trotsky likewise associated habits of the past with disease.[69]

The description of inappropriate behaviors as illnesses made infection with dirty, old ideas debilitating rather than just defiling. The past became contagion. For his part, Lenin depicted capitalism as a disease plaguing the entire world—and fatal to the revolution. Dread for this infection saturated Soviet propaganda in the 1920s.[70] Ideological deviation was medicalized as a perversity that endangered both the individual and the entire social body; the capitalist simultaneously became a degenerate and a symptom of social degeneracy. Party actives may have compromised themselves by living in close contact with the old order, but in the language of party policing these diseases were also communicable. Sick party actives needed to be rehabilitated. If they could not be reeducated, they would have to be excised before they endangered the party body. The primary method used to accomplish this was the purge, or *chistka* (literally "cleansing"). Purging the party of those subject to "illnesses" allowed the party to remain pure and inviolate.[71] The dismemberment, or disunity, of the party inspired horror since a fractured party was depicted as open to disease.[72] Eliminating the fractious members and cleansing the party of contrary elements was preferable to disunity. The Soviet government treated society as a body, hunting out those who might be tainted by the past or pose a threat to the future and depriving them of Soviet citizenship.[73]

The use of the body as a metaphor for the party was not surprising, given the scientific mindset of the Marxists. Corporeal metaphors, used since ancient times to describe the health of a society, became a mainstay of the social sciences in the nineteenth century, with the organic nature of the state the dominant metaphor.[74] Social scientists, concerned with regulating this social body, diagnosed behaviors and individuals as pathological or normal.[75] Since the actions of every individual contributed to the health of the entire society, antisocial behavior became an assault on the social body, with criminality assuming the status of a plague assailing all of society.[76] Just as Lenin charged the bourgeoisie with parasitism, so Soviet, German, and American elites reified entire groups as cancers, vermin, or parasites.[77] This identification was but a first step. Once diagnosed and identified, malignant individuals could be singled out, treated, forced into compliance, or excised.[78] Hygienists, already interested in eradicating dirt, gave concrete political impetus to their fight by arguing for the cleansing of the individual body as the means to effect political change. By creating individual Soviet bodies, hygienists moved forward the production of the larger corporate state—the body Soviet. The dirt of the past had ethical and even medical implications in addition to its political meaning. By assigning all aspects of life—political, social, cultural, and personal—to the categories of clean and dirty, hygienists equated excess in any aspect of life—sexual, gastronomic, or sensual—with filth and sickness. Visible dirt, already connected by metaphor to the past and imperfection, became a manifestation of poor politics.

Hygienists described a quick progression from ideological illness to physical degradation due to the connection between mind and body, arguing that in materialism there was no room for the distinction between body and soul. In 1926 Commissar of Health N. A. Semashko reflected: "Among us, even now, we have taken to talking about the 'soul' and the 'body' as in olden days and to separate and contrast the spiritual and physical life as if the 'soul' and the 'body' settled in our different pockets." Semashko argued that such a division was impossible. He insisted, however, that ancient philosophers were not altogether wrong in their explanations of the connection between body and mind: "When the ancient Romans said: 'in a healthy body there is a healthy soul'—they incorrectly separated the soul from the body but correctly noted the connection and dependence between the 'spiritual' and 'bodily' phenomenon. They said: 'the physically healthy man displays a healthy mental life: whoever is generally sound of health is also sound of mind.'"[79] Semashko agreed with the ancients and concluded that the state of the body manifested itself in the state of the mind. Other Marxists believed in a close connection between physical and mental health. Lenin held that body and mind were connected, maintaining that physical training tempered the character.[80] For these political leaders manipulation of the body led to enlightened communist behavior.[81] The health of the body became evident in the workings of the mind; the condition of the body was consciousness. As Lenin told Zetkin, "Healthy bodies, healthy minds!"[82]

The idea of bodily strength leading to mental fitness has classical roots and greatly influenced nineteenth- and twentieth-century activists. In Russia the interdependence of body and mind was evident in some of its oldest traditions. For example, the bathhouse (*bania*) was intended not only for the cleanliness of body but also for the purification of the spirit.[83] In nineteenth-century literature the assumed relationship between bodily restraint and mental preparedness led to detailed depictions of the "new man" of literature whose mental and physical preparation served as a model for societal change.[84] The assumed connection between mental and physical health buttressed discussions of national power. European philanthropists and activists fretted that women in the mines lost the markers of their sex, and that children harnessed to the machine became twisted, dehumanized creatures. Heavy labor hurt the weak, but lack of physical activity imperiled male vigor. Stuck behind desks, denied fresh air, and engaged in mental, not manual, labor, the bourgeois male became flaccid and neurasthenic according to alarmist, Social Darwinist, and nationalist critics.[85]

Fears of declining male potency brought on by the debilitating frenzy of modern life and the sad necessity of bureaucratic inactivity saturated European society and filtered into Russian popular culture.[86] In Germany these anxieties resulted in an entire "life reform movement" focused on vegetarianism, regimentation, and a variety of pseudoscientific therapies to attack the disease brought on by civilization, urbanization, and industrialization.[87] In Russia the disease was viewed as part of a general critique of society that couched political and social disquiet in the language of health—and nervousness in particular.[88] To combat nervous diseases brought on by physical and environmental hazards, Russian health advocates recommended physical activity, fresh air, and cold baths to temper the body and character.[89] These concepts appealed across a wide political spectrum, if not to all classes. Both Nicholas II and Lenin believed in the positive effects of fresh air and exercise.[90] The equation of modern life with physical decline bridged the revolutionary divide. A 1926 article emphasized how conditions of the modern urban world dragged down the Soviet man: "It is beyond doubt that the consequences of the events of the past years, such as the imperialist and civil wars, the revolution, and the current standards of daily life—unemployment or overwork, foul living conditions, the sharp contrast between the old lifestyle and the new forms of social construction—have markedly increased the number of neurotics."[91] Whether or not there was a crisis of nervousness, the perception of one led to a great deal of disquiet and underscored the anxiety over NEP with health authorities worrying that physical and political conditions contributed to the individual's mental downfall.[92]

Emphasizing the close interrelation of body and mind, health experts argued over the origin of disease as part of the social hygiene debate. Activists sought to bring certain problems—such as alcoholism, suicide, and crime—into the realm of hygienic inquiry.[93] The state, in turn, made health a political issue in 1926–27 by disenfranchising victims of venereal disease and drunkards.[94] Artists turned the correlation of health, cleanliness, and mental transformation into major themes in their works. In his dystopia *We* (1920), Evgenii Zamiatin toyed with the concept of diseases of the mind being manifested in one's appearance by having his politically compromised hero plagued by a spot on his otherwise pristine overalls. Even children's literature, such as the popular nursery rhyme "Wash Until There Are Holes" (1923), by Kornei Chukovskii, played on themes of cleanliness and transformation. In the short poem a giant washbasin calling itself the "washbasin boss and the Loofah Comander" chased a young boy until he submitted to a good scrubbing and proclaimed "Eternal Glory to Water!"[95] A popular obsession with hypnosis grew out of the discussion of the mind/body connection. The library for the journal *Hygiene and Health of the Worker and Peasant Family* included A. L. Mendel'son's works on hypnosis and memory.[96] Lectures in clubs often focused on hypnosis, and Bogdanov included it in his Martian doctor's treatments.

The marriage of body and mind divorced consciousness from class; political purity was a condition of the physical body. This allowed workers, peasants, and women to be sullied by retrograde attitudes while still being martyrs of capitalism.[97] In his "Report at the Second All-Russia Trade Union Congress in 1919," Lenin argued that workers were impure themselves even as they worked to purify society. He noted that "the workers were never separated by a Great Wall of China from the old society. And they have preserved a good deal of the traditional mentality of capitalist society. The workers are building a new society without themselves having become new people, or cleansed of the filth of the old world; they are still standing up to their knees in that filth. We can only dream of clearing the filth away."[98] While members of the laboring class were theoretically purified by their labor, years of contact with capitalism had left them vulnerable. Significantly, the workers remained passive and needed to be cleansed by an outside force. Workers remained incapable of ordering themselves, or their world, without guidance.

Lenin's passive, dirty workers were the subject of hygiene propagandists' expert recommendations. Discontented with the workers as they were, revolutionaries wished to transform the workers' politics by organizing, civilizing, and acculturating them.[99] This "inward turn" connecting personal with political behavior echoed the "civilizing process" of European society. It also reflected the prerevolutionary Russian emphasis upon restraint and control as a means of cultural attainment.[100] Behavior that strayed from these ideas took on both moral and social connotations. Following prerevolutionary and European examples, Soviet health propaganda linked citizens' behavior to the state's stability.[101] Workers who ordered their lives and avoided political unorthodoxy ensured their individual health. In turn, this benefited society by decreasing costs for care, increasing worker productivity, and providing examples to others.[102]

Health experts backed state power with science and united rationalization and hygiene in their exhortations.[103] During the 1920s, 1930s, and 1940s the Soviets encouraged orderly citizens as part of the campaign for cultured behavior (*kul'turnost'*), which fit in with the Bolshevik values of rationality, orderliness, and utility. In close approximation of the model that Norbert Elias put forward in *The Civilizing Process,* Soviet state-sponsored propaganda touted model citizens as rationalized and regulated, in contrast to those who posed a threat of disorder and infection for all of society.[104] The Russian process, however, was complicated by an expansive notion of proper behavior and the confusion of class upheaval. The pursuit of *kul'turnost'* entailed a broader range of behavior than in Europe, encompassing an entire lifestyle of consumption, leisure, politics, and personal hygiene. For example, in his 1923 recommendations for the Red Army Trotsky noted the need not just for political awareness and literacy but also the fact that the military man must "acquire habits of tidiness, punctuality, and thrift."[105]

Even as the Soviets declared worker rule, prejudices against worker order, or disorder, bled through.[106] Soviet advice literature took on modes of address that distanced author and reader.[107] This distance between leaders and followers was also evident in more pointed commentary. In a note attributed to him dating from the days of the revolution, Lenin worried about the poor grammar of the incoming recruits and decried their "spoiling" of the Russian language.[108] Others echoed this condemnation of the vulgarization of Russian language. Trotsky composed an entire commentary on foul language.[109] In their equation of poor language with defiling influences, Lenin and others betrayed their distaste for those workers or peasants who exposed their poor education and somehow degraded the revolutionary process.

This diagnosis of the uneducated, politically unconscious working class as past contagion revealed itself in popular literature. Vladimir Maiakovskii, an enthusiastic revolutionary, futurist poet, and energetic provocateur, involved himself in the revolution and concerned himself with propaganda and the acculturation of the masses in particular. He made attacking symbols of the old the centerpiece of many of his works, utilizing the language of cleanliness and purification in them.[110] In his strident prerevolutionary futurist manifesto entitled "A Slap in the Face of Public Taste" (1912), he advised readers to "wash" their hands of the "filthy" literary works of the past. His infamous play *The Bedbug* (1928) told the story of the worker Ivan Prysypkin, who, despite his worker status, held dangerous attachments to the banalities of bourgeois life (including a curious, fur-lined brassiere). Transported fifty years into the future, Ivan is responsible for infecting the now perfected future with problems of the past.

Ultimately scientists identify him as a *bourgeoisius vulgaris*—a name that plays with the scientific classification of the all-too-common bedbug of the 1920s—and lock him and his foul habits away. Not only did Maiakovskii carry over the concept of capitalism as contagion, but he also made the worker harboring capitalist sentiment an infectious agent capable of derailing the future with societal and health problems.

In his play *Mystery-Bouffe* (1918) Maiakovskii again used the language of purity to express his distaste for workers' past habits while contrasting them favorably with the bourgeoisie. Maiakovskii retold the revolution as a story of the "clean" and the "unclean," with the bourgeoisie representing the clean and the workers the unclean. His description of the workers as unclean reflected their physical state under capitalism, his wordplay voicing the poorly disguised paternalistic sentiments of the leadership. The workers were capable of revolt but not sufficiently cultured to rule. In the play the unclean passed through many lessons before they entered the earthly paradise of the commune. As the workers traveled along the path from disaster, to hell, to paradise, through chaos, and into the scientifically engineered heaven on earth of the commune, they faced the tricks of the clean bourgeoisie, who first attempted to get them to accept a king and then, in turn, a representative government. Only after the unclean disposed of the bourgeoisie and purified themselves through hard labor did they enter the commune. Maiakovskii's description of the commune confronted the irksome contradiction of a utopia on earth. The idealistic utopia lacked substance, and the promised future had still not materialized. As if to underscore the distance between the commune and reality, the characters questioned its existence and ran bits of dust through their fingers to be certain of its authenticity.[111]

At least workers *could* become clean. For the grimy peasantry, long an object of intervention by the state and intellectuals, the path to purity was fraught with peril.[112] In prerevolutionary contemplations of Russia, dirt clung to the peasant as a symbol of the barbarous nature of the country.[113] In both propaganda and fiction the ignorant peasant served as a foil to the politically conscious urban worker. Hygienists showed peasants making poor choices, with disastrous consequences. Peasants went to faith healers instead of doctors. They traveled to the city and caught venereal diseases. Peasants did not understand the value of science.[114] This denigration of the peasant allowed the urban workers to feel superior and may have made urbanites more receptive to the message hygienists wished to convey. The interpretation of data on sexually transmitted diseases further infantilized the peasantry by distancing them from conscious, mature, urban workers. Doctors insisted that syphilis in the countryside was spread through nonvenereal means, such as the sharing of towels or silverware, in contrast to infections in the city, which were caused by sexual licentiousness.[115] According to this nosology, doctors emphasized the diseased and corrupting influence of urban life, implying that the peasantry was untouched by civilization, being too immature to participate in illicit sexual relationships. Medical authorities continued this paternalistic, condescending idea of the peasantry even as letters and questions addressed to medical authorities by peasants challenged the stereotypes.[116]

The campaign against peasants penetrated deep into the traditions of prerevolutionary populist sentiment and popular medicine. The foulness of the peasantry signified their ignorance and illiteracy as well as their grooming.[117] Prerevolutionary campaigns, like Soviet efforts, emphasized the transformative, beneficial powers of education and science.[118] In the case of the peasantry, darkness, dirt, and backwardness denoted a group beyond the reach of Soviet order. This attack upon the peasants ignored the meaning of dirt to the peasant, for whom it symbolized labor and productivity. Russian peasant concepts of purity allowed for ritualized, spiritual purity independent of the presence of visible dirt. Peasant ideas did not filter upward into the world of specialists and medical practitioners; peasants were largely absent from the practice of power and the active formulation of ideology.[119] Instead, hygienists' perception of the peasant as filthy, disordered, and ignorant held sway. Acting upon this conception and bolstered still further by Marxist disdain for agriculture, Lenin pushed electrification as essential to the revolutionary awakening of the countryside and a way to transform the dark life of rural Russia. Electrification, the most visible manifestation of the modern, would make way for modern thought and life in the countryside and transform even the most forsaken hut into a Soviet home and the most backward peasant into a proletarian.[120]

Though there was disagreement over what constituted order, Soviet ideologues' and peasants' concepts both denigrated the peasant female as quintessentially impure.[121] Peasants depicted woman as the essence of darkness, referring to the stove and its surroundings as the "black" area of the hut. Obscured by soot and smoke, it remained the province of the wife.[122] Soviet propagandists continually showed peasant women endangering their husbands, children, and society through ignorance and obstinacy. For example, in B. S. Ginzburg's agitational play *Trial of a Mother Who Abandoned Her Child* (1924), the house surgeon for the State Institute for the Protection of Motherhood and Infancy told of a mother who ignored Soviet institutions and advice, with dire consequences.[123] In another agitational play a woman newly arrived in the city caught syphilis and spread it because she refused Soviet help.[124]

Painting urban women with the same broad strokes, propagandists continued their vilification. These attacks shared much in common with the prerevolutionary period, when women's connection to procreation, and thus to the cycle of life and death, defiled them and made them unacceptable as objects of transcendence in Russian millenarian discourse.[125] Their connection to birth and decay made women incompatible with purified, utopian spaces, which banished illness and death; women defiled utopia through their very existence. Though Bolshevik writers condemned the church for its association of women with sin, they argued that women were befouled politically by an unhealthy interest in privacy and personal comfort, which turned them away from the collective. Women's putative impurity was transformed from the sin of Eve to the worship of Mammon. This discomfort with the feminine translated into a portrayal of women as willfully—and often stubbornly—ignorant and therefore dangerous to socialist construction.

Since women resisted this conversion to Soviet life, they dismembered the social body. Women served as a convenient metaphor for describing the flaws of the revolution. According to Lenin, women were, "little worms which, unseen, slowly but surely, rot and corrode" the men in their lives.[126] The association of woman with earth, and a creature which ate and disgorged earth, intimated the dirty nature of the female being as well as connecting woman to the process of putrefaction. Lenin's further diagnosis of prostitutes as a "diseased excrescence" made them not just individually filthy but morbid protrusions and growths on the social body.[127] The Bolsheviks, however, did not despair of their ability to cleanse women. Even as they defined women as dirty and backward, they celebrated the malleability of their childlike, unformed consciousnesses. As they infantilized women and emphasized their lack of sophistication, they created an ideal canvas for social transformation. Women's education would be of particular import to the new regime; to transform women would be their greatest achievement.[128]

Just as peasants and women carried the connotation of dirt and disease, reformers deemed certain ideas of the past as contaminants. According to hygienists, the Russian Orthodox Church presented a pernicious danger.[129] Marx's description of religion as an "opiate" for the masses fueled conceptions of society as a body and religion as a destructive substance. In propaganda the dangers extended to individuals. I. D. Strashun's pamphlet entitled *The Battle for Health Is the Battle with Religion* (1925) opened with an attack upon the religious mindset and its deleterious effect on health.[130] According to Strashun, who served as director of the Sanitary Enlightenment section of Narkomzdrav, the danger of religion was systemic.[131] Russian religious leaders resisted science, discouraged personal initiatives, and argued that sin, not microbes, led to disease. Strashun concluded that they were "the greatest reason, the greatest culprit in the ill health of the working masses!" He further attacked the church's glorification of people who did not bathe or refused to cut their hair, asserting that the association of the flesh—particularly female—with sin contributed to great ignorance about women's health. Strashun blamed religious attitudes toward work, alcohol, women, and hygiene for the poor health of Russia, especially in the countryside.[132]

Didactic tales in health magazines implied that participation in religious rituals caused illness. Icons became the sites of infection, either through the transfer of saliva in rituals, where the observant kissed them, or by attracting tuberculosis-laden dust in the home.[133] In Central Asia health activists claimed the wearing of a veil caused birth defects and even aged wearers prematurely.[134] Posters attacked religious holidays as the reason for mass drunkenness and resultant absenteeism.[135] The magazine *To a New Life!* picked up the theme. For example, in the 1927 story by O. Stepanova entitled "From the Opiate to a New Life," the heroine, described as a politically conscious woman, still believed in priests and God. Her political illness resulted in infection for her family. She attended church and took her son with her, where he became infected with scarlet fever when he took communion. Wracked by guilt, and panic-stricken, the mother confessed all to her politically conscious husband, who immediately placed their son in the hospital and chastised his wife for taking him to church "because in church you can pick up any type of infection." The husband's admonition could not have been about proximity to crowds because his political meetings presented no danger to his health. The objection centered on the lack of communist content.[136] The author underscored this message when the hospital doctor chided her: "Let us agree that you will never set foot with him in the church again."[137] This heavy-handed prescription brought medical authority to the battle for political conversion.

Hygienists linked religious ritual and observance to illness, lauding the powers of sanitary education to combat the opiate. A 1923 publication of the Moscow Department of Health even termed it the "best method for battle with religion and other superstitions." This tract did not, however, consider that the eradication of religion would leave a void. The needs of the solitary soul would be met by sanitary culture, which "also entails hygiene and the spiritual and moral [*dukhovno-moral'nyi*] improvement of daily life in its entirety." According to the author, there was "not one important question from that complex of issues of 'lifestyle' that the sanitary organization may pass by nonchalantly as not its affair."[138]

Not everyone welcomed this intrusion. Dystopias—from Zamiatin's *We* to Mikhail Bulgakov's *Heart of a Dog* (1925)—parodied the obsession with order, arguing for the implacable desire of humanity to rebel against structure, categorization, and even its best interests. With these authors the contemplation of order was a way to view the evils of the state and its control mechanisms. Rebellion against the tightening noose of state control led to challenging the correlation of cleanliness with political readiness. Different interpretations of revolutionary behavior led to resistance and manipulation. Youthful enthusiasts exposed their pristine politics by sporting disheveled appearances. Some even considered the glorification of a worker image—notably a lackadaisical attitude toward hygiene—the height of revolutionary consciousness.[139] While youth saw a "worker" style as the epitome of revolutionary activism, others cynically adopted worker costumes in order to be identified with the proletariat. One traveler noted that in the chic restaurants of Moscow men of authority dressed in workers' clothing during the day but met their fashionably attired mistresses for expensive dinners in the evenings. He concluded cheekily: "The truth is that a well-cut waistcoat, just like a well-shaved face, gives the men of Moscow that hated appearance—middle-class. So each dresses himself like a workman and swings his arms like a blacksmith, even if, during the whole of his life, the only hammer that he has seen is on the Soviet coat of arms."[140]

Although the general population found room for differing interpretations, the language of cleanliness permeated Soviet political discourse. Lenin labeled his enemies as filth, vermin, or disease and described those of different mindsets as suffering from illness. Workers, peasants, and women—liminal beings who stood on the brink between old and new—were splashed with metaphoric muck for their lack of political consciousness. The danger of dirt was more than rhetorical. Political unorthodoxy, religious belief, and acquisitive attitudes were viewed as infectious agents that could contaminate the environment, the body, and, most injuriously, the future.[141] By cleansing the population—male, female, peasant, and worker—of the past and training it to accept cultured behavior, the Bolsheviks ordered society, cleared the way for utopia, and made Russia conform to the Marxist ideal.[142] Since they attacked diseases of both mind and body, hygienic measures resonated with the images of literary utopias, which had appeared before the arrival of the Marxists. Utopias exist nowhere but in the mind. If purity of mind was predicated on purity of body, and if the former was a necessary step toward Marxist utopia, then cleanliness was not an aesthetic consideration but an essential political component of revolutionary life.

Although the subjects for intervention were identified and the ideal was clear, popular resistance and poor conditions conspired to hamper the implementation of utopian plans. The economic policies of NEP meant suturing the Marxist ideal onto an imperfect reality. Attempting to force pure ideas into concrete programs and policy further complicated the issue.[143] Utopias (literally "no place") are generally not subject to stories of construction but appear fully formed outside of reality or rise ready-made and perfected from the ashes of an obliterated past. Still rarer is a depiction of a utopia populated with citizens who display human frailty. Instead, people immune to weakness, greed, lust, and other vagaries of character tend to form the basic building blocks of these idealized futures. For the intrepid hygienists of Narkomzdrav, this meant that not just the problems of NEP but also the variability of human capital would plague their programs. For the Soviets the question of the past lingered, transporting the utopia from its hermetically sealed universe into the tainted present.[144] Even in F. V. Gladkov's idealized *Cement* (1924), the process of moving from War Communism to NEP and the restart of the factory was complicated by violence, corruption, and moral ambiguity.[145]

By focusing upon massive change, these reformers neglected to articulate the banal path needed to get there. The image of the sparkling future may have blinded reformers to the more humble steps needed to achieve reform. Svetlana Boym argues that the opposition between the spiritual and the everyday contributed to a certain disinterest in articulating the mechanisms of change; Russian and Soviet intellectuals found the description of daily life mundane and wished to focus upon monumental change.[146] Disinterest in the small was belied by the attention of leaders and cultural figures to seeming minutiae. The calls of Lenin for eliminating body lice or Maiakovskii's politicized diatribes against filth and bourgeois paraphernalia indicate that attention to seemingly dull details infused plans for Soviet construction.[147] Trotsky argued that attention to daily life was essential to revolutionary change.[148] He discussed revolutionary behavior, speech, and dress and made calls for cleanliness a regular theme in his writings. The call for shoe shining which opened Trotsky's 1921 *Pravda* article "Attention to Trifles!" suggested leading figures saw a grand political meaning in even the most banal personal grooming decisions. Arguing that "Trifles, accumulating and combining, can constitute something great—or destroy something great," Trotsky railed against "spitting and dropping cigarette butts in public corridors and stairways" equating such actions with a lack of attention to "economic significance." He further noted that with such a citizen there was no hope for triumph: "We can never revive the economy on the basis of the likes of these. Such an individual breaks glass out of sheer carelessness, never polishes a boot, and is certainly a carrier of typhus lice."[149]

In this one slovenly character Trotsky smoothly merged political, economic, social, and bodily disorder:

> If we really intend to develop institutions based on communal living, it is imperative that every man and woman devote full attention to order and cleanliness and the interests of the house as a whole. Otherwise, we end up (as happens all too often) with a foul, louse-ridden pit, rather than a communal dwelling.
>
> We must wage a tireless and relentless struggle against such slovenliness and lack of culture—by word and deed, by propaganda, and higher standards, by exhortation, and by calling individuals to account for their behavior. Those who tacitly overlook such things as spitting on the stairs or leaving a yard or house looking like a pigsty are poor citizens and unworthy builders of the new society.[150]

Trotsky concluded, "In order to implement great plans, you must devote great attention to very small trifles!"[151] He would have found ready agreement with theorists of the modern state. As Foucault concludes concerning the disciplinary process, "And from such trifles, no doubt, the man of modern humanism was born."[152]

In 1928 Commissar of Health N. A. Semashko argued that hygiene was the measure of the revolution's success: "Cultural revolution means not just the spread of literacy through the population but the refashioning of all life along new, pure [*svetlyi*], 'cultured' foundations. Without a cultured way of life there cannot be culture in general. And our way of life will not be cultured if it is not healthy."[153] Semashko's rhetoric placed hygiene at the cornerstone of all future progress. With so much at stake, the battle for hygiene became the revolutionary struggle.

Semashko's impassioned plea for health undoubtedly stemmed from his embattled position in the late 1920s. But as Lenin's and Trotsky's remarks show, in the early years Semashko did not stand alone. In his rhetoric Lenin linked cleanliness and political purity. Cleanliness was essential for contrasting communism with capitalism and vital to the development and articulation of the revolutionary state. The metaphoric equation of capitalism with dirt led to a broad conception of hygienic cleansing eventually encompassing daily life, the body, home, family, leisure, the city, and much more. Controlling the penetration and pollution of the body by other substances—food, alcohol, tobacco—became necessary for the creation of the utopian body of the future.

The transition to utopia required the rationalization of behavior, the reorganization of environments, and the disciplining of the body as a way to condition consciousness. The prophylactic emphasis of NEP-era Narkomzdrav fit in with this utopian drive for control, balance, and rationality. Living a healthy life meant living a Soviet life, or at least a life that might hasten the coming of the socialist utopia. This wedding of the political and the physical made healthful behavior indicative of politically correct Soviet behavior. Only purified citizens could come together to form a new perfected nation—a body Soviet that could act out the revolution's success on the global stage.

Hygiene prescriptions provided easily interpreted models of behavior for those who, unable to negotiate the new terrain, sought manuals of proper comportment. Disorder reigned in the world, the state, and the city. The power to create monumental projects was absent. It was at the individual level that an activist could combat the chaos of NEP, urbanization, and industrialization. Hygiene gave hope to those who wished to proceed with the revolution post haste and believed that it was only on the individual level that transformation was possible. Trotsky noted the difficulty of transition rather than creation: "New daily relationships must be built with the human material we have at our disposal."[154] It was this very difficulty, however, that brought individual behavior into such sharp relief. By maintaining a clean body and a regulated life, citizens could create their own personal utopias and perhaps experience a little of the pristine future in the horrid present. Propagandists supported this interpretation of the power of the individual and implied that washing hands could well be the most political act of a Soviet citizen.

2 The State

Diagnosing, Monitoring, and Disciplining

The densely layered poster "People's Health Care in the USSR" (1926–29) presented the primary methods and goals of an idealized Narkomzdrav (plate 2). A red scroll across the top emphasized that though the workers had rights as citizens, they also had duties, declaring: "The protection of the health of workers is the responsibility of workers themselves." Underscoring this dependence upon prophylaxis over treatment, the most prominent spot on the poster featured education in the person of a doctor lecturing to a group of workers. Beneath the doctor a scroll unfurled to disclose the merits of sanitary enlightenment in the creation of a new life. The layering of the poster and its didactic friezes imitated the style of iconography. Whereas an icon might have shown Christ the teacher, the propaganda poster glorified a new savior and his gospel: the doctor and the message of science. Taken together, the slogan and pictures indicated that the state's most important programs were packaged in the least expensive forms available—self-help, prophylaxis, and propaganda—rather than being accompanied by a slew of new facilities or expensive therapies.

The second and third rows of the poster showcased those programs, which sought to bring health propaganda into the insular life of home and family. Under the slogans "Children Are Our Future" and "The Nursery Frees the Woman Mother," the second row featured the all-encompassing care promised to children by the state. In the center the newly founded Soviet institution, the consultation for mothers and infants, monitored children's health and offered preventative care. To the left toddlers benefited from the professional care provided by the nursery, and on the right youth enjoyed the opportunity to build Soviet life as members of the Pioneers. At bottom-center a nurse-inspector, pictured visiting a peasant home, called to mind the work of thousands of women who went door to door spreading the message of health. In both the efforts of the consultation and the nurse-inspector, the emphasis was on providing lasting change to daily life by urging citizens to take care of themselves and thereby prevent illness.

At the very bottom of the poster, charts revealing birth and death rates reflected the international concerns spurring Narkomzdrav's programs. The poster's borders, however, suggested that not all health progress was so easily measured. In the margins glimmered the hoped-for political and cultural results of health education and the justifications for state expenditure in health. Smokestacks belched out the promise of a strong industry in the upper-left corner. In the upper-right corner a rally showcased a populace engaged in the highest form of culture—political participation. The pantheon of worker and peasant, soldier and national minority, man and woman tied health care to the leveling, unifying forces of the revolution. Narkomzdrav programs educated the population and linked health care to the cultural, industrial, and political transformation of the state.

Though the poster emphasized worker self-help, Narkomzdrav created a series of institutions to guide the Soviet citizen's transformation through universal, prenatal-to-grave care. Utilizing international example and exercising their paternalistic desire to order and perfect workers, Narkomzdrav doctors experimented with natal care, outpatient education centers, residential treatment facilities, and outdoor care. Consultation and dispensary doctors, nurses, and inspectors educated their patients and entered their homes even as they monitored pregnancies or treated illnesses. For those whose condition required more drastic intervention, the sanatorium system provided treatment, supervision, and education. To spread the message to even the healthy, the House of Leisure was designed to allow workers to vacation in doctor-supervised, hygienic surroundings during their state-mandated two-week break.

With the victory of the Bolsheviks, prerevolutionary authorities and revolutionary activists united in a quest to cleanse the population and join the order of modern, industrialized nations. Due to its importance to political orthodoxy and the creation of communism, the spread of hygienic ideas could not be left to chance. Narkomzdrav used the disciplinary techniques of the modern state to extend medicalized hygiene to all aspects of life, thereby joining an international movement for multifaceted state power in the late nineteenth and early twentieth centuries. Because of the peculiar mating of politics and purity in Soviet ideology, however, the strength with which these ideas were applied, and the pervasive methods of observation, were uniquely Soviet. While the Bolsheviks, like their European and tsarist counterparts, implemented health programs to strengthen the state, hygiene had a more central role in revolutionary Russia. It was an integral component in the transformation of the masses into a politically conscious population capable of leading the world revolution and creating the socialist utopia.

This universal, comprehensive, institutionalized system of health care presented in the poster and outlined in other propaganda was never realized. Though Narkomzdrav's goals were grand, its means were few. Propaganda, not institutions, became the foundation of Narkomzdrav's work as NEP budget cuts and calls for self-sufficiency made other types of care difficult to provide. Within Narkomzdrav statistics and comparative studies provided a source of propaganda and a tool for bureaucrats seeking funds. In the city posters, pamphlets, lectures, plays, magazines, and films spread the message of prevention and urged workers to take the initiative to care for themselves, their fellows, and their neighbors. Unlike trained personnel or specialized institutions, propaganda could be supplied by the state at bargain prices and distributed to the public for free or for a few kopecks at a book vendor.

While Narkomzdrav managed hospitals and sanatoriums for the very ill, the focus of its work would be prophylaxis—staving off illness rather than treating it. Workers who took care of themselves cost the state less than those who had to be cured. Medical personnel could barely provide care in major urban centers, but the virtual saturation of the cities with propaganda ensured that many more would see a poster than a doctor. Faced with shortages in funding, personnel, and goods, prophylaxis was more than just a prudent strategy for the future; it was about all the state could provide for the present.

While the October Revolution provided activists with the opportunity to categorize society's disorder and plan for the future, the Enlightenment framed the techniques for control that the Soviets would use to spread these ideas to the population. Force was not incompatible with utopian thought or with Marxism, which preached the violent overthrow of an alien class.[1] The use of force originated in a willingness to sacrifice individual liberty for the collective well-being, reflecting a disinclination to champion individualism inherent in the German-influenced, antibourgeois philosophies of nineteenth-century Russian intellectuals.[2] Indeed, more prevalent in Russian intellectual discussions was reverence for society—specifically a hierarchical society with a delineated group in charge who worked for the public good—rather than the individual. The rest of society would be subject to its prescription.[3] This combined veneration for social progress and indifference to the use of force was evident in the social programs of earlier days. Peter the Great's grand vision of St. Petersburg featured a prison at its center, and Alexander I modeled his experiments in social engineering on the military discipline of Alexander Arakcheev's soldiers' settlements.[4] Public health advocates, who depend upon the concept of individual liberty being subsumed by societal needs, were bolstered in Russia and, later, the Soviet Union by these concepts.

This movement toward intervention in the private sector for societal growth was a gradual development throughout Europe as the conflicting Enlightenment impulses of fostering liberty and protecting society fought for supremacy. Epidemic disease, however, forced the first confrontations between the individual and the state well before the concept of liberty was articulated. The earliest public health reforms addressed epidemic disease and the threat to domestic order following in its wake. In the late Middle Ages the rise of urban culture made outbreaks more frequent, deadly, and unruly. Municipal health boards, funded by emergency taxes, were established to contain epidemics through quarantines, registration, and the health police. Even as states looked to health reforms to maintain order, humanitarian concerns led to the rise of philanthropic initiatives such as private hospitals and care for the indigent.[5]

Provisions for public health changed as the concept of enlightened rule forced a reexamination of the idea of the state.[6] As rulers connected the economic and political power of states to the management of populations, public health became associated with more than the containment of disease or some humanitarian impulse. Societal health expanded from the individual body to encompass issues of defense and economy. Inspired by the work of the Marquis de Condorcet (1743–1794), the French mathematician and social scientist, states engaged in social mathematics to evaluate their progress. European governments used investigations, censuses, and statistical analyses to study health questions and then justified the creation of health police based on their conclusions.[7] The centralization and increasing power of governments ensured states a greater ability to intrude into the private affairs of citizens and augured the new era Foucault has called the age of "biopower."[8]

The interconnection between the political and individual condition forced a reconceptualization of the relationship between the citizen and the state. Enlightenment philosophers converted the social compact into a healthful contract by asserting that citizenship entailed individuals caring for their own health even as it involved the state working toward protecting its citizens. Thomas Jefferson (1743–1826) posited that in a democracy health could be a state duty as well as a citizen's responsibility. He argued that the health of the political system was visited upon the bodies of its subjects and that democratic governments produced the soundest citizens. The Frenchman Constantine Volney (1757–1820) stressed that because popular health made such an important contribution to the state's power, maintaining one's health was a duty of citizenship. The revolutionaries of 1848, alive with the rhetoric of liberty, also called for health reform as a facet of democratic citizenship.[9]

Public health in Russia followed a similar path of development, spurred on by international influences and domestic needs. On his grand tour Peter the Great (r. 1682–1725) indulged his interest in science by visiting medical centers and observing dissections in Amsterdam, Leyden, and Paris.[10] After his return, he created Russia's medical infrastructure by establishing the first hospital, medical study, and medical museum.[11] The first hospital, built in 1706, was modeled on Greenwich Hospital in England, which Peter may have seen in 1698. Doctors from Holland provided the first medical instruction.[12] Though medical dissections and dentistry were private passions, as with European monarchs, Peter's interest in popular health grew out of a desire to manage and increase the Russian population as an economic and military resource.[13]

The growth of the medical infrastructure in Russia slowed after Peter the Great's death, but Catherine the Great (r. 1762–96) continued Peter's project by founding departments of social reform, expanding medical instruction, financing medical administrations, establishing foundling hospitals, and promoting treatment for victims of venereal disease.[14] In addition to her attempts to expand the circle of those served by public health institutions, an outbreak of plague encouraged an increase in public health precautions.[15] In her instructions on public health and hospitals, Catherine carefully outlined provisions for the education of both men and women and emphasized the links between mind and body. She also forged connections between citizens' lives of cleanliness and health and their duties to the ruler.[16] Strong ties between Europe and Russia continued throughout this era. Many scientific discoveries of the West were quickly adopted in Russia. Catherine the Great was vaccinated for smallpox within a year of the publication of this treatment in London. After determining that it was safe, she had her son and others vaccinated.[17]

In addition to identifying health and hygiene as questions of political order, both Peter and Catherine betrayed an interest in the condition of their subjects' behavior and embarked upon campaigns to civilize the populace. Peter instituted dress reform to make Russians look more European and encouraged travel so they might learn to act more European. Catherine's educational programs for both sexes stressed the virtues of order and efficiency. Just as she did not target one sex, the empress did not focus on one class. Manuals instructed the lower classes in the new virtues and counseled the upper classes to serve as examples.[18] For both classes she emphasized hygienic balance as the basis for an ordered citizenry. The later reforms of Alexander I (r. 1801–25) and Alexander II (r. 1855–81) regarded health care as one aspect of population control and looked to Europe for inspiration.[19]

In the West the findings of statisticians such as France's Louis-René Villermé (1782–1863) and England's Edwin Chadwick (1800–1890) spurred public health reform and gave it new direction. Using social mathematics, Villermé drew up elaborate tables showing the discrepancies in mortality between Parisian neighborhoods of different classes. His analysis established statistically supported links between economic conditions and health and inaugurated discussions of the "social question" among French reformers.[20] In England Chadwick, a follower of Jeremy Bentham (1748–1832), concluded that investigation into disease and its prevention made good political sense. In 1842 he published the fundamental document of modern public health, *Report on the Sanitary Condition of the Labouring Population of Great Britain*.[21] Chadwick established that disease—especially communicable disease—flourished in the filth of modern cities because of bad drainage, poor water supply, and piles of muck that characterized crowded urban centers. Through statistical analysis, Chadwick turned dirt from a private matter into a public enemy. His findings provoked interest in creating a healthier urban environment and inspired many to consider the health of all urban residents across class lines and geographical divisions.

Prompted by Chadwick's reports and goaded by public pressure, in the 1840s the British government enacted legislation to alleviate what it considered the greatest problems for the laboring class.[22] Statistical analysis joined with humanitarian impulses, the desire for civic improvement, and an emphasis on self-help to spread interest in public health across Europe.[23] Even as states came to recognize problems, revolutionary activists developed theories to explain the fundamental causes of poor health in worker dwellings. European socialists argued that overcrowding, substandard living conditions, and the high incidence of social disease were logical outgrowths of capitalist economic relations.[24] In tracts such as Engels's *The Condition of the Working-Class in England* (1845), Marxists made the connection between health and political action. As socialists strengthened their appeals, bourgeois governments fought back with social welfare. The idea spread throughout European governing circles that health benefits undermined the appeal of the socialists even as they strengthened the state.[25]

Although concern over the volatility of the working class furthered state support for health reform, other motivations—including military, political, and economic necessity—figured prominently in the adoption of public health programs. States needed healthy citizens in order to obtain stronger recruits, create effective armies, and increase productivity in the war industries. Military needs stimulated all types of reforms, from interest in natal care, to improved workplaces, to battlefield hospital sanitation. For example, American reform gained momentum following the Civil War and British reform was motivated by the Boer War.[26] The same forces influencing public health worldwide propelled Russian reform. In Russia the connection between health care and military needs had been evident since the time of Peter the Great, who had made his top military medical inspector the highest-ranking medical official of the empire.[27] Reform of all aspects of Russian society, including provincial health care, followed Russia's humiliating defeat in the Crimean War (1853–56). The poor performance of the military and the low number of fit recruits necessitated action.[28]

Partially in response to the war, Alexander II pursued his "Great Reforms" by addressing the "cursed questions" of Russian difference and development. After abolishing the legal basis of serfdom, Alexander turned to the question of governance. He established local assemblies, called *zemstvos,* which were placed in charge of governing the provinces and providing social services. As part of their numerous duties, the *zemstvos* were charged with caring for public health. Although they never received full financial support (the authoritarian center feared their power), the *zemstvos* used their limited funds to introduce many standard programs of public health, including nurseries, dispensaries, water systems, school sanitation, and registration of disease.[29] These programs did not even come close to meeting the regional needs of their citizens, let alone the entirety of the empire, but they were a crucial first step.

Young, idealistic people involved with Russian populism or other reform movements were drawn to the medical wings of the *zemstvos.*[30] Perhaps because of their enthusiasm, but most definitely because of their ties to radical politics, the *zemstvo* physicians met resistance from the government as they attempted to institute substantive changes. Authorities feared the intentions of their radicalized physicians, and successive tsars worried that independent organizations might form the basis for popular resistance.[31] This did not stop *zemstvo* physicians from meeting in the 1880s and forming the Society of Russian Physicians in Memory of N. I. Pirogov. As members of the Pirogov society and as *zemstvo* activists, many doctors pursued social reform. As proof of their commitment, some even established free clinics.[32] International institutes, hospitals, journals—even a Moscow conference attended by seven thousand doctors in 1897—furthered Russian medicine's ties to worldwide research and troubled authorities even more.[33]

Community medicine, a philosophy popular in Germany and England, formed part of the goals of Pirogov physicians.[34] The effect of the European sanitary movement was evident in the actions of *zemstvo* doctors, who attempted to investigate and eliminate disease at its source, involving physicians more closely with the daily life of the patient.[35] Influenced by studies from abroad, many Russian physicians held that poor, filthy, urban environments encouraged disease; they attacked the developing city as too dangerous a place to live.[36] Reports presented at the meetings of the Pirogov society underscored abysmal sanitary conditions, which caused deaths to exceed births in many Russian cities.[37] By the late 1800s doctors, public health officials, statisticians, and reformers warned of severe consequences to the state if urban problems were not addressed.[38] As a result of pressure by public health advocates and problems of industrialization, the areas of urban development, sanitation, and housing all received government attention, intervention, and investment at the turn of the century.[39] Though their professional powers were circumscribed, these activists accomplished a great deal.[40]

Although Pirogov physicians portrayed themselves as a progressive force besieged by a hostile state, the tsarist government also expressed concern for the health of its citizens. The tsar, however, wished to have reform come from centralized institutions under the direction of the state.[41] For example, in the early years of the twentieth century, tsarist laws provided for security in case of industrial-related injury or sickness.[42] According to progressive physicians, these efforts fell woefully short of substantial reform. In 1907 only a third of all mills had some type of organized health care.[43] Other efforts encountered even less success. For instance, a commission approved by the tsar to consider the creation of a centralized health administration in Russia was stymied by the outbreak of war.[44]

The natal campaigns of Russia and Europe in the late nineteenth and early twentieth centuries reflected the confluence of political and humanitarian goals. At the end of the nineteenth century, governments and societal groups worldwide expressed concern over birth rates as a result of humanitarian considerations for mothers and children, the need for military recruits, and the desire to ensure an increase in "pure" racial stock for Social Darwinist agendas. A perceived depopulation crisis led to the institution of natalist programs in France in the 1870s.[45] The British and Americans showed greater interest in natal health after encountering difficulties in finding fit military recruits at the turn of the century.[46] Private, humanitarian initiatives preceded government programs, which began in England in 1918 and in the United States in 1921.[47] The Italians began state intervention in the 1920s.[48] Russia followed a similar pattern. Doctors and private individuals organized the first natalist programs in Russia in the early 1900s, with the state taking over these programs after about a decade.[49] The large number of female physicians involved in professional development in Russia contributed to the increased attention to children and women's health.[50] In addition to natal programs, tuberculosis-related activities and famine relief were areas of public welfare that interested private organizations and volunteers.[51]

The need to ensure public compliance was a question of return on investment, as well as a political, military, and economic requirement, and it led to more and more invasive programs. Health became a right, but citizens had the duty to maintain their health for the benefit of the state. Even as countries such as Britain preached a liberal agenda, they permitted increased intervention in the home to ensure public health. Encouraged, in part, by concerns over tuberculosis—which was viewed as a disease of social interaction—the British invested in new techniques of surveillance and social control to bring public behavior in line with governmental requirements.[52] At the other end of the political spectrum, socialists and utilitarians pursued public health reform and emphasized the importance of individual behavior—hygiene, diet, and exercise—to progress.[53] Both sides justified intrusion in the home as necessary to protect society as a whole. The overall objective of this surveillance and discipline was to fashion bodies that were docile, productive, and ready for recruitment.[54]

The fall of the tsarist regime in 1917 left behind a poor record on public health. Doctors had been oppressed and their professional organization was weak. The *zemstvo,* charged with caring for public health, received little material help. Government distrust of independent groups had thwarted philanthropic development; however, the emphasis on a well-ordered state had resulted in medical surveillance of the population. Monthly medical reports of all treatments were required of health care practitioners.[55] Revolution did not lead to immediate change. The Provisional Government had little success because of its brief term of office and low funding.[56] With the arrival of the Soviets there would be a massive turnaround in public health. The Soviet interest in controlling populations meant a proliferation of measurements, diagnoses, and prescriptions that addressed natal questions alongside all aspects of personal hygiene. Soviet leaders recognized the crucial need to manage their population and its health in preparation for industrial and military competition with the West. Hygienists harnessed the state's interventionist tendency in their desire to save the workers from themselves.

Narkomzdrav analyzed the population through a central bureaucracy, created new programs, and drafted citizens as inspectors and organizers for health care.[57] Soviet reliance upon categorizing, surveilling, and controlling its citizenry arose just as these techniques and concerns were becoming part of the modern state elsewhere. While Bolshevik techniques mirrored those of other countries, their more ambitious goals for transforming all aspects of daily life resulted in differences in how and to what extent the Soviets used these tools.[58] Trotsky argued that intrusion into the worker family could be done for hygienic or pedagogical reasons. As the transformation of culture became a quest to change even the most mundane aspects of behavior, these two entrees into the worker home became gaping doors to state penetration.[59] In addition, Russian traditions that emphasized the collective over the individual opened the doors more widely for health inspectors and medical investigators to charge the individual family with maintaining the health of the entire society.

It was not just Soviet activists who proclaimed Narkomzdrav unlike any other program in the world and only possible in a communist state. Contemporaries noted the unique nature of Soviet public health and the amazing intersection of political and hygiene agendas. In his 1937 study Henry E. Sigerist, founder of the *Bulletin of the History of Medicine,* concluded: "The Soviet system of protection of the people's health is basically different from all other public health systems. It is a socialist system. The weapons used in the war against disease are very similar to those used in other countries, but the whole strategy and tactics are different."[60] The promise of health care served as a symbol of the unique communist agenda. The Bolsheviks founded Narkomzdrav in 1918, claiming that it was the first ministry of its type in the world.[61] Health figured prominently in the rhetoric of revolution, with the Bolsheviks loudly broadcasting their commitment to worker care. In the *ABC of Communism,* N. Bukharin and E. Preobrazhensky's popular version of the party platform of 1919, the provision of good housing, the campaign to eradicate epidemic disease, and the fight against social diseases received top priority.[62] As testimony to their commitment and their revolution, the Bolsheviks insured all workers, promising them treatment and medicine free of charge.[63]

N. A. Semashko, the first head of Narkomzdrav, served as the People's Commissar of Health from 1918 to 1930, coming to the post after many years of political activism and medical practice. He entered the revolutionary life early, joining a Marxist circle at Moscow University in 1893. In 1895 he was sent into internal exile for his political activities. While serving his sentence in Kazan, he attended medical school and engaged in Social Democratic actions. He finished his medical degree and graduated with distinction before moving on to work in provincial posts. His involvement in revolutionary upheaval in Nizhnii Novgorod in 1905 led to his incarceration and subsequent exile to Switzerland, where he fell in with Lenin. In 1917 Semashko returned with Lenin on the sealed train for the October Revolution. Forced out of office in the late 1920s—the Stalinist great turn meant new priorities and different leadership—he lived on until 1949.[64]

Semashko's conception of health problems and plans for Narkomzdrav drew upon his revolutionary experience and medical training. The organization developed as an amalgam of past institutions and international concepts. Though Soviet reformers decried the efforts of the tsarist government and contemporary bourgeois states as ineffective, prerevolutionary goals for hygiene and bourgeois techniques meshed well with the ideals of the new state and its priorities.[65] Indeed, Narkomzdrav benefited from the foundations provided by prerevolutionary organizations and institutions.[66] Not only the institutions but also the personnel were similar. Many radical Pirogov physicians helped establish Narkomzdrav.[67]

In 1918 Semashko set out an agenda for Narkomzdrav dependent upon the concepts of social hygiene. Social hygienists combined the fields of sociology and biology to address the circumstances that gave rise to disease, arguing that instead of understanding disease as a condition of the body, medical specialists would be better served by studying the condition of society. Under Semashko's urging, social hygiene became the guiding principle of Narkomzdrav. Semashko came to his understanding of social hygiene through such German pioneers of public health as Alfred Grotjahn, a Social Democrat who popularized the concept during the late nineteenth century. Narkomzdrav officials borrowed heavily from the Germans in this and many other areas, translating German works and maintaining links with German journals.[68]

While social hygiene informed policy and propaganda, other practitioners argued for different approaches. Narkomzdrav sheltered both social hygienists and eugenicists in the 1920s; even social hygienists differed in their teachings from university to university.[69] In fact, social hygiene would never gain as much acceptance with students and practitioners as it had from the commissar of health and would founder once he was removed from office.[70] Thanks to its official sponsorship, during the 1920s the rhetoric of social hygiene would color medical teachings, general hygiene lessons, and the vast amount of propaganda that emerged concerning health questions.

In order to change society, modify behavior, and prevent disease, Semashko wanted Narkomzdrav to provide centralized, universal, and prophylactic care.[71] Conditions for change were less than auspicious, but a commitment to these three principles still determined Narkomzdrav policy. Despite opposition from some physicians, centralization occurred quickly. Because of budgetary constraints, shortages, and pressure to privilege workers, universal health care never became a reality. While Semashko and many of his fellow Narkomzdrav physicians and hygiene propagandists were committed to the revolution, they were also set apart by their particular goals, which did not always coincide with those of economic or worker organizations. Prophylaxis was still important for Narkomzdrav but proved difficult to achieve in the environment of war, famine, and disease that greeted the new commissar of health.[72]

Even before 1914, Russia had been a land of epidemics subject to devastating outbreaks. Internal disruptions from war and revolution only worsened health conditions. Between 1919 and 1923 three quarters of the population suffered from famine. The American Relief Administration (ARA) stepped in to feed nearly eleven million Soviets daily, but it was still not enough. Hunger weakened immune systems, and Spanish influenza, cholera, smallpox, and plague tormented Russia. Other infections raged because of the disruptions of war. Malaria became a significant problem after 1922 when Allied forces blocked the flow of quinine. In 1923 there were more than four million cases registered. The total number of deaths from disease and famine soared as high as ten million between 1916 and 1923.[73] Semashko would have to address these critical health issues even as he tried to realize his goals in "the fight against tuberculosis, venereal disease, [and] professional diseases; the protection of mothers and infants; the protection of the health of children and youth; sanitary statistical analysis; and measures for physical culture and sanitary enlightenment."[74]

Conditions were dire. A visitor could not fail to notice the awful situation of the majority of the population. H. G. Wells, staying in Petrograd in 1920, described horrendous material circumstances where medicine was unattainable and minor problems spiraled out of control. He observed that a "buoyant, healthy person is very rare in this atmosphere of discomforts and petty deficiencies" and painted a bleak picture of hospital conditions: "There was an appalling lack of every sort of material, and half the beds were not in use through the sheer impossibility of dealing with more patients if they came in."[75] Wells's description of "petty deficiencies" merely hinted at the depth of the problem. Doctors left the country. Pharmaceuticals were nearly gone.[76]

Within this atmosphere of deprivation, epidemic disease blazed. Particularly prevalent were typhus and cholera—illnesses characteristic of rapidly urbanized populations with poor water supplies, bad food, and overcrowded housing.[77] Typhus, by far the worst of the epidemics, spread quickly throughout revolutionary Russia along rail lines. According to some estimates, one in four adults suffered from typhus and relapsing fever after the revolution.[78] Famine, especially in the Ukraine and Volga provinces, aided the spread of the disease.[79]

From 1918 to 1920 five million registered cases of typhus claimed almost three million lives.[80] Estimates put the total number of cases at anywhere from sixteen to twenty-five million.[81] The numbers are staggering when compared with the rest of Europe. For example, England had only 390 typhus deaths from 1899 to 1913.[82]

Typhus epidemics and their itchy handmaidens, lice, were the chief impetus to reforming health policy. Indeed, Lenin singled out typhus as a major threat. At the Eighth All-Russia Conference of the Russian Communist Party (Bolshevik), held in December 1919, Lenin lamented, "A third scourge is assailing us, *lice,* and the *typhus* that is mowing down our troops. Comrades, it is impossible to imagine the dreadful situation in the typhus regions, where the population is broken, weakened, without material resources, where all life, all public life ceases."[83] Lenin's emphasis upon the disruption caused by the disease showed his concern for more than people's comfort. By silencing public life, typhus threatened the population as well as the government. A broken population without public life would fall rather than fight. Lenin linked disease prevention to political necessity, thus ensuring that louse control would become a major focus of Narkomzdrav from 1918 to 1922.[84] So prevalent was the connection of Narkomzdrav to the control of lice that one observer quipped that people called the parasites "Semashkos" after the commissar of health.[85] Of course, this flippant, mocking comment may indicate that the population trivialized these campaigns even as they recognized their ubiquity.

Only after several years of desperately trying to turn the tide of epidemics did Narkomzdrav turn to Semashko's third goal—prophylactic work. Since Semashko considered "lifestyle" (*bytovoi*) illnesses to be the main threat to the health of the population, he sought to create healthier citizens through social engineering.[86] In *The Foundations of Soviet Medicine* Semashko tied prophylactic medicine to the goal of changing the way Soviet citizens lived: "'Lifestyle' illnesses are to this day the misfortune of our country. They still mow down both the adult and youth populations. Therefore Soviet medicine sets itself the task for the sanitation of life and labor of the population, that is, the improvement of those conditions in which the population lives. The prevention of illnesses (preventative maintenance) is the main task of Soviet medicine."[87] Semashko's campaign to eradicate illness by changing behavior made private behavior a public issue. He did not, however, heap all the blame onto the victims. Acknowledging social hygiene's dependence on social conditions, he argued: "Alcoholism, degeneration, crime and similarly all other deadly sins depend, above all, on living standards."[88] Semashko's inclusion of crime and degeneracy linked individual care to the prevention of social problems. By grafting the fight against disease onto the cause of reform, Narkomzdrav echoed the arguments of tsarist Pirogov physicians, replicated the health programs of bourgeois governments, and furthered their own case for state support.[89]

To combat "lifestyle" illnesses, Semashko and the physicians, workers, and volunteers of Narkomzdrav used new institutions as distribution points to provide care. The most prevalent of these—the dispensary, the consultation, the sanatorium, and the House of Leisure—combined treatment and education to improve public health. The principle behind the prophylactic approach was simple and naïve: inform people of the consequences of their actions and they will choose the healthy path. Doctors and inspectors treated patients, dispersed information on preventative medicine, and monitored progress. Organizers expected both the ill and the healthy to leave with the knowledge of how to improve their lives and the motivation to do so.

In theory dispensaries served the health care needs of all workers and attempted to monitor both the sick and the healthy. Dispensary doctors visited workers on the shop floor and received the ill at the clinic. The doctor had the authority to treat the body and manage the life of the patient. He could prescribe conventional treatment, move the patient to a new apartment, urge him or her to change jobs, arrange a sanatorium stay, or recommend more extensive treatment at a specialized facility. In addition, the patient learned about the disease through educational literature and private consultations with the doctor. Doctors instructed patients regarding how to alter their home, diet, leisure activities, and work habits to prevent a relapse. The ideal, full dispensary treatment included home visits by a doctor or nurse as a form of direct intervention and to determine if anything in the home hindered the healing process. The home inspectors, most often nurses or volunteers rather than doctors, carried out sanitary enlightenment within the home, made the inhabitants aware of housekeeping "errors," counseled balanced personal behavior, and in extreme cases found hygienically designed apartments for patients.[90] As a result of factory visits, home investigations, and medical consultations, the dispensary spread new ideas about health and consequently became associated with the sanitary enlightenment of the population.[91] For difficult cases organizers envisaged a vast support network—including ambulatory clinics, spas, special dietary cafeterias, and night sanatoriums—to join the dispensaries.[92]

Given their combination of surveillance, treatment, and education, dispensaries became involved in the life of the patient as well as the illness. They also accumulated reams of documentation on the physical characterisitics of citizens, comparing and classifying in the hope of constructing an ideal.[93] Nurses and doctors then used the statistics to identify problems. Narkomzdrav, the first centralized system for observation of health needs, was uniquely positioned to apply these figures and calculations to disciplinary techniques. Statistics provided an important tool in the management of the population. According to one later theorist, Lenin considered statistics "one of the most important weapons of social knowledge" and an invaluable "tool of socialist construction and state management."[94] Even in the truncated form it assumed during the NEP, the dispensary provided both the observational tools and the disciplinary structure to carry the Soviet mission for cultured, politicized living into individual homes.

The Fifth All-Russia Congress of Health Departments, held in 1924, emphasized the centrality of the dispensary and its prophylactic contribution to Soviet health.[95] While Moscow claimed to be the "first in the country and the first in the world" to introduce the practical dispensary method, the dispensary's foundation rested deep within European state traditions.[96] England developed the first dispensary for the poor in 1769. The perceived usefulness of the institution can be appreciated in their rapid spread. By 1840 twenty-three existed in London and eighty were scattered throughout the provinces.[97] Dispensaries permitted treatment and observation to work in tandem, thus extending medical supervision to social interaction.[98] Dispensaries figured in later European utopian thought as well. Bentham conceived of his industry houses as functioning dispensaries, serving as sites for experimentation, the gathering of statistical information on the population, education, and treatment.[99] In Russia the dispensary system was a late-nineteenth-century phenomenon, although its adoption was rapid.[100] On the eve of war, the All-Russia League for the Fight against Tuberculosis put the dispensary method at the center of its system of care.[101]

The Soviets developed dispensaries for the treatment and prevention of tuberculosis in 1919 and four years later opened special dispensaries for venereal disease.[102] Some dispensaries retained a specialized focus, whereas others treated all types of health problems. Dispensaries did not come near to providing for the entire population; although modest in number, they had a long reach. In 1925 the eighty-four dispensaries of the Russian federation devoted to the treatment of venereal disease saw some three hundred thousand individuals and did nearly three million follow-up investigations.[103] The capital benefited most fully from this system. In 1926 dispensary doctors in Moscow visited factories and examined two hundred thousand workers, recommending medical treatment for more than half.[104] By the end of the 1920s a large number of dispensaries for general illness, turberculosis, venereal disease, and even substance abuse served the population. In 1927 Moscow dispensaries numbered over three hundred and claimed to have admitted over seventeen million visitors in the years 1925–26.[105]

While the dispensary concentrated on changing personal habits, the programs of natal health focused on changing the care given to others. Mothers, viewed as the responsible parent, received instruction stressing their importance and were blamed when things went poorly. The consultation used elements of the dispensary method but provided for the special needs of mothers and children as a way to ensure the health of the next generation. Consultations for pregnant women, nursing mothers, and small children served development, infancy, and childhood. In addition, they functioned as sites for the distribution of propaganda on child care and home management. In association with the consultation, nurses investigated the home to diagnose domestic problems, provide instruction, and, in severe cases, request material assistance. By 1927 the Moscow Department of Health oversaw more than sixty consultations of various types.[106] Included were thirty-five consultations for breast-feeding children, which claimed to have logged over 630,000 appointments in 1925–26. Birth homes numbered twenty-one in Moscow, with 62,046 served in 1925–26.[107] In addition, a number of specialized institutions aided Soviet consultations with further care for children and new mothers. The Subdepartment for the Protection of Children's Health inspected children in Moscow schools, visiting 510 schools in 1921 and progressively more with each new year. They also visited children's homes and institutions for sick children. In addition, the Department for the Protection of Motherhood and Infancy oversaw nurseries; milk kitchens; homes for youth, mothers, and children; and summer nurseries.[108]

The consultation, like the dispensary, first appeared in the West. Inspired by humanitarian, political, and Social Darwinist concerns, nineteenth-century European and American communities shifted from providing aid in milk kitchens to children's clinics with supervision and instruction for mothers. Some British officials argued that infant mortality resulted from poor maternal care and intervened in the home for the protection and observation of children.[109] In the United States, beginning in 1908 the New York City Health Department united a concern for infant health with a push for prevention. Using birth records to target new mothers, the health department sent the public health nurse to visit and teach the mother "what to do to keep the baby well." Organizers believed a change in the mother's attitude was as necessary as medical attention for children's health. To aid the consultation, American public health officials established milk distribution points, baby health stations, and foundling hospitals; it also initiated school inspections.[110]

Possessing similar networks, the Soviet dispensary and consultation attempted to instruct workers and families in familiar settings. For those who did not benefit from this system, Narkomzdrav developed companion institutions. The sanatorium and House of Leisure placed patients in isolation to treat and educate them.[111] The sanatorium sheltered the ill from poor living conditions to aid recovery. The House of Leisure offered healthy workers an alternative during their annual vacations. In both institutions a strict, doctor-recommended and doctor-enforced regimen defined life.

Such treatment facilities were not new to Russia. Following his Grand Tour, Peter the Great developed the first spas in Russia. In imitation of European grandeur, he ordered a palace built at Petrozavodsk to take advantage of the mineral springs and their "curative" properties. Sanatoriums for tuberculosis cures arrived in Russia in the last half of the nineteenth century, focusing on manipulation of hygiene and diet to cure the body. The Soviets took over the sanatoriums, as they had taken control of the lands sheltering them, adding the spas of Crimea in 1920 and soon moving eastward.[112] Spas, sanatoriums, and Houses of Leisure attended to increasing numbers of patients and visitors during this period. By 1925–26 351,045 Soviet citizens had experienced the benefits of the system and organizers anticipated that in 1926–27 these facilities would serve over 500,000 people.[113] In 1925 nearly forty Houses of Leisure and sanatoriums catered to the needs of over 60,000 Muscovites, of which thirty sanatoriums served nearly 20,000 ill.[114]

While the sanatorium had a long history, especially for tuberculosis treatment, the House of Leisure was fully a creation of the Soviets, as propagandists never failed to mention. Health authorities constantly noted that their programs could exist only in a worker state, thus underscoring for the population and foreign visitors the benefits of their new government. Working-class delegations and distinguished visitors invariably toured an impressive, experimental health institution that highlighted not only the vigor of the new state but also its public priorities. Enthusiastic visitors noted the degeneracy and weakness of capitalism in contrast to vigorous, worker-centered government, and even the more cautious were impressed by the scope of the experiment.[115]

The dispensary, consultation, sanitarium, and House of Leisure all received significant press coverage that far exceeded their scope. Indeed, the coverage for all health care institutions was disproportionate in terms of their numbers. During the latter half of the 1920s, Narkomzdrav expanded at a greater rate of growth than any other branch of government yet still came nowhere near meeting the needs of the entire population. Although they nearly met the medical needs of the capital, they fell ludicrously short of providing for all of Russia and, later, the Soviet Union. Existing facilities remained in a poor state, salaries were lower than before the war, and personnel were still few in number.[116]

A lack of state support exacerbated these problems. Health care had been a priority during the various epidemics, but when they faded so, too, did government interest. With the introduction of NEP, the entire country turned to the belt-tightening measures required for efficient enterprise. Health care suffered, with much of the financial responsibility for public health institutions shifted to already strapped local budgets. The May 1922 transfer of responsibility for medical needs to local authorities, however, was not universal. The funding for the campaign against social diseases and for essential services remained the responsibility of the central authorities. Though no group really had the money, after 1922 Narkomzdrav did expand its personnel and programs.[117]

It was clear that the working class would receive the lion's share of medical resources. The social insurance fund maintained by workers provided most of the support for public health. Unions pressured Narkomzdrav to ensure preferential coverage for workers by threatening to withhold their contributions—representing 30 percent of the total health budget—if Narkomzdrav did not follow the 1922 decree giving priority to workers.[118] Narkomzdrav officials, however, pushed for need-based care. Narkomzdrav retained control, but this would prove to be a brief victory. Union agitation plus other factors led to inequities in care between urban and rural citizens. The insured had much more money spent on their care and greater access to doctors rather than physicians' assistants.[119] By the late 1920s transfer of care to the insured was nearly complete. This meant that, compared to prerevolutionary figures showing about 20 percent of workers insured, now about 90 percent of wage earners received care.[120] Still, only a small percentage of the population had insured care. By 1929 10.9 million workers received insurance benefits out of a population of around 150 million.[121]

The policies of NEP and insurance medicine held a number of consequences for medical practice. Economic problems entailed replacing universal health care with fees for services, which severely limited the ability of many to seek medical care and led to closings. Because of the pressure to insure workers, programs remained concentrated in urban areas. Moreover, the use of class to allocate benefits led to a great deal of political intrusion in the distribution of health care.[122] The uninsured population was hit hard. Local budgets provided funding for peasants and uninsured urbanites, who accounted for about 90 percent of the population, but preferential treatment meant that by 1926–27 the uninsured rural resident saw an expenditure of 1.05 rubles for health care, while 20.31 rubles were spent on the insured urban worker.[123]

Semashko's task was further complicated by a significant decrease in the number of doctors in Russia and the low opinion of medicine held by the general population. Before the revolution the majority of the population had only been exposed to folk medicine, having dealt with faith healers or, at best, doctors' assistants. Doctors' assistants, known as *fel'dsher,* had grown in number during the nineteenth century, first as military doctors and then as regular health care providers. They were scorned by the public.[124] The increase in poorly trained medical professionals stratified medicine and led to an opening of the field to women during the late nineteenth century. The medical profession in revolutionary Russia was further plagued by a reputation for disloyalty. The relationship between the prerevolutionary community physicians and the Bolsheviks had been a stormy one. A number of Russian physicians rejected the revolution, and the Bolsheviks alleged that the majority plotted against them.[125]

The Bolsheviks desperately needed the help of doctors and nurses even if they did not trust them. In 1919 Lenin argued that only with the help of persons trained in science could the revolution triumph in Russia. Narkomzdrav recruited all those available. The doctors of the department were small in number but highly educated, older, and middle or upper class in terms of background. Although they had a great deal of expertise and a genuine, long-standing interest in public health, preventative medicine, and government action, they could not make up for the dearth of resources with enthusiasm. Doctors survived difficult conditions in the 1920s. The state paid them little, and their morale was low. Most gravitated toward the major urban areas; in 1924, 80 percent of all physicians lived in the city. While the periphery languished, Moscow had more doctors than it could afford to employ.[126] Some set themselves up in private practice and proved important as abortion providers, but they were subject to harsh crackdowns in the late 1920s.[127]

Many doctors chose to leave. Russia had long experienced a shortage of health care practitioners. On the eve of 1917, European Russia could only boast 13,475 doctors, well below England (22,105), Germany (16,270), and France (14,380). If the ratio of doctors to inhabitants was taken into account, Russia stood in even more stark contrast.[128] The loosening of requirements and the recruitment of large numbers for the medical profession—especially women—constituted an attempt to rectify the problem. On the eve of World War I Russia had a larger percentage of female physicians than any other country. By 1913 10 percent of physicians and 28 percent of medical students were women.[129] Even with the influx of women, the number of doctors for the population remained low, with about 11,000 doctors (13,000 fewer than before the war) available in 1921.[130] Under NEP the number of women in medicine increased; by

1926 women constituted 52 percent of Soviet medical students and by 1934 they accounted for 71 percent.[131] By 1928 52 percent of doctors were women and more were well on their way to receiving their degrees.[132] The increase in personnel did not translate into better care. Many of these new medical professionals had taken abbreviated courses and emerged woefully unprepared and unwilling to move to the countryside.

In the face of a shortage of institutions, practitioners, and supplies, sanitary propaganda represented the linchpin of Narkomzdrav's prophylactic program. According to one historian of public health, it had developed in the Soviet Union more than in any other country.[133] In 1918 sanitary enlightenment became a formal concern of Narkomzdrav with the formation of the Department of Sanitary Enlightenment, headed by A. N. Sysin, under the Sanitary-Epidemiological section.[134] The first All-Russia Conference on Sanitary Enlightenment took place in Moscow in March 1921, when 203 delegates met to discuss sanitary education in theory and practice.[135] This attention paid to propaganda as a force for change fit in with the Enlightenment-inspired faith of the Soviets in the didactic power of newspapers, magazines, and posters. It also served as a powerful merging of science, health, and humanitarian concerns in the area of population control.[136]

Sanitary enlightenment emerged significantly in the 1918–20 fight against epidemics.[137] For the general population sanitary enlightenment took the form of pamphlets, lectures, railroad-car exhibitions, and weeklong campaigns devoted to cleaning out hot spots of infection.[138] The Red Army organized its own work and launched a massive education campaign to fight epidemic diseases. In 1920 86,000 sanitary presentations reached 6.4 million military listeners, and nearly 4 million attended health lectures.[139] In 1921 Moscow province claimed to have hosted over 800 lectures in just the period up to June 1.[140] In 1926 there were 227,984 sanitary presentations reaching 1,052,002 people.[141] Although these lectures and performances drew in a limited number, considering the size of the country, they still dwarfed contemporary international efforts.

The introduction of NEP hampered Narkomzdrav's abilities to publish, but in 1922 the department reached an agreement with Gosizdat and by the next year the Medical-Scientific section of Gosizdat was in charge of medical publications. Over 13 million pieces of literature relating to the fight against syphilis, typhus, and other diseases were released between 1919 and 1927.[142] Between 1925 and 1927 Narkomzdrav presses printed 40 titles in print runs of 600,000 copies and produced 50,000 slides to accompany medical lectures.[143] The Moscow Department of Health had its own publishers, who were particularly active, including a special press devoted to natal issues that printed 90 titles, while private presses, such as Practical Medicine, put out 522 titles during the same period.[144] Newspapers and magazines joined in the production of health care articles. Many of the foremost authors and artists participated; Deni and Dmitrii Moor created posters, while Maiakovskii penned slogans for sanitary enlightenment.[145]

Narkomzdrav did not produce all health-related material intended for the public. As Frances Lee Bernstein shows in her study, the sex question in particular attracted many authors with varied reasons for producing pamphlets. Semashko became irate over materials he felt were intended merely to titillate or those that were based on politics thinly disguised as science, but these were unique cases. There was general unanimity on most hygiene questions, probably as a result of the medical community's shared ideas and training. Bernstein notes the "overwhelming sense of sameness" in the literature on the sex question, whether from Narkomzdrav doctors or private presses. The same degree of unanimity is found in the less controversial advice on cleanliness.[146]

Health propaganda authors attempted to reach a semiliterate or newly literate population with simplified prose and pictures that did not stray too far into avant-garde presentation. The sheer number of titles and high print runs indicated that even though in theory Marxist cultural transformation was predicated on changing the material bases of society, leaders were confident that a well-intentioned pamphlet could move the process along.[147] Small, portable, and easy to read, with drawings on the covers and inside, pamphlets were designed to grab the attention of barely literate readers. Magazines used simplified prose and short articles to appeal to those who might have trouble with long, detailed offerings. They contained cartoons, games, and photographs to draw the eye. Despite all these efforts, pamphlet literature reached only a limited audience of the interested and educated. In 1926 only 44 percent of the population of Moscow province was schooled, even though the city was more literate than the countryside and Moscow province was more so than the rest of Russia.[148]

Although written materials reached a limited audience, posters made greater inroads thanks to the strong visual tradition in Russia and the necessity of reaching an illiterate population. Political posters came out in the millions after the revolution and were affixed to every conceivable stationary object—in some cases they even adorned mobile displays on boats, trains, and cars. When paper supplies proved inadequate, stencils were used to apply slogans directly to buildings, walls, and fences. Until 1921 political posters espousing the civil war had predominated. After 1921 national priorities changed and general tasks—such as industrial and agricultural buildup, literacy, and public health—came to the fore.[149] Among these pleas and exhortations were posters supporting health care and the fight against epidemic diseases. Health-related posters were generally representational and easily interpreted. Instead of lengthy scientific discussions, they often settled for catchy slogans with simple text and visuals rather than cutting-edge art.[150] Posters recalled such traditional art forms as the *lubok* woodcut and the icon.[151] This style broadened the appeal of posters to people missed by written propaganda or the more experimental aesthetic of monumental propaganda.

Posters for health-related propaganda remained largely unsigned, making it difficult to establish authorship. Most posters were the product of health departments and were produced under the supervision of health professionals. In pamphlet literature the tendency for doctors and medical candidates to claim authorship and establish their authority was strong. The title page often included the author's professional credentials. The authors' political affiliations were not always apparent. Although private presses were active and some authors did not support the entire Bolshevik agenda, publications generally had to to be approved by Soviet censors.[152] Despite questions, it can probably be assumed that the authors of advice literature belonged to an elite group whose mission was to educate the public.[153]

The didactic health poster and pamphlet borrowed techniques from Europe and the past. European activists issued pamphlets in the mid-1700s that appealed to individual reason for the improvement of health. The publication of health care pamphlets exploded during the Enlightenment period. According to scholars of European health movements, these works increased elite society's interest in health but had a negligible impact on the masses. Even as the message spread, the effects of the industrial revolution upon workers' health and lives ensured that despite the working class's inclination to follow prescriptions, the actual capacity for change was limited. The prescriptions of the pamphlets had limited therapeutic value in the face of extremely poor living conditions.[154]

Despite such problems, health advocates continued to rely upon educational efforts—and not always as a last resort. For reformers fighting tuberculosis in the United States, education was a preferred tactic, not a fallback when other initiatives failed. Americans emphasized educational work in late-nineteenth-century campaigns against tuberculosis because it was cheap and inoffensive.[155] In 1914 the New York City Health Department organized the first bureau for health education within an official agency. By 1929 there were over eighty municipal and state health department bulletins being published in the United States. World War I accelerated health education initiatives, especially with respect to providing information about venereal disease. American women's clubs and workers' unions functioned as important allies in the movement. Europeans employed education in their battle to change common harmful practices. Germany began spreading health propaganda to the public in 1908. The English founded the Central Council for Health Education in 1927. In France education was a recognized duty of official agencies, but private organizations were also heavily involved.[156]

Health professionals worldwide spread their message in different and innovative ways, utilizing educational techniques, new technologies like the moving picture, and even advertising approaches. For instance, in the United States tuberculosis activists employed staple premises of advertising rhetoric—shame, responsibility, or reward—in their appeals to pursue healthy lifestyles. They published human-interest stories in the popular press that emphasized personal triumph over tuberculosis. They printed anti-spitting messages and dispensary addresses on streetcar transfer stubs.[157] By the 1920s American public health advocates had popularized their message with pamphlets, leaflets, and newspaper stories. In Louisiana authorities even mounted a train exhibition.[158]

Though health propaganda was used heavily in Europe and the United States, foreign visitors were astonished by its ubiquity among the Soviets. Horace Gantt, an American doctor who worked with the American Relief Administration and later with Ivan Pavlov, concluded: "There is no corner in Russia which propaganda in the public health campaign against disease has not reached."[159] Others commented upon the omnipresent didactic poster. Educational theorist John Dewey observed the prevalence of instructional propaganda in the Soviet Union in 1928, saying that nowhere was it so consistently employed for "the universal good of universal humanity."[160] During a visit to the country, novelist Theodore Dreiser was amazed by the waves of propaganda devoted to hygiene topics:

> Wherever I went, there they were. Pictures or charts relating to every conceivable type of thing—cooking, washing, exercising, cleaning the house, getting rid of fleas and dirt, packing fruits or vegetables for shipment or preservation; mixing different kinds of grain or vegetables for animal or human food; pruning trees; running the automobile or caring for the house; making the right sort of roof for the winter; arranging the right sort of ventilation in summer; showing the right sort of clothing for baby or school child; showing the proper arrangement of a new town; showing methods of building a cellar or a silo—a thousand and one things in connection with the life of the people.

Dreiser concluded: "I sometimes wondered how the poor Russians made out under all—why they were not smothered under the downpour."[161]

Since the time of Catherine the Great, advice concerning comportment had included health recommendations. In the late nineteenth century hygiene propaganda came into its own and gained institutional support. The *zemstvo* physicians conceived of their work as enlightenment rather than treatment, employing teachers or clergy and distributing pamphlets urging better housing, clothing, diet, summer nurseries, and kindergartens.[162] In 1894 the Pirogov society founded the Commission for the Spread of Hygienic Knowledge to the People, which was charged with distributing popular medical literature and visual aids. The commission published over 2 million leaflets and nearly 300,000 brochures. In 1919 A. V. Mol'kov, then head of the commission, turned over its stock and equipment to the Department for Sanitary Enlightenment under Narkomzdrav.[163] Mol'kov continued to be an active figure in the 1920s, and this continuity of personnel and equipment suggested the melding of pre- and postrevolutionary messages for public health.

Glorious visions of the future, threats of public humiliation, and promises of economic prosperity—all prominent in Western health propaganda and prerevolutionary advertising—also appeared in Soviet sanitary enlightenment.[164] In addition to advertising techniques, native art and folk traditions framed appeals. Rhyming couplets and slogans set to popular song lyrics graced the pages of Soviet magazines, with the occasional quiz, crossword puzzle, or rebus on health themes to amuse and draw in readers. Like their foreign counterparts, Bolshevik health propagandists relied upon a variety of mediums, including plays, films, and exhibitions. Inspiration could come from anywhere. One traveler recounted a conversation she had with a Russian journeying to the United States. When the Russian spied the decoration of the ship's matchbooks with the name of the line, he exclaimed: "'What a splendid idea! . . . I shall send some of these home. We should adopt this idea. Only we would not use them to advertise private boat companies. We would write on each match: 'Wash your hands before eating' . . . 'Take a bath every day' . . . 'Eat slowly' . . . 'Keep your dining rooms neat.'"[165]

Hygiene propaganda saturated Soviet society and appeared in surprising venues as well as in multiple forms. Youth groups, schools, and clubs all contrived to refashion people as part of their mission to create the new, Soviet citizen. Films, posters, and traveling exhibitions got out the message. Many of these efforts were aimed not at health education but at the broader mission of refining citizens. Often staged in former private mansions or museums, these exhibitions combined with posters to define an ordered lifestyle.[166] In their recommendations and tables, authors delineated a life, a home, and a body that was regulated and purified. By making certain habits part of a sound life and vilifying others, they accentuated balanced behaviors that underscored the classical conception of hygiene.

Hygienists attempted to integrate their message with the entire culture of creation around youth groups and workers' clubs. Particularly popular with these audiences was the theater, both professional and amateur. With its combination of sensory experiences and involvement between audience and actor, the theater was considered an especially powerful tool in cultural efforts.[167] Acting troupes performed plays with social and political content, often with didactic agendas. Plays attempted to be both informative and enjoyable by presenting important social issues in an entertaining format. For instance, *The End of Happiness* featured singing microbes and other amusing elements.[168] The "living newspaper" acted out events of the day. "Blue Blouse" theater groups presented songs and skits in cafeterias and workplaces to address questions of daily life. The group in Moscow attracted avant-garde authors and was extremely popular with audiences. By 1924 fourteen such groups were on tour, giving thousands of performances. Some even took their shows abroad.[169]

The agitational mock trial, based on prerevolutionary peasant rituals, emerged as a method of propaganda during the civil war period.[170] The mock trial was first used to attack enemies of the people, foreign dignitaries, and political foes. After the civil war, the focus shifted from enemies without to enemies within—the prostitute, the bootlegger, the drunkard. These short, verbose, formulaic dramas mixed the concepts of poetic and proletarian justice with all the trappings of the regular trial. A judge, witnesses, defense, and prosecution all toyed with a specific theme. Audience members were encouraged to serve on the jury and even pass judgment at the end of the play. By involving the audience, organizers perhaps hoped that the experience would be more vivid and the lessons more permanent.[171] According to laudatory articles in the press, mock trials so excited their audiences that they often mistook them for the real thing. In a rather suspicious episode, the newspaper *Pravda* reported on a sanitary agitational trial as if it were a real trial, later explaining that it had made the mistake because the play was so true to life. Adding fuel to the fire, some actors reported that they felt threatened if they played the villain.[172] This dramatic take on the tribulations of actors was particularly self-serving since they portrayed themselves as victims of their own verisimilitude.

The theater's popularity made it an ideal locus for propaganda. In 1923 more than twice as many people attended the theater than went to lectures and discussions.[173] Amateur groups had the additional benefit of drawing crowds of participants as well as spectators. Club organizers noted that theater circles enjoyed special popularity with club members, and theater groups sprang up everywhere. Some groups devoted themselves to health-themed productions. Ukraine had eight sanitary-enlightenment theater groups that toured both city and countryside. The club of the medical workers' union had a theater group that did "living newspaper" productions. The Theater Institute of Sanitary Culture employed professionals to stage plays on alcoholism, venereal disease, and tuberculosis, even plundering Chekhov and Tolstoy for dramas dealing with health and medicine. The Moscow *oblast'* (regional) Department of Health organized a special institute devoted to issues of sanitary culture. It published a journal called *Theory and Practice of Sanitary Enlightenment* and organized a special theater collective that spread propaganda on hygiene.[174] In the latter half of the 1920s critics began to chip away at the amateur nature of agitational trials and "living newspapers" by pushing for a more diversified repertoire in theaters. During these early days, however, participants likely learned as much as spectators as they read and memorized their lines.[175] The performance pieces of sanitary theater attempted to grab the attention of an urban, semiliterate audience, which was attracted to multiple entertainments. Still, these pieces could only reach those who had the time to attend a club or could find a place in these often limited, almost always crowded spaces.

Other forms of propaganda aimed to entertain as it educated. The public craved variety in its leisure activities and propaganda workers catered to this desire with films on hygiene themes. The first films appeared in Russia in 1896 and the first native features were produced in 1908.[176] During the 1920s sanitary workers tailored this form to fit their own message by producing films on the health sciences, contagious diseases, and alcoholism.[177] Hygiene films such as *Fight for Life* (on malaria), *Life's Truths* (on syphilis), *Dispensary—Work and Life,* and *Abortion* were shown in clubs and factories.[178] These cultural films were a specialty of the clubs, whereas commercial theaters relied on light entertainment, and (usually) foreign films. Nevertheless, an English observer deemed the Soviet hygiene films "excellent," noting that they "seemed to excite the greatest interest in an audience that did not differ in externals from the ordinary 'movie' crowd."[179] In Leningrad film seemed one of the more popular pastimes for youth and women. By the end of the 1920s over 90 percent of both groups regularly attended films during their free time.[180]

Museums devoted to sanitary education, such as Moscow's House of Sanitary Enlightenment, presented workers with a different type of evening out, a concrete vision of a new, healthful life. In January 1919 Narkomzdrav founded the Museum of Social Hygiene and chose as its director A. V. Mol'kov, formerly of the Pirogov society's educational wing. In just its first month the museum greeted forty-five hundred visitors, with a total of nearly forty thousand by the end of the year.[181] Visitors seemed impressed with the museums, leading one traveler to remark,

> These institutions, with central headquarters and local branches in different parts of a large city and in the smaller provincial cities, prepare exhibitions of wax figures, pictures, charts, and lantern slides of epidemic, industrial, and venereal diseases. This material is open to the public, and is also sent out to such institutions as clubs and reading-rooms as part of a general propaganda of hygiene and health measures. . . . Through excursions a large number of workmen and peasants, also of students and pupils, are able to get the deeper impression given by the large exhibits of the directing Museum of Social Hygiene and its branches.[182]

The writer noted that social hygiene enjoyed greater exposure than just the programs of Narkomzdrav and focused on the many styles of learning promoted at the health museum.

By 1921 these two permanent exhibitions in Moscow were joined by fifteen *uezd* (district) museums, six traveling exhibitions, and two shop-window displays.[183] There were eighty-five permanent exhibitions in 1927.[184] Petrograd opened its first health museum in 1919 and already had two thousand visitors during its first month of operation, claiming nearly forty thousand over the course of the year. Petrograd also boasted a train exhibition and a tramcar display.[185] Although there is no denying the number and variety of propaganda venues, their quality may have been suspect. A photo included by Horace W. Gantt, an American doctor with the ARA, features a crowd of doctors posed in front of a rather unimposing facade belonging to one unfortunate House of Sanitary Enlightenment (figure 2.1). Not only does the establishment appear to be in a sorry state of disrepair, but its small size could not have accommodated more than a wax display or two and a smattering of posters.

These techniques reflected foreign influences. Specialized health museums and exhibitions made their first appearance in the nineteenth century in the form of a tuberculosis exhibit at the London World's Fair. In 1906 the first tuberculosis exhibit toured the United States. It was manned by specially trained guides who employed leaflets, slides, and movies in their presentations. A similar Toronto exhibition managed to attract thirteen thousand people in two weeks. The first permanent health display was mounted by German health authorities. The German Hygiene Museum was established in Dresden in 1912. The United States did not open a permanent exhibition until the 1940s.[186]

The Soviet exhibitions built upon these examples but eclipsed them in number and variety. The sanitary enlightenment activities of Moscow's Sokol district covered a typically diverse range of efforts. According to records of the district's health department dating from 1925, sanitary enlightenment activities included lectures, films, mock trials, and permanent exhibitions. During the first six months of the year, lectures on the themes of "work, life, and health" reached 161,306 listeners in the district. Traveling and corner health displays informed 54,292 people about hygienic living, though how this figure was tabulated remained a mystery. In addition, the department presented 117 films and 30 plays on sanitary themes, sponsoring 142 excursions to health-related spots. It distributed 6,162 leaflets, 3,208 brochures, and 627 books. It also maintained 25 traveling libraries, each with 50 to 70 books on health, and nearly 9,000 slides. The department assisted 17 labor circles and 51 study groups. Finally, officials opened a House of Sanitary Enlightenment on February 1 that saw nearly 9,000 visitors. It had over 800 items on exhibit, including 258 posters, 87 models, 20 wax models, 58 lesson exhibits, and a library containing over 1,000 books.[187] Even if only one person was touched by each effort, this would have affected nearly a quarter of a million people. This large array of activities focused on the needs of just one Moscow district—for only half the year.

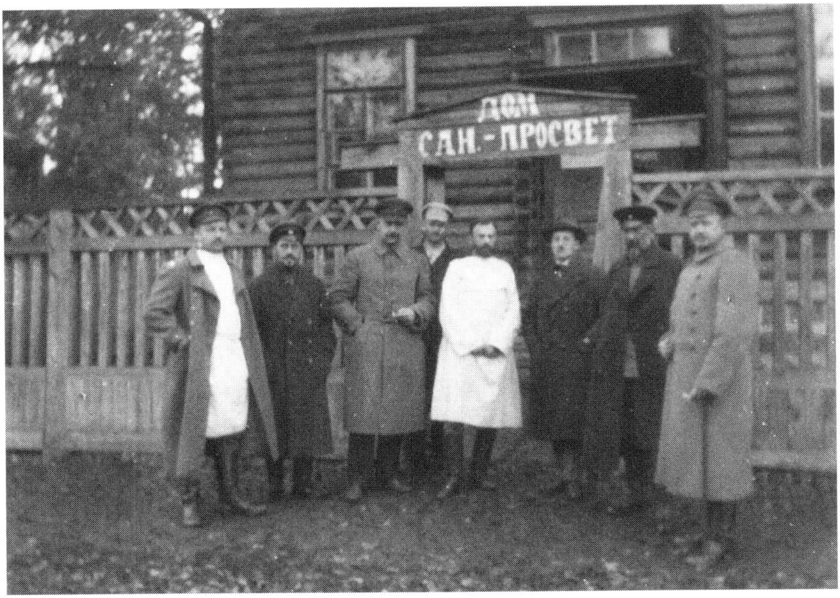

FIGURE 2.1. "House of Sanitary Enlightenment." Whereabouts unknown, 1920s. Gantt Papers. Courtesy of the Alan Mason Chesney Medical Archives of the Johns Hopkins Medical Institutions.

As the above litany of numbers suggests, statistics, figures, and lists formed an important base for propaganda. This reflected a belief, both inside and outside Russia, in the descriptive, didactic, and prescriptive value of numbers. Arising in tandem with the social sciences, statistical analysis became not only a weapon in the battle for influencing populations but also a measure of progress in their control. At the turn of the century statistical comparisons of birth and death rates were undertaken by all of the major industrialized countries. In the late nineteenth and early twentieth centuries, nations throughout the world looked to health statistics as a way to publicize their progress and proclaim their merits over their rivals. Statistics fueled French concerns over depopulation and became integral to forging a national identity in the United States. Given their intimate knowledge of clients and records of weights, measurements, births, and deaths, medical professionals played a major role in collecting, interpreting, and compiling data. The dispensary and its attendant medical surveillance provided a ready base of figures, comparisons, and ranges for the quantification of the normal.[188]

Tsarist statisticians had likewise examined Russian development in the late nineteenth century. Given their faith in science as a means of social engineering and their centralized system of health provision, it was not surprising that Soviet leaders counted and quantified the population for the purpose of controlling it.[189] Doctors charted chest sizes of sanatorium patients, the weight of consultation children, the percentage of dispensary patients who brushed their teeth, and the ratio of women who chose the doctor over the midwife. A 1923 national health survey of worker youth devoted great attention to comparative height, weight, and chest measurements for pre- and postrevolutionary development with over fifty pages of analysis on this topic.[190]

The Soviets used these figures to diagnose problems in the population and allocate resources. They also deployed these figures in their domestic propaganda, although these numbers should be regarded with suspicion. Statisticians created a world in numbers by manipulating questions, analysis, and even the figures themselves to present a desired picture. Rather than being a reflection of reality, statistics are a political tool used to depict a hoped-for reality.[191] Dispensary doctors created and gathered statistics for government consumption. This presents interesting questions of interpretation because of their bleak outlook. Those who used the statistics for reporting supposedly supported the programs on which they worked and wished to show them in the best light in order to receive increased funding. The picture is often so disappointing, however, that they may have been underscoring the depth of the problem as a way to bring greater attention to health. Given these difficulties, all such statistics should be regarded in the same way as any political utterance—with circumspection.

Gauging the effect of propaganda is also difficult. Play performances, acting troupes, and museum outings were part of club work, but clubs were overwhelmingly urban, young, and male, leaving many outside their walls. Propaganda performed in clubs, distributed in dispensaries, or affixed to walls as broadsheets reached an audience limited to urban areas because of distribution problems and literacy rates. The peasant, already considered more backward than workers for political reasons, was further distanced from the civilizing mission by illiteracy and geography. In general, women were not as literate as men and attended clubs, the Komsomol, and other propaganda sites less frequently.[192] Reaching them was difficult. Even with special attention, women's involvement remained low and interest lukewarm. Young women had other commitments that made participation difficult. Health care institutions such as the dispensary and consultation conceivably made up for the lack of women's attendance at club sites by cornering them during illness and pregnancy. The Pioneers and Komsomol also made it a point to encourage their members to look toward change in the home as part of their mission in an attempt to reach women outside regular paths of communication.

Teaching women held special importance. Even before the revolution women were considered more backward than men in relation to modernization, Westernization, and politics, yet this perceived backwardness made them attractive as an object for transformation—a blank canvas untainted by opinions or political ideas. Activists believed that women could be molded in a way men could not.[193] Women figured prominently in magazines, especially the journal *To a New Life!* Lengthy stories on women's health initiatives, charming biographies of female activists, and fiction about domestic issues filled the pages of these journals—most probably intended to entertain and encourage female volunteers.

Even as they saturated society with the message of health, hygienists realized the limits of their appeal. Faced with what was diagnosed as individual lethargy, even the best programs withered. A 1925 pamphlet aimed at worker youth hammered the point home that government programs could only do so much: "All those achievements may not be enough if every individual person in their private life does not follow the rules of hygiene. On the contrary, the infringement of these rules by individuals may weaken significantly the results of social-sanitary works."[194] This pamphlet emphasized that personal behavior extended beyond the home and individual to all of society. According to organizers, appealing to individual worker initiative could bridge the gap between the message of health and its reception. Narkomzdrav encouraged grassroots efforts; maintaining personal health took on the added meaning of agitating for societal health. Prerevolutionary health authorities had pursued public support for health care as well. During the 1905 revolution physician activists campaigned for the reduction of centralized authority as a way to make room for citizen groups to pursue health initiatives. Pamphlets and posters featured the slogan "The maintenance of worker health is the duty of workers themselves." The 1924 conference on sanitary enlightenment in Leningrad promoted worker self-help. This was in line with Lenin's hope, during the early days of Narkomzdrav, that health initiatives would come from below.[195]

The push for voluntary organizations had not just arisen in 1917 but originated in concepts and policies of the prerevolutionary period. Welfare organizations emerged in the late nineteenth century in response to the considerable problems associated with rapid industrialization and urbanization. Voluntary efforts took place in a contested field of governmental authority, municipal responsibility, public charity, and bourgeois femininity.[196] Although the Soviets viewed these private philanthropic efforts with derision, they were interested in the concept of worker self-help and organic creation. Beyond mere rhetoric, volunteer work proved very important to Narkomzdrav. The latter could not provide the forces needed and therefore depended upon volunteers. According to the 1927 survey *Health Care in Soviet Russia for Ten Years,* both government and volunteer groups carried out sanitary enlightenment work that included Committees for the Sanitation of Labor and Life, housing sanitary representatives, and health cells sponsored by schools, factories, and apartment buildings.[197] The authors emphasized the importance of these cooperative organizations: "Through these, with these, among these, sanitary enlightenment is carried on in the home, factory, and elsewhere."[198] Other groups exemplified worker self-help. The Workers' Commissions for the Fight for Cleanliness in the Red Army and other district departments devoted their time to health work in Commissions for Cleanliness or sanitary troops (*santroiki, sanpiaterki,* etc.).[199]

These surveillance bodies were aided by Soviet conceptions of privacy and the crowded conditions of the 1920s. The Soviet emphasis on the collective over the individual and the transparency afforded by overcrowded conditions blurred the line between bodily health, domestic health, and societal health. Perhaps the prime example of this, the most pervasive form of involvement by individuals, and the most written about by contemporaries was the health cell. The health cell consisted of a small group of men and women in an apartment building, factory, school, or club that carried out grassroots efforts to improve health, educate the populace, and inform on miscreants. Most apartment buildings had a housing association responsible for maintenance and budget. Often the health cell linked up with this organization. Moscow dispensaries claimed over nine thousand specialized cells in 1925.[200]

Aside from these groups, the Octobrists (up to age 9), Pioneers (9–14 years), and Komsomol (14–23 years) were charged with bringing the revolutionary message into the family by way of the children, including ideas on hygiene. Activists believed that youth could be molded more easily than adults since their transitional status made them more susceptible to outside influences—both good and bad. They envisioned clubs and physical culture activities as vehicles for guiding youth toward proper behavior and protecting them against negative influences. The Komsomol started off in 1918 with a few thousand members, but by the close of the decade the youth organization swelled to almost twice the size of the party. Though this represented a small percentage of eligible youth, in areas like Moscow this meant that 60–70 percent of youth were involved.[201]

Like youth groups internationally, the Octobrists, Pioneers, and Komsomol attempted to guide the development of children by means of militaristic ritual and strong adherence to state-supported values. This included not only political advice but also lifestyle guidance. Pioneer and Komsomol membership was not automatic but rather was conferred on the basis of merit, which gave children an incentive to accept educational and moral instruction.[202] As an American contemporary noted, "In the first place the Pioneer becomes the champion of cleanliness and particularly of fresh air. He or she sees that the younger children wash their hands and faces before eating." The writer concluded that "the low standards of living of Russian workmen and peasants give a real importance to these homely tasks."[203] Pioneers also helped with housework; notified the doctor when family members fell ill; attended the club; promoted volunteerism; spread news of collective institutions like the nursery, laundry, and cooperative; and reported all their work back to the brigade leader, thereby adding another opportunity for state surveillance.

Public health and its centrality to the creation of strong states was a connection made by Enlightenment philosophers and transmitted to Russia by Peter the Great and Catherine the Great. Humanitarian influences spurred public involvement in health care in the West and in Russia. Autocratic pressure, however, made it difficult to organize private initiatives. The tsarist government did not express a great deal of interest in putting money or effort behind public health. Following the revolution, Soviet propagandists announced to the world their programs for clean, healthy citizens as evidence of the state's commitment to its people, in contrast to the cruelty of tsarism and the defiling influence of capitalism, and as a way to promote communism at home and abroad.

Narkomzdrav built on previous efforts and applied new techniques to the old problems of epidemics and social diseases. In the dispensary, consultation, House of Leisure, and sanatorium, patients saw a medical professional, learned healthful habits, and received extensive care. Dispensary and consultation doctors and nurses visited the homes of patients in order to diagnose problems and propose solutions. These techniques were derived from abroad and built upon the belief of pre- and postrevolutionary physicians that behavior influenced disease. The conception of health as a social problem led to inspection of the home and resulted in surveys and examinations of individuals and their domestic conditions. Investigators and institutions targeted propaganda on domestic care and leisure choices at the citizenry. Much like advertising, health propaganda sought out new forms to spread its message. Although the content was new, the propaganda retained a traditional look. Between the emphasis of Bolshevism on enlightenment and the budgetary problems of Narkomzdrav, the shift from universal care to worker self-education made sense, as did the state's encouragement of grassroots efforts. Volunteers could provide free service in troubled times, in addition to serving as intermediary figures between state and home. Health recommendations from an acquaintance might be more forceful and result in greater feelings of shame.

Hygiene propagandists attempted to invade all fields of daily life. Narkomzdrav posters blanketed the city, factory, and apartment building with dire warnings. Visiting nurses and health cell inspectors arrived at the home armed with pamphlets and admonishments. On every front the Soviets battled to control private behavior. This show of force, however, was also an admission of weakness. The very prominence of Soviet propaganda—an indication of the impulse of the state to reach into and control social life—was itself an acknowledgment of the inability of the Soviet state to reach its intended level of control through institutional surveillance programs. Volunteers were urged to step in when the state could not provide sufficient professionals. Propaganda was meant to take up the slack where institutions, doctors, and volunteers could not reach. Sanitary enlightenment was a weapon of the weak in a state that could provide little beyond persuasion.

3 The City

Instruction, Regulation, and Isolation

In May 1920 reports glorified the transformation of a mortar-and-stone reminder of tsarist oppression—a palace on Kamennyi Island in Petrograd—into a House of Leisure.[1] In this revolutionized palace, as well as others like it reclaimed all over the former empire, workers spent their annual two-week vacation learning how to rest rationally, for in the workers' state even leisure time had to be productive. Doctors, dietitians, and health practitioners guided the vacationers and educated them for their return home with a simple yet rigid regimen consisting of nutritious food, timed naps, edifying activities, and physical exercise. Sutured together from the palaces of the past and electrified by dreams of the future, the House of Leisure provided a retreat for workers poisoned by the capitalist-tainted, urban environment or by workplace stress.

These therapeutic centers received a considerable amount of attention both for their ideological and curative potential. Organizers confiscated palaces, monasteries, and summer retreats for the benefit of workers.[2] Socialist concepts redeemed these former bourgeois mansions and church properties. White paint and light colors transformed grand ballrooms into lecture halls and reading rooms, although gilded furniture with satin upholstery remained. Propagandists crowed that where formerly a family of 8 had resided now 150 children and staff lived and convalesced.[3] The confiscation and resurrection of these buildings served as visible testimony to the state's goals, while also articulating power in new, modern ways. Rather than displaying power, as in edifices of old, these buildings were meant to transform and, in the style of Bentham's panopticon, disperse power throughout the population. They reflected the efforts of governments around the world where reformers believed, as Foucault so cunningly put it, "stones can make people docile and knowable."[4] These structures, used to contain and tame, showed the power of the Soviet state to change the physical environment, reflecting the hope that it could manipulate human behavior, as well as the faith of the hygienists that physical change precipitated socialist consciousness.

Hygienists argued that leisure did not come naturally. While the term for leisure, *otdykh,* can be translated as "rest," this was not Soviet leisure.[5] Instead of leaving workers free to determine their time away from work, these hours had to buttress the eight hours of labor. Hygienists attributed low worker productivity to slovenly leisure. Drinking and carousing all night on the dangerous streets of the city weakened workers. Proper leisure—such as club activities, physical culture, and excursions—restored and invigorated workers. For those already ill, organized leisure provided a cure. In urban night and day institutions, as well as in sanatoriums in the countryside, doctors tailored leisure time and sleep regimens to patients' illnesses, theorizing that adherence to such regimens would prove a cure-all. Healthy leisure, together with home and bodily care, would mold citizens into a modern industrial force—strong of body and politically sound of mind. If the people gave themselves over to the institutions of leisure, hygienists argued, productivity and culture would rise and the revolution would triumph. Writers recommended that workers exploit their leisure time and use it to rejuvenate their body and enrich themselves. Healthy leisure served as a basis for further cultural activity and expanded, challenged, and informed the mind as well as the body. Cultural leisure spaces provided political enlightenment through entertainment. A healthy, informed, and rested population would lead the way to the socialist utopia. By encouraging workers to use their leisure time wisely, reformers sought to mobilize men and women for revolutionary goals.

For those who could not abandon their old forms of leisure, new institutions were created to isolate them after work, buffering them from the pernicious influences of the city and engaging them actively in living healthfully. Within the city, night and day sanatoriums, day squares (outdoor day camps), and prophylactory (rehabilitation and reeducation facilities) took sickly workers and children and surrounded them with therapeutic influences in the hope of reworking the mind and body. The extremely ill stayed in sanatoriums tailored to their needs and located well outside the stifling confines of the city. In these institutions doctors promised full recovery to patients who followed the regimen and rested in a proper way.

Not all workers welcomed instruction. They held their own ideas of what constituted good leisure. Much to hygienists' dismay, many workers continued to drink, dance, and play cards. For women, obligations of home and family prevented them from joining the Soviet leisure movement, and what little time remained was used to attend church or visit friends. Although authorities continued to look for ways to attract workers and get them involved, their ability to do battle was hampered by a lack of funds and facilities. The arguments between government agencies for funds and between institutions and citizens over definitions of leisure were just further battles in the quest for orderly citizens. Since leisure could influence productivity and politics, it could not be left to chance. The Bolsheviks did not trust workers to find their own forms of leisure, just as they had doubted their ability to create their own revolution.

"The inactive organ dies," declared Doctor I. Gel'man in his 1925 book *Labor, Fatigue and Rest.*[6] Gel'man, a clinician and professor at the Obukh Institute for the Study of Professional Illnesses, considered labor essential to life, not just because Engels had noted that it was the source of riches but because it was indispensable to man the "machine."[7] Atrophy caused muscles and even bones to deteriorate. To function properly, he argued, the body needed to engage in labor. He admitted, however, that work alone did not meet man's needs. Man also required rest.[8]

Commissar of Health Semashko concurred, saying that while others often likened man to a machine, this analogy was incomplete: "Food for a human is the same as fuel for machines. But the comparison of man with machine is incorrect in that a machine, in contrast to a human, may work long periods without breaks. A man without rest cannot work a very long time."[9] The prolific pamphleteer Doctor B. S. Sigal agreed regarding the necessity of leisure: "Weariness and ruin are the outcomes of exhausting work." The doctor went on to chart the correspondence between work hours and accidents, underscoring both the detrimental effects of too much work and the essential role of leisure in increased productivity.[10] In his popular prerevolutionary utopian novel *Red Star,* Bogdanov made the case that the desire to engage in labor was so strong in man that it had to be monitored. During a factory tour the hero, Leonid, heard of the near death of a worker so entranced with his position on the floor that he had nearly thrown himself into the maw of the machine. The Martian guide informed Leonid that the position was monitored lest the worker fall victim to a "convulsive fit of madness that may irresistibly draw him under the hammer."[11]

The Soviets passed labor legislation guaranteeing workers rest in the form of breaks during the day, over the weekend, and an annual two-week vacation.[12] Hygienists emphasized the physiological necessity of enforced breaks. Doctor A. G. Kagan gave a lengthy account of the system of rejuvenation wherein special cleansing nutritives moved to the organs and purified them of the "poisons of fatigue."[13] L. M. Vasilevskii, a former *zemstvo* doctor and sanitary-enlightenment activist, stated that the body needed leisure so that the organism could recover and labor "without danger."[14] According to A. G. Kagan, without leisure the laborer could not work and became difficult to control in social settings: "Languorous, lackadaisical, irritable, impatient, suffering from headaches or fainting spells, reduced appetite, insomnia, etc.—this is what the overworked person feels and presents to others."[15]

Though Semashko argued that the best rest was sleep, he and others were not content to leave workers to enjoy passive leisure.[16] Leisure time had to be utilized and exploited rather than whiled away. Kagan pointed out that just staying in bed was not enough since the body had to move in order to flush poisons out of the organs.[17] Gel'man, Director of Housing Sanitation for Narkomzdrav, lamented the fact that too many workers spent their leisure time at home, "passively awaiting the next workday." Gel'man further noted that nonlaboring time should be "spent expediently and carefully" to ensure health. He also recommended the "rational" use of this time: "Sufficient time in the fresh air, sufficient movement, which is indispensable for the development of all parts of the body—these are what must be used first of all during the nonworking time regimen."[18]

Good leisure did more than tone the body; it cultivated the mind. Kagan insisted that "the rest time of youth must improve them, be filled with cultural content, and be collective."[19] Physical fitness served this purpose admirably. Games provided both mental and physical conditioning. A good game strengthened muscles with "elements for mental development, for the development of the senses, and also elements for the development of the will (self-control, alertness, courage) and aesthetic feelings."[20] "*Just as there is an art of labor so, too, is there an art of leisure,*" declared Gel'man.[21] L. M. Vasilevskii recommended the American "art of leisure" as a model and further insisted that "one must remember that leisure and laziness are far from being the same thing. Leisure is a necessary preparation for labor and for a higher level of its completion."[22]

In his definition Kagan emphasized regimentation: "*Rhythm saves energy, accelerates the restoration of processes, and increases the 'accumulation' of stores of energy for the future!*"[23] He concluded that because of the importance of leisure, the day should be organized and the vacation period strictly planned. The emphasis on rationalization and the medicalization of leisure allowed Soviet hygienists to present required leisure as a productive, acceptable policy. It also defined Soviet leisure as different, better, and more worthy then the decadent leisure of the bourgeoisie. Soviet leisure tempered and fortified the body.[24]

According to Semashko, constructive leisure was unavailable to industrial workers before the revolution. Since clubs and theaters closed their doors to the poor, only the privileged classes enjoyed physical exercise. Censorship ensured that lectures could never enlighten or even interest the working class. Both men and women suffered under this system. Semashko continued, "Naturally, the ordinary worker lived numbed by the hard labor of an unenlightened life and on Sunday drank to a stupor, beat the wife, scared the kids, and went to bed a little early." The wife spent her time at church, "looking at golden icon screens and icons and hiding in the corner lamenting a nonexistent god." Semashko contended that instead of respite such leisure provided "heavy rest without any enlightenment or pleasure." He noted that with the coming of the revolution there had been "a complete turnaround in leisure." By 1928 workers had clubs "in order to broaden their knowledge, in order to define their needs, in order to understand how they must fight and work for a better future." Leisure activity had evolved from drinking and carousing to learning and political agitation. Now a significant number of workers enjoyed the club, theater, and movies. Semashko boasted: "Many have become so used to this kind of cultured pastime that for them it even seemed odd to contemplate spending leisure time at home in bed in a smoky room, staring at the ceiling instead of at a general meeting."[25]

While Semashko exaggerated the effects of the club, he was not alone in seeing the club as the base of effective leisure. Other reformers contended that by being cooped up in overcrowded and stuffy apartments, workers could not begin to rest properly.[26] As one reformer lamented, "The crowded nature of our dwellings, the inconvenience of our kitchens . . . the expense of entertainment for the workers, the dirt and discomfort of pubs" meant workers required a space for proper leisure.[27] The club built upon the nineteenth-century concept of the people's house. By 1913 there were 147 in Russia. The Moscow city government founded a people's house in 1904. It combined a theater with a library, tearoom, and lecture hall. The city planned to have 24 houses by 1915, but the war disrupted this process.[28] Soviet clubs, people's houses, and houses of culture shared analogous goals. While on a visit in the early 1920s, the British Trade Union Delegation marveled at the effect of the Soviet version of the workers' club: "The clubs are also very influential in the campaigns of Communism for cleanliness and clean living. In fact, the clubs play the same part for the adult worker as the schools do for the children."[29] Moscow leaders readily pushed forward. In 1924 there were 107 clubs in Moscow, and by 1925 they numbered 450.[30]

Sanitary enlightenment activists saw great potential in the club. The model club provided "healthy relaxation, healthy laughter, songs, good conversation, games, dancing, and sports."[31] The club, however, did more than just entertain. According to one official, "The club must affect and influence the rebuilding of everyday life." Furthermore, the club had to serve as a model in terms of organization and structure: "It must be noticeable for its cleanliness, comfort and order of its strongly regimented life. Lectures and frequent bad talks, noise and racket are not very attractive and do little."[32] Not just a space for healthful leisure, the club educated workers to healthful living. Doctor I. D. Strashun, head of the sanitary enlightenment publishing house, recommended in his article "Sanitary Enlightenment in the Club," that clubs be sites for healthful relaxation and spreading sanitary enlightenment's message: "Without sanitary culture there cannot successfully exist any other culture. The club should become a basic item shaping consciousness of the circular nature of responsibility and the collective care of health for all and consequently for every one."[33] Club evenings consisting of physical culture, question-and-answer sessions, spectacles, as well as planned excursions to museums and scientific institutes, became part of enlightenment work.[34]

While hygiene figured heavily in most club offerings, not all activities involved the subject of cleanliness. Any lecture—political, scientific, or cultural—was still hygiene-related if the intent was to draw the workers to enriching pursuits. Many activities made up the club calendar, and some simply replaced an hour's entertainment with one not detrimental to physical or political health. For example, in December 1923 the club connected to the Hammer and Sickle factory presented thirty-two different events, including: lectures on religion, gonorrhea, and literature; spectacles entitled "Life and Hard Alcohol," "For the Red Flag," and "Crime and Punishment"; and movies such as "Orphans" and "The Bourgeoisie in Hell." They hosted meetings of different groups, such as physical fitness and youth groups. In all, they entertained 14,216 spectators.[35] While this was one of the more active clubs, in 1924 Moscow clubs entertained 87,698 attendees in all at 564 lectures and by 1927 clubs sponsored 2,955 events for 623,498 patrons.[36]

The connection between the club's cultural mission and the furtherance of hygiene stood out in the commentaries of Narkomzdrav authorities. According to Semashko, the club needed to be "attractive and interesting" to carry out cultural work, indicating his inclination to sacrifice some content in order to increase attendance.[37] Club circles appealed to a variety of interests. One 1924 club included groups for literature, union work, billiards, choir, drama, chess, graphics, youth, tourism, book lovers, newspaper clippings, and NOT (the time league).[38] A 1925 article in the journal *Klub* recommended a "lifestyle" circle as a desirable part of club activities. The writer conceived of a group that would investigate problems of daily life by undertaking excursions and then creating exhibitions.[39] Youth associations abounded. Pioneer troops attached themselves to clubs, as did representatives of the Komsomol. One theorist insisted that "the workers' club without Pioneers is like a family without children."[40] A 1924 survey found that 293 physical culture groups brought 13,000 members to Moscow clubs.[41] Organizers were not content. According to a 1927 report, although workers attended family nights and joined chess clubs and physical culture circles, attendance at lectures was dropping.[42]

Clubs offered attractions to keep workers off the streets and away from the taverns. Libraries provided a space for reading and housed political and classic books as well as periodicals. The library of the Astrakhov club at the Hammer and Sickle factory grew steadily throughout the 1920s. In 1923 the library held only 1,183 books for 870 readers. In 1927 the number had increased to 9,332 books, with 13 journal titles. A total of 1,102 adult patrons and their 243 children enjoyed the library, with the average daily attendance being 47.[43] Libraries hosted readings, rhythmic gymnastics, and even magic lantern shows.[44] In addition to club libraries, other repositories dotted the city, some of which had been established by the city government in 1916.[45] By 1921 Moscow's 161 libraries contained 1,197,594 books.[46] The central workers' library and reading room had 4,300 books when it opened in 1918; by September 1921 it had over 50,000 volumes.[47]

Workers' clubs also made a practice of arranging excursions and walks to sites around the city and the surrounding countryside. Doctor Gel'man, who envisioned the excursion as a way to fight the debauchery that accompanied holiday weekends, lamented that if only holidays could be utilized as they were in England, where excursions were planned for such long weekends, "the huge, beneficial influence of such mass excursions of the workers [would be] visible to all hygienists."[48] According to a report presented at a Komsomol conference, a trip to an approved leisure site could combat the pernicious influences of street culture, pulp literature, and sex.[49] Excursions in Moscow could involve visits to a museum, palace of the people, or outings to special parks. The first public parks in Moscow opened before the revolution, and in 1912 the city began offering special recreation for children.[50] A decree issued shortly after the revolution looked toward the preservation of orchards and green spaces. Many club excursions found these spots to be ideal destinations.[51] Museums provided an alternative during poor weather. The State Museum of Social Hygiene opened in 1919 as a source of health information and leisure. Guides set out in increasing numbers to these and other places, growing from 261 excursions in 1921 to 1,194 in 1927. Organizers worried, however, that many workers still preferred individual outings to the collective experience.[52]

Although these club outings provided relief from the overcrowded club building, making the club more attractive was a major concern of organizers, who lamented the low attendance by women and older workers. In 1926 most Moscow club members were male and 40 percent were under twenty-three.[53] Organizers urged clubs to attract older workers by providing entertaining offerings instead of dismissing older workers and women as uninterested and unreachable.[54] Though activists admitted that women were overburdened—some clubs established day care facilities and communal kitchens—it was still the club's unattractiveness that activists blamed for turning away women.[55] One writer noted that although women complained of being too busy to attend clubs, they still found time for religious observance, dances, and hosting guests. He concluded that the club "must fight for this time."[56]

Reformers explained the club campaign as a battle for worker interest. Semashko insisted that the biggest task of the club was "to distract the worker from the streets. For this the club should be not only objectively useful but also subjectively interesting to visitors."[57] This was particularly important to organizers because the club combated "drunkenness and absenteeism."[58] As one reformer noted, "If we do not give the worker relaxation in the club, he will go to the beer hall, to the inn, and to the boulevard."[59] One writer attributed drinking among hooligans to the shortage of leisure space, asserting: "In the evening after work, they look for a place, a place where they can forget, and not finding any other means, they drink [to forget]."[60] Others concentrated on how to inject enlightening messages into those activities that workers enjoyed, such as linking science lessons to club work. To appeal to these groups, activists recommended new spaces and greater attention to different interests. Some even went so far as to recommend alcohol in the club, but most seemed to regard this solution as Trotsky did when he quipped, "To lure [the masses] away from the tavern with the help of beer is tantamount to driving out the devil with the help of Old Nick."[61] To attract women, writers advised introducing more lectures on women's themes and taking over sewing circles by infiltrating the discussions with political issues.[62]

Theorists argued about the nature of clubs but never about their import. Transforming daily life was so significant that activists created supplemental institutions to fill in where clubs could not reach. Since club premises were insufficient and the building of new clubs progressed slowly, the Red Corner provided a spot where workers could meet for games and lectures.[63] A room or even a corner of a cafeteria could be made over with a table, some posters, reading materials, and games. A sample set of lectures for a Red Corner in 1926 included several evenings devoted to such health themes as drunkenness, sexual promiscuity (venereal disease), and absenteeism (usually associated with drunkenness).[64] Red Corners presented a popular alternative to the club and multiplied rapidly. In 1926 there were 2,199 in Moscow and only a year later there were 2,680. Those that existed struggled with shortages of materials and space. One Red Corner reported that workers had to use benches as tables for checkerboards and chess while sitting on the floor since the tables overflowed with books and magazines.[65]

Although Semashko insisted that the revolution had transformed the workers, the journalist René Fülüp-Miller contended that increased leisure time only allowed workers more time to drink.[66] Reformers found that they not only had to educate the public in the area of wholesome leisure but also had to attack existing worker activities. Semashko presented poor leisure as unhealthful: "If the relaxer carries on an irregular way of life, staggers about at night but does not sleep, drinks, etc., . . . he does not restore his strength but, on the contrary, destroys it. If he uses rest on binges and debauchery, he directly damages his health. Instead, taking advantage of a regular way of life during leisure time is necessary for a healthy person."[67] Semashko spotlighted drinking and carousing as poisonous. Enthusiastic revolutionaries agitated to wrest workers from the clutches of alcohol and late-night binges.[68] Pamphlets cited the rise in work-related accidents and lower productivity following weekends as evidence of social danger. Holidays, traditionally associated with drinking, merited special attention in the literature and posters.[69]

One symptom of these problems, according to commentators, was the rise in hooliganism. In a 1926 article published in the journal *Klub*, Semashko framed hooliganism as an issue of health. He emphasized the need for clubs to organize "societal opinion" against hooligans and held great faith in the power of collective action to shame individuals into proper behavior. For those who blamed hooligans for closing clubs, Semashko countered that such clubs had marked themselves for failure by not mobilizing the neighborhood in favor of the new Soviet lifestyle. "The creation of societal opinion is the most trusted way to fight against hooliganism and against poor behavior, drunkenness, [and] work skippages."[70] Other activists similarly cited community opinion as vital in the fight against hooliganism.[71] For organizers of hygienic worker leisure, the hooligan was the embodiment of the dangers of individualism and the unordered private lives of the urban working class.[72]

Authorities hoped to mobilize public opinion to counter a perceived increase in antisocial behavior. In a 1927 mock trial of two young men of the streets, an expert testified to the rising number of hooligan-related incidents and diagnosed the people that created such problems.[73] Those activities authorities deemed hooliganism—including drunkenness, fighting, and disruptive behavior—often overlapped with traditional worker culture and youth behavior.[74] A list of activities associated with the term "hooliganism" in an article on club problems reflected this confusion:

> There is the drunk kind, where the hooligan brings in wine, gets drunk on the club premises, curses his mother, sings bawdy songs, hangs onto the women, fights in the club and on the street at its entrance, practices petty theft, defaces a wall, door, or window with inscriptions, spoils furniture, portraits, musical instruments, fans, and in general destroys the property of the club. They also do not take off their coats in the club. They smoke if they have cigarettes, litter and drop sunflower seeds, create a row, clog up or create noise in places where people congregate, and hinder the work of the masses with conversation, bustle, preening, laughter, and with comings and goings during the lectures and reports.[75]

The author recited a litany of antisocial, disruptive behavior; some were violent, others merely rude, and a few simply evidence of high spirits ("laughter"). As challenges to order and rationality, the offenses took on a political tinge, linking them to impolitic views and economics.

Reformers viewed hooliganism as an urban social problem that fed off the fetid atmosphere of capitalism and bred in rank, metropolitan environments. Magazine writers portrayed the city as the source of poverty and negative influences. Critiques of the city can be found as far back as Genesis's depiction of the city as a den of iniquity, but anti-urbanism grew vociferous as industrialization brought crowds and disease to municipalities in heretofore unknown numbers. Edwin Chadwick's studies provided scientific bases to these biases on the Continent. Nineteenth-century Italians had identified the city as an incubator of disease; by the 1920s they had connected it to demographic problems.[76] Although Marxists had decried the "idiocy" of rural life, this did not translate into a wholehearted acceptance of urban life by revolutionary Russians. The city, with its symbolic edifices of the modern—the factory, the streetcar, the apartment building—was not only a vision of the future but also an example of the taxing life required of the modern individual. While the city provided the communal circumstances necessary for the socialist self, it was also the object of continued disparagement. Moscow and Petrograd were the soul and site of revolution, but they had to be reconstructed. Architects envisaged a new world to be created out of the present city—a "materialized utopia"—but for the present people had to live in the cities of the past.[77]

For Soviet hygienists the existing city could not be redeemed even by the great opportunities and the promise of modern advancement it held out.[78] Cities were overcrowded, filthy havens for disease. One author lamented: "According to modern standards of labor and life, and especially in big cities . . . [the worker is] in danger at work, in danger at home, and in danger on the streets from 'cold and rain,' filth and dust and, finally, the risk of infection from many diseases."[79]

Two physical conditions of the city made it especially hazardous for workers, namely, overcrowding and filth. Overcrowding resulted in filth but also led to the breakdown of barriers between individuals, revealing the sexualized subtext of anxiety.[80] One doctor commented on the prevalence of sexually transmitted disease in the city, arguing that it was easy acquaintances and life under the unflagging gaze of others that led to promiscuity: "Acquaintance in the theater, the trolley bus, the cinema, meetings at parties, at lectures, close work in a circle of some kind—all of that serves as enough base for the start-up of a sexual relationship."[81] In addition to the easy contacts of overcrowding, the filth of the streets came in for special attention. Writers detailed rituals to prevent workers from bringing street dirt into their homes. The article "The Street and Hygiene" described at length the dangers of urban dirt and how to combat it.[82]

NEP Moscow endangered workers with more than just physical conditions. According to reformers, it tempted them to be consumers, indulge in illicit behavior, drink, patronize prostitutes, and generally to indulge in "bad habits."[83] Intellectuals of the late nineteenth century had also railed against what they saw as the irrational nature of urban amusements—especially the rowdy theater, rough entertainment, and drinking culture associated with the boulevards. Their condemnations extended to the capitalistic development of the city, which they considered alien and corrupting.[84] This distaste for the urban and the commercial city carried over into conceptions of the NEP metropolis and the NEP man. NEP men spoiled the city during the day with their commercial activities and at night they further ruined it as they indulged their craven tastes for cabaret entertainment, loose women, and raucous dinners.[85] Characters in plays, posters, and poems lost their health—and sometimes even their lives—in pursuit of dangerous leisure in bars and along the boulevards.[86] Doctors associated depravity with the city to such a degree that they insisted syphilis in the countryside was spread by nonvenereal means, such as the sharing of spoons or towels, whereas in the city it was spread by prostitutes and through casual sexual encounters.[87]

The glitz of the city streets may have attracted some workers, but other factors also lured them off the path of healthy leisure. Many neighborhood pubs offered more comfortable forms of relaxation. Activists worried that the beer hall was more accepting of older workers than clubs, where they felt isolated and confused because of the overwhelmingly youthful membership.[88] The pub also had stronger roots in workers' lives.[89] In the play *The Trial of an Illiterate* (1924) two politically unconscious workers, one male and one female, used heckling and the allure of the beer hall to tempt students away from their literacy classes.[90] "Go to the beer hall and you're equal to all," declared a politically backward husband in an agitational trial, emphasizing the tavern's leveling aspect.[91] In a 1926 "sanitary agitational trial" of a hooligan, the fictional prosecutor brought in a string of older workers who had left the club because of the pub's tranquil atmosphere.[92] To encourage workers to avoid the tavern, one article advocated free movie and theater tickets, noting: "It is clear that the more people who are in the club, the fewer patrons there are in the beer hall and the fewer still 'going visiting' or 'to parties.'"[93]

Whereas bars endangered older workers, health care advocates depicted dances as a baneful influence on youth.[94] They warned that dancers took the first step onto a slippery slope where "NEP-man music" like the tango and its temptations to promiscuity could lead to objectionable behavior. The tango came to Russia before the revolution and—to the horror of activists—reemerged as a favorite of the younger set during the postrevolutionary period.[95] Pamphlet writers combined hygienic and moral concerns to justify their objections. Instead of condemning clothes as too revealing, they argued that the dresses hampered the body since "dancers breathe poorly, particularly in those special, tight dresses." Likewise, the chilled drinks at dances encouraged colds.[96] Others viewed dancing as a means to lure youth into the clubs. The topic provoked a debate at the 1922 meeting of the Moscow Komsomol. Given the dearth of organized physical activities for the young, one activist proposed dancing as a solution.[97] The topic was still sensitive in 1926, when another activist recommended that informal dances be infiltrated by agitators, who could change the character of these gatherings and thereby influence the young.[98]

Theorists constantly worried about youth leisure choices—apparently with good reason. Organized leisure found a less enthusiastic welcome than organizers had anticipated. The most popular options were those that appeared to offer the least political content—dances, theater, and the cinema. Activists, working with printers, lamented the need to follow political lectures with films to guarantee attendance and the popularity of free theater tickets over all other forms of activity.[99] According to a 1929 study, 75 percent of young men and 77 percent of young women had not read a single political book over the course of the year. Instead, the overwhelming majority of the population viewed films, visited country houses, and played cards.[100] The Komsomol, intended to put youth on the true path, had only affected a small percentage of the population by the mid-1920s.[101]

Despite all their problems, authorities considered clubs sufficient in theory, if not in number, to meet the needs of the healthy, urban denizen. For the ill they designed new institutions based on their biases regarding the harmful effects of the city and built upon a faith in isolation and regimentation as the foundation of health. In these part-time sanatoriums (either day or night) the sick found sanctuary. Doctors referred sick workers or children to the sanatoriums and the special squares, where patients came to spend their time healthfully rather than in home environments that, medical workers believed, worsened their conditions. Authorities hoped to control workers, teach them correct habits, and hopefully restore the patient's health.[102] According to Narkomzdrav theorists, the idea for the night sanatorium came from the Americans and the German Red Cross.[103] The night sanatorium resembled the New York preventorium, which housed undernourished, tubercular children and treated them with nutritious food, constant fresh air, excursions, and educational training.[104] In 1921 four night sanatoriums opened in Moscow, thus importing the tradition to Soviet Russia.[105] In 1923 the Petrograd Department of Health opened its first night sanatorium.[106] By 1926–27 the tuberculosis dispensary system in Moscow maintained ten day sanatoriums (two for adults), eleven night sanatoriums (three for children), and fourteen physical therapy squares (nine for children).[107]

The night and day sanatoriums combined treatment with a healthful environment. Authorities considered the day sanatorium the "simplest and cheapest" of the sanatoriums. Intended as a surrogate parent for sickly children, it often held classes in addition to providing day care.[108] The night sanatorium, directed at adults, provided a cleaner, less crowded environment than worker homes. The institution did not take the patient from his work station, which one writer considered "both its weakest and strongest point. . . . The patient, continuing his professional work, during his stay in the night sanatorium severed his connections with his family and usual conditions of life." One worker reportedly called the night sanatorium a refuge from a hectic home: "My apartment is poor. I live in a corridor . . . but the night sanatorium is exactly what workers need."[109]

Separation permitted the patient to glimpse a different way of life and make requisite changes in his or her own behavior. As one observer noted, "The sanatorium gives him a convenient place, answering to his needs for food and those cultural boons that are necessary to help the organism triumph over illness. At work he is the same as the others, but, returning to the sanatorium, he discards his work clothes, washes off the dust and dirt, and, refreshing his body after hours of work, changes into light, clean, sanitary clothing and turns into the patient who submits to the obligatory regimen of the sanatorium."[110] The description emphasized how the patient completely altered himself for the night sanatorium; stripping away the grime of the city, he entered this new realm and transformed himself from a worker into a patient and from a source of infection to a cleansed inhabitant of a perfected space.

The squares (*ploshchadki*) used similar techniques but were distinguished by their outdoor sleeping arrangements. The special health squares occupied urban green spaces and had little overhead—just beds and personnel. One descriptive article entitled "On the Square," stressed the ways in which—even without a roof and walls—they provided sanctuary. "Quiet. The sounds of street life barely reach here. Only a bell's toll occasionally breaks through with its tone." As the muffled sounds of city life indicated, the square buffered workers from the temptations of the boulevards and the stress of the streets. One patient testified to the way in which the square provided a world apart: "How can I not like it? Is it possible to relax at home? The air is stale, the children are loud—how is that rest?"[111] Worker testimonials in the press praised the squares for lessons learned and the haven they provided. Most did mention their initial reluctance: "It was quite cold at the beginning of winter. Everyone laid down and shivered . . . [but we] got used to it—the same for the regimen and the discipline."[112] This mild criticism spoke volumes, but supposedly the patients grew used to the cold, just as they did the inescapable forces of discipline and regimen.

The scheduling of the day and night sanatoriums and squares adhered to the tyranny of the clock. Propaganda highlighted the schedule's rigidity. A 1926 report on a night sanatorium specified that workers entered the institution at 5 p.m.; showered, changed, and rested in bed until dinner at 7 p.m.; engaged in cultural enlightenment work until 9 p.m.; at which point they had tea before retiring at 10 p.m. The mornings started at 6:30 a.m.; the patient rose, washed, and breakfasted at 7 a.m.; he or she left for work at 7:30 a.m.[113] In addition to the supervision during waking hours, sleeping practices merited detailed attention. Organizers kept windows open, even in winter, to provide healthful air. Evidently people resisted this and attempted to close the windows since some facilities found it necessary to nail the windows open.[114] Sanitary issues took center stage in discussions, readings, and physical culture. In the *Moscow Department of Health Weekly* Doctor Kagan suggested the following themes for nightly lectures: bodily hygiene, labor and rest, diet, home life, sex, alcohol, smoking, and narcotics use.[115]

Equally important as to how patients lived within the facility was how they conducted themselves once they left. One doctor maintained that this "school for healthful practices" encouraged patients to take their lessons home.[116] To gauge the effectiveness of the treatment, night and day sanatoriums offered statistics on weight gain and more detailed investigations into the lives of those who left. Anna Haines, an American nurse who had been greatly impressed by the Soviet night sanatoriums, observed: "Needless to say, the records show almost all the cases improved on discharge, but the authorities felt that the education value of the treatment to the patient and to his family is of even greater benefit than his immediate gain in health."[117] Haines remarked that the institutions seemed to be popular. Testimonials from workers filled the pages of health magazines and showed either the heavy hand of an editor or the workers' internalization of health care rhetoric. One worker noted, "The night sanatorium shows us that work is not all that harmful if we live that time when we are not at work sensibly [*po-chelovecheski*]." According to a worker from Moscow's AMO factory, the night sanatorium provided a special space for relaxation: "After the day's filth and hard work, you fall into a true place of relaxation where all is clean and good. The nervous system, after carrying on healing and after a break, calms and increases the capacity for work."[118]

Although the sanatorium organizers anticipated great immediate consequences for the individual's health, they hoped to change the family life of the patient as well. An article on a children's health square stated that while the children listened avidly, the lasting reform came later: "When they go home they talk to their parents about the same things—open the transom, do a wet cleaning, and brush their teeth." The article further argued that these changes reached into all aspects of the patient's life. Not only does the children's health improve, but they also "study better, are more disciplined, develop hygiene skills, and grow accustomed to an amicable, collective life."[119] In short, their experience transformed them into good citizens. The statistical evidence did not show tremendous lasting effect, instead testifying to the difficulties still facing Narkomzdrav. A 1925 investigation of one hundred former patients of the night sanatorium for the factories of the Rogozhsko-Simonovskii district found more humble results. Of the one hundred patients surveyed only forty-three began to brush their teeth, nine obtained individual plates, six got bedding, twenty-one began to do rub downs (*obtiranie*), and six quit smoking.[120]

Occasionally even the lessons of these hygienic institutions proved insufficient and reformers called for the complete removal of the worker from the city. In a 1926 article A. Lipets described the startlingly destructive home environment of most industrial workers, arguing that political work was impossible without recognizing "that the worker family loses the quiet and restorative forces of sleep because of bugs, that cockroaches float in the soups of our restaurants, that in the countryside there are no lavatories, and that in cities people are not able to use them." Lipets contended that it was unfair to ask workers to fulfill even the most basic cleanliness strictures in such situations: "It is impossible to write 'wash your hands' and not provide a clean, dry towel and soap. It is also impossible to be reconciled . . . [to] the naked, sad walls of our dwellings and public places."[121]

While concentrating on the utility of the club, Lipets could just as easily have been discussing the necessity of the night sanatorium or the House of Leisure. Reformers decried the baneful influences of modern life and looked for places to isolate workers for rest and recovery. As one hygienist lamented,

> What is the sense of lectures, posters and slogans when the lectures about hygiene are conducted in stuffy and dirty rooms? What is the sense of hanging posters on the walls about the dangers of smoking and the necessity of bodily cleanliness when on the floor there is so much trash that it must be scraped up with a shovel, when one cannot even enter the lavatory and the single water faucet does not work because of filth? The House of Leisure teaches not by words but by the mere fact of its existence—its example. It shows the necessity of living and building one's home rationally and hygienically.[122]

Workers could not find health in the city because the conditions of modern life ensured that they had to escape in order to be healthy. In the anti-urban vision, perfected leisure took place outside the city in the clean air of the countryside.[123]

Two types of institutions—the sanatorium and the House of Leisure—provided respite. Both were opened to workers following the October Revolution and both struggled to obtain limited resources.[124] For the ill, the sanatorium was designed to provide shelter, to educate, and to spur recovery. The House of Leisure sought to isolate healthy workers from the city and educate them to hygienic norms, keeping them for just two weeks during their annual vacation. Though they differed in terms of their setup, they coincided in their goals: "In sanatoriums as well as in the House of Leisure, attention is paid to the patient learning new skills with which he learns to struggle with illness."[125]

Like other programs, health resorts borrowed ideas from abroad and built on native traditions. Russian health resorts grew out of Peter the Great's travels. Throughout the eighteenth and nineteenth centuries spas increased in number and sophistication, becoming especially numerous in the Crimea. On the eve of

1917 there were about 350 spas in Russia. In 1919 Lenin nationalized such institutions and in 1920 he decreed that Crimean resorts should be reserved for workers. In 1920 the first House of Leisure was set up in the former home of Count Polovtsev, located on Kamennyi island in Petrograd. Following a visit, Lenin issued a decree calling for more such facilities.[126] Unlike spas and sanatoriums, Houses of Leisure were "facilities for workers to restore their strength and energy under the most favorable conditions, during annual leave." Rather than places for treating illness, they were palaces for building up health.[127]

The creation of the first House of Leisure in a former count's estate established a precedent. Country estates of the wealthy—and even their city homes, with large, airy, sunny rooms; beautiful furnishings, surrounded by nice parks—proved an ideal setting for healthy leisure. They also highlighted the revolution's power and avowed purpose. The land and property of the old bourgeoisie were taken over for the good of the people. Undoubtedly, the opulence of the surroundings was used by propagandists as a basic lesson in Marxist principles to remind workers of the exploitation under the former system. Across the Soviet Union it meant converting 22,500 buildings into workers' clubs and 543 country palaces into vacation resorts; on an individual level it meant healthier vacations for workers, with built-in political lessons.[128]

Patients of these institutions were selected through the Central Council of Trade Unions and by Narkomzdrav.[129] After a brief decrease following the introduction of NEP, spas, sanatoriums, and Houses of Leisure served more patients.[130] By 1924–25 the twenty-six sanatoriums of Moscow cared for 14,000 patients, completely healing almost 9 percent, according to their own statistics, and providing 79 percent solace.[131] By 1926–27, thirty-one sanatoriums cared for 16,655 patients.[132] The Moscow House of Leisure system increased greatly throughout the 1920s. In 1920 only 240 people attended the House of Leisure. In 1921 some 7,213 workers enjoyed stays, and by 1924–1925 the twelve Houses of Leisure greeted 50,000 vacationers.[133]

Prescribing a sanatorium, in contrast to other institutions, constituted a drastic step taken only when doctors decided that "to return a worker to health, they must isolate him from that sphere where he is surrounded by harm, where his organism is in such a state as to be unable to fight the illness."[134] The House of Leisure used the same techniques but worked toward a different goal, namely, prophylaxis. Organizers attempted to create a different world for healthy workers, who would be indoctrinated though its didactic agenda: "The House of Leisure teaches not with words but with the very fact of its existence, its example, how to live rationally and hygienically and build your home."[135] The House of Leisure functioned as an ideal space in which workers were surrounded by images of the world to come. As the slogan stated, "The House of Leisure, with its regimen, not only sanitizes and strengthens . . . but also teaches through the environment. . . . It agitates for a new life by its very existence."[136] These "school[s] for new life" had two major components: sanitary enlightenment and the regimen. Sanitary enlightenment proved integral at one sanatorium, where "concerts, spectacles, evenings of question-and-answer, living newspapers, and movies were organized. For men and women they put together special segregated lectures on questions of hygiene and sexual life."[137] In the House of Leisure the worker learned skills. As one couplet quipped, patrons learned "something about cleaning the body and home, something about drinking and smoking / About how the sun and water nourish / And even how to go to the bathroom."[138]

The regimen introduced in the House of Leisure and sanatorium attended to those trifles of behavior ignored by the law. Details concerning care for the body came out in prescriptions for sleep, leisure, and food intake. Workers learned of the need for regimentation from lectures and from the example of the sanatorium's scheduling.[139] Organizers credited the regimen with positively changing workers' lives: "The day of the patient in the sanatorium is precisely divided by hours. The patient rises at a determined hour and goes to bed at a determined hour. At certain hours he eats, goes for a walk, takes sun and air baths, etc. Furthermore, the patient becomes accustomed to careful care of his body—regularly cleaning and rinsing the mouth, keeping the skin clean, breathing correctly, growing accustomed to clean air, sensibly clothing himself, and accustoming his body to cold water."[140]

Doctors compared the regimen of the sanatorium to a druggist's prescription. Strict adherence to the rules served to cure all problems. One medical tract went so far as to present the same simple regimen as equally applicable and effective for all illnesses. Patients filled their schedules with sun baths, mud baths, waters cures, dietary therapy, and koumiss treatments.[141] Every aspect of the patient's life "had to be done according to a special timetable, based on scientific factors, and should be for one purpose: to put the patient's organism in the most fortuitous conditions for the struggle with the illness."[142] If patients followed the prescription, the sanatorium functioned like a medication: "If the patient eats well and spends a lot of time in the sun and, in general, strictly fulfills the hygienic instructions . . . the 'ill' in practice will live his entire life as 'healthy.' But if the patient returns to live in poor conditions—crowded apartments, poor nutrition, works in dust, etc.—and in addition forgets the advice of the doctor to not smoke or drink, stay in the fresh air, etc., then the organism will gradually weaken and the [tuberculosis] bacillus will again live, awaken, and get back to work."[143] The writer presented the sanatorium as a cure but did give himself an out. If the patient returned to crowds—a certainty given housing conditions—then the cure would not hold up.

The House of Leisure provided both escape and education for the worker. According to Doctor Kagan, the House of Leisure served as a "two-week practical school of a healthful and new life."[144] In this school the lessons learned applied to more than just the individual. The vacationer needed to take these ideas home and apply them to domestic life. In this respect the facility was a "factory of health" that was "favorable and [provided] the cheapest protection from mass social illness, against which the struggle is considerably more difficult and more dear." The new environment also allowed the worker to rest "physically and mentally [*dushevno*]."[145]

One Moscow Department of Health poster made the point (figure 3.1). "Workers in the House of Leisure Learn and Build a New Life" (1926–29) depicted the pristine, orderly setup of the House of Leisure, with a red arrow directly connecting it to the reordering of the worker home. The disordered, crowded, dark, and airless room of old worker life was presented in the hell-like position below. The red color connected the House of Leisure to the communist path and consequently to political consciousness. The color and contrasting visions of worker life revealed the political, social, and cultural changes organizers hoped to provide with just a two-week window. Another poster taught citizens not just to bring home the lessons but to change the domestic situation completely. In "The Spa at Home" viewers were shown how to transform their home by opening windows while sleeping, eating meals outdoors, and even napping outside. The poster concluded: "Everyone can build for themselves a spa at home. They need only to live, work, and rest correctly [*pravil'no*]."[146]

While anecdotal evidence touted great changes resulting from Soviet care, surveys revealed the small numbers of vactioners who had actually transferred their House of Leisure experience to their home life. Organizers wished their patrons to pattern their lives after their vacation or sanatorium experience, but for many it was impossible or too bothersome. According to a 1925 survey of 1,000 vacationers, only 23.5 percent had improved their personal hygiene, nearly 12 percent had bettered their home lives, almost 12 percent made more rational use of their free time, a little over 6 percent ate better, about 2.5 percent changed their sleeping habits, nearly 9 percent began doing morning gymnastics, and nearly 74 percent would readily move to a communal apartment.[147] These self-reported figures probably reflected inflated results. Concrete changes were slight in scope and duration, but nearly everyone agreed that any type of new apartment was a good idea.

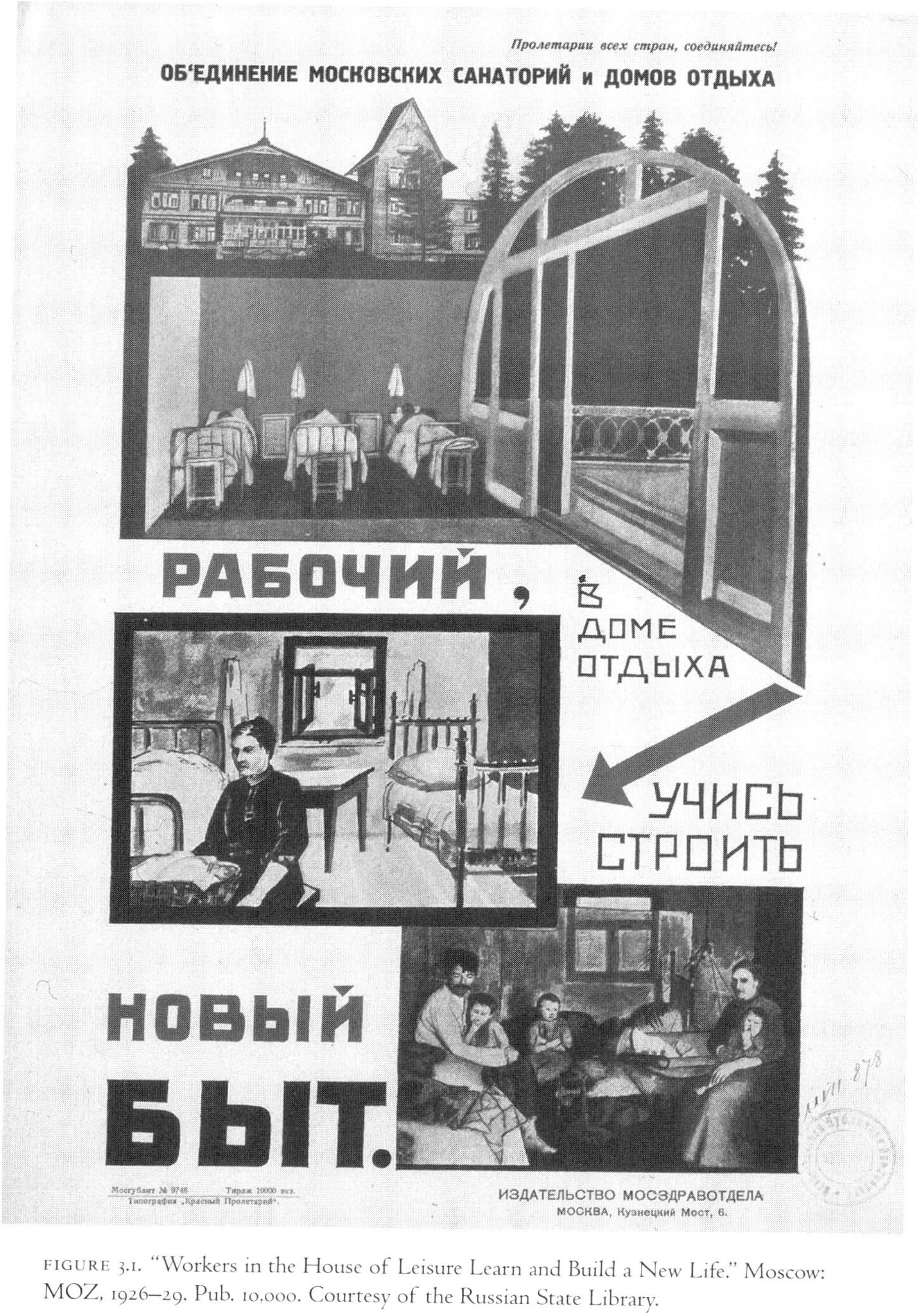
Пролетарии всех стран, соединяйтесь!
ОБ'ЕДИНЕНИЕ МОСКОВСКИХ САНАТОРИЙ и ДОМОВ ОТДЫХА
РАБОЧИЙ,
В ДОМЕ ОТДЫХА
УЧИСЬ СТРОИТЬ
НОВЫЙ БЫТ.
Мосгублит № 9746 Тираж 10000 экз.
Типография „Красный Пролетарий".
ИЗДАТЕЛЬСТВО МОСЗДРАВОТДЕЛА
МОСКВА, Кузнецкий Мост, 6.

FIGURE 3.1. "Workers in the House of Leisure Learn and Build a New Life." Moscow: MOZ, 1926–29. Pub. 10,000. Courtesy of the Russian State Library.

The numbers were depressingly low despite the fact that the goals for transformation remained high. One article admitted that most of the workers relaxing at the House of Leisure were not used to washing or bathing. The writer explained that this was not due to reticence but rather to a lack of soap and clean water in the city. He then acknowledged that poor, crowded, unsanitary conditions would not be remedied anytime soon. Rather than expounding upon the problems of contemporary life, or even postulating solutions, he chose to look to the future, ultimately concluding that the House of Leisure would change working-class lives by showing workers how they *could* live: "The House of Leisure gives a worker such a dwelling temporarily, which introduces him to the necessity of a new dwelling, to the need for striving to build cooperative housing and, to a certain extent, adjusting him to the habit of cultured living in a healthy dwelling. . . . On the whole, familiarizing the worker with a normal, healthy life is the purpose that the House of Leisure serves."[148] The writer assumed that exposure to a perfected life would kindle the desire within vacationers to live a rational life.

Lenin expressed his own worries about the Houses of Leisure in a 1921 memo to Commissar of Health Semashko, in which he decried "abominable . . . bribe taking, privileges for the bourgeois, and a disgusting attitude toward the workers." He concluded that these problems were small in comparison to the "total disorder" in treatment and, worse still, the "complete lack of supplies."[149] Not all problems were structural. Activists did recognize popular resistance to the House of Leisure. A 1925 article published in the journal *To a New Life!* claimed that many older workers and working mothers distrusted the very idea of these institutions and went unwillingly. These wary types were suspicious of a "strange, unfamiliar house where, according to the rumors, there was 'bolshevik order' and they lived communally, where they have some kind of 'physculture' and where men and women go around the whole day in 'shorts and wide trousers . . . with bare legs.'"[150] These popular attitudes cloaked disquiet with the House of Leisure that reeked of sexual anxiety in its emphasis on half-naked men and women engaged in physical antics. Authorities battled these images of health institutions as pleasure palaces. "About no other type of medical institution does there exist so many incorrect assumptions as those of sanatoriums," claimed one article. The author further challenged the idea that the sanatorium visit should be "pleasant," saying that while it was often enjoyable, the main purpose of the sanatorium was to heal, with the principal method being the regimen. According to hygienists, workers came not for sex, rest, or pleasure but rather for their health.[151]

As might be expected, not everyone accepted the transformation of their yearly vacation into a seminar. Resistance took on active forms, as complaints about poor behavior attest. At a meeting in the Khamovnicheskii district, the participants were highly interested in the workings of the House of Leisure and sanatorium. They called for a longer stay for the ill but saved their vitriol for a discussion of problems. One member said, "The regimen of the House of Leisure must be strengthened [in order to] liquidate the flirt once and for all."[152] The reputation of the House of Leisure as a site for sexual transgression appeared in the worker press as well, underscoring if not the reality of the House of Leisure then its potential danger, as well as the prevailing idea of a society on the verge of sexual chaos.[153] Other types of behavior also annoyed organizers. A 1926 article entitled "There Need Not Be a Place for Drunkenness and Hooliganism in the House of Leisure" detailed problems involving discipline: "Now, we must take note of the unhealthy phenomenon that is being observed on the part of a small group of workers. We are referring to cases of drunkenness, hooliganism, and incidences of malicious infringement of the regimen." The article noted a case where five workers had to be "thrown out by the militia from a House of Leisure."[154]

Bad behavior might be less extreme. A 1925 article by the head of the Krasno-Presnenskii insurance office noted that conversations and fights disrupted the quiet nap time and that people who insisted on eating lunch in their rooms threatened the collective experience. Enlightenment work allowed authorities "to mobilize a social opinion among the working masses" and brought power to bear against the hooligan and the flirt.[155] A letter published in *To a New Life!* called for corrective, collective shaming of misbehaving vacationers, such as reporting them to the factory committee, publishing their names in wall newspapers, and publicizing their crimes throughout the community.[156]

If workers challenged the regimen or resisted the House of Leisure, propagandists blamed ignorance. "There is a worker contingent that does not understand the importance of the regimen," insisted one writer, "and this incomprehension leads to their restless behavior and disturbing the others' relaxation." To fight ignorance, the article recommended instruction in the social responsibility of the patron to the House of Leisure. Finally, sanitary enlightenment within the House of Leisure should be increased to fight the problem and to underscore the "meaning of the regimen."[157] Hygienists argued that workers resisted this orchestration of their free time due to political ignorance.

Organizers were convinced that workers required guidance during their yearly vacation because of their innate need for productive leisure. If this need was not met, hygienists warned that workers' energies would be misdirected:

"Workers by their nature cannot spend two weeks in a state of 'doing nothing' even in a state of leisure. . . . Those hours of rest not taken up by eating, sleeping, or physical culture must be filled with cultural work; otherwise the flirt, drunkenness, *buza,* or at best boredom will flourish in the House of Leisure. In those Houses of Leisure where cultural work is not carried out or is poorly executed, the worker cannot have proper rest."[158] Organizers argued workers could not rest without direction. Without instruction they would turn to destructive behaviors.

Vacationers mouthed propaganda-laden phrases testifying to their enjoyment of the House of Leisure. Following a 1928 meeting, on the last night of a stay at the House of Leisure telegrams were sent to the Moscow Soviet and the Moscow Trade Unions singing the praises of the House of Leisure. One missive noted: "Only the October Revolution gave the working class the ability to use royal palaces and forests for the health of the workers."[159] Another group of vacationers enthused that "hundreds of thousands of workers now rested in a spot where the Iusupov princes and their fellows held their orgies." Now workers relaxed not just for their own health but for "the construction of socialism in our country."[160]

Another group of telegrams attested to the way in which patrons had "used" their rest time intensively to "restore their organism" thanks to the "skillful organization of leisure, the careful supervision and management of relaxation, the fulfillment of the regimen, conversations with the doctor about the rate of progress, the filling of the entire day with excursions and sessions of physical culture."[161] They also mouthed the hopes of the organizers: "We promise that we will take into our own lives that which is rational and applicable and which we have learned in the House of Leisure"[162] In articles workers used similar language to describe their experiences and echo the propaganda. Worker P., a forty-year-old, nonparty female janitor with three children, praised the House of Leisure for teaching her "a correct life" and vowed to "attempt to carry out that which I have seen." The article spotlighted another worker who wanted to start the "normal relaxation" he had learned. Worker Po-ov, a married forty-three-year-old, insisted, "the House of Leisure taught me everything good and I will put my home in the same order."[163]

An article in *To a New Life!* contended that the very existence of sanatoriums and Houses of Leisure provided proof of the power of the revolution: "The House of Leisure is wholly and completely a work of the October Revolution. Not only did it not exist earlier; even the idea for it did not exist."[164] The writer gave a history of the houses, which had been transformed into sanatoriums. The Ogarev sanatorium had once been the palace of a Romanov prince. The home of a wealthy merchant became the Chekhov sanatorium.[165] Another House of Leisure took over a former monastery.[166] Rehabilitation of buildings was a constant struggle. An article on the Sverdlov House of Leisure argued that the building had not been sufficiently renovated. The writer decried the presence of pictures that "could not be interesting to a worker" and called for a Lenin corner filled with portraits, books, and biographies. He concluded, "Where workers relax the worker spirit must prevail" and took the House of Leisure to task for retaining a bourgeois aura.[167]

The guarantee of leisure and the attempts to rationalize its use became a pillar of Soviet propaganda at home and abroad. Trade delegations and other foreigners could not complete their visit to the new state without a tour of one of the miracles of Soviet power, namely, a sanatorium or House of Leisure. The British Trade Union Delegation noted the conditions of the House of Leisure and the opulent surroundings left by the wealthy. They particularly marveled at how little wear could be noticed on the original furniture of these bourgeois estates. In predictions that echoed organizers' hopes, the delegation praised the House of Leisure: "A worker or a peasant after a month's holiday in these surroundings returns to his own home armed with duster and pots of paint, which he utilizes in his spare time by cleaning and decorating his own quarters."[168] Not all visitors were as easily convinced, but so proud were authorities that they presented the House of Leisure as an answer to all criticisms. One visitor noted: "When we dragged into bright conversations captious questions about low wages or high prices or the cramped life of the worker in the 'toilers' garden,' as one of our guides liked to call it, we were always reminded of his unique compensations, above all of his rest houses and his vacations."[169]

For H. G. Wells the magnificence of the former estates was "at once rather fine and not a little absurd." Life within was refined: "The meals are served on white cloths with flowers upon the table and so forth." Wells, however, found the surroundings and clientele incongruous. Ensconced in splendor, workers still indulged in habits of the street. Wells's incredulity at the contrast of old and new was evident in his attention to worker behavior: "If in a forgetful moment he [the worker] clears his throat in the good old resonant peasant manner and spits upon the floor, an attendant, I was told, chalks a circle about his defilement." The chalk circles over parquet flooring must have been an appalling reminder of how much had still not changed. Even with these reservations, Wells seemed won over: "But after all," he concluded, "the idea of civilizing your workpeople by dipping them into pleasant surroundings is, in itself, rather a good one."[170]

Hygienists found the modern city a dangerous place where proximity to social disease and political corruption led to weakened bodies. Faith in the power of buildings and schedules to transform flesh and consciousness was a cornerstone of Soviet health policy. Faced with the reality that they could not police workers after they left the factory floor, authorities developed a host of institutions to provide workers with alternative leisure, healthy sleeping quarters, and a place of respite for two weeks a year. While patients were selected because of their weak bodies and poor living habits, they were expected to leave as strong citizens. Clubs and day/night sanatoriums graced the city. Parks and museums sprang up to provide hygienic alternatives.[171] The spa, sanatorium, and House of Leisure provided respite in the countryside and became features of the Soviet landscape. They also provided a strong symbol of Soviet power for reticent citizens and skeptical visitors. By 1928 thirty-seven Houses of Leisure served Moscow and thirteen served Leningrad. Their popularity and numbers only increased with time. By the 1970s more than ten million people took advantage of leisure institutions every year.[172] Hygienic slogans continued to grace these palaces of productive leisure, but the regimen slackened in severity.

For those who attended leisure activities, the reaction was mixed. Not every patron of the club ran to listen to a political discussion. Many preferred movies or music circles. Older workers and women chose not to attend. In the House of Leisure not every guest came to live communally and relax healthfully. Resistance was prevalent. Finally, while hygienists hoped that these sites would provide for all citizens, their numbers remained too small to accommodate all comers. Large portions of the population outside the cities, as well as those not members of unions or engaged in factory work, never had a chance. For those few who had access to hygienic leisure, made it into the cramped spaces, and were receptive to the message, the clubs, museums, and institutions of Narkomzdrav presented a healthy alternative to overcrowded apartments or the NEP streets. Many of these institutions even provided a double dose of health by including sanitary enlightenment content during the night's entertainment.

4 The Home

Housekeeping, Social Duty, and Public Concern

When the curtain rose on the 1925 play *Our Life: An Agit-Lifestyle-Buffoonery in Two Acts,* the stage set resembled the audience's apartments—crowded, filthy, and disordered. In the midst of the muddle, an infant squealed, an older girl sang loudly, and twin boys splashed in a washtub. Another boy, sprawled on the floor pretending to read, bellowed a demand for quiet. Amid this chaos, a woman worked doggedly on one of the innumerable piles of laundry. Referred to only as "mother," her labors went unnoticed while the children screamed. The pandemonium continued as the curtain fell on the brief first act.

The second act provided a startling contrast. The curtain rose to the sound of "cheerful music and white light. It is the same room, only sparkling clean and orderly. . . . The wall is covered with portraits of revolutionary leaders. A Pioneer corner. Shelves with books." At center stage the older girl, Liza—with a cheery, red kerchief around her neck—cleaned the room with her brother's help. The mother entered and set the table with Liza's eager assistance. The father appeared and was admonished not to touch the children until he had cleaned up. Only after he and the family had washed and dried their hands—on separate towels—did they sit down to dinner. When the mother announced her election to public office, the father objected that she already had too many duties, but she crowed that her obligations had never been so light because her children had become "such heroes [*eagles*]!"

In a jaunty tune the players revealed the reasons for this transformation:

ALL: In the scene we have just shown you,
The connection we've not told you.
MOTHER: Listen, comrades, here's the deal,

I have joined the *zhenotdel.*[1]
I do not cook a luncheon
Our home has not a kitchen.
From now on that room must be
Communal for you and me.
For me it was two in one,
A slave cell and prison.
SEVEN-YEAR-OLDS: Brother and I did smarten.
We go to kindergarten.
MOTHER: My dearest little kiddies
Will soon be *Oktiabristki.*[2]
VANIA AND LIZA: To Pioneers we did sign
A year ago and we're fine.
MOTHER: Treasure your children, believe me!
And let them Pioneers be!
ALL: We are all a little gladder
'Cause mom's a *zhenotdeler*[3]

These scant seven pages of script found in a 1925 issue of *Workers Club* contained almost all of the Soviet reformers' critiques of the home, their recommendations for more rational domestic organization, and their predictions for the political and social benefits of Soviet planning. Hygienists predicted that if women would take advantage of Soviet institutions, everything would improve and their homes would be transformed from a living hell to a haven. In the play, once the children entered nursery school and enrolled in the Pioneers, the daughter worked in the factory kitchen, and the mother participated in the *zhenotdel,* laundry disappeared and toil vanished. The children helped with chores.

While touting the benefits of Soviet institutions, the play also revealed the biases and naïveté of reformers. The playwright displaced certain labor-intensive tasks from the home while ignoring the many new chores hygienists recommendations required of women. In the play, simply removing daytime child care and food preparation from the home resulted in a clean apartment. The play depicted a single-family dwelling. In a city plagued by overcrowded, dilapidated apartment buildings and a lack of basic services, reformers seemed ignorant of or ambivalent about the drudgery of maintaining a house. For example, in the play the laundry disappeared even as the family switched to the use of individual towels. The daughter ate at the factory, but the wife prepared the husband's meals at home in the "cell-like" kitchen she declared herself free of in the song.[4]

Inattention to detail did not translate into a lack of concern for the questions of home and family. Basing their concepts upon the works of Engels, Kollontai, and others, Soviet theorists argued that under capitalism the burdening of women with unpaid household labor had led to their inequality. Following the revolution, women's rights activists—often working in association with the *zhenotdel*—hoped to overthrow the oppression of the hearth through collective institutions and the increased use of technology.[5] While hygienists taught women more involved regimens for cleaning their homes and provided more expansive reasons for doing so, political activists argued that housework was insignificant in the face of social activism. Hygienists joined their concern for cleanliness in the home with calls for women's liberation in an uneasy and often unworkable relationship where yet-to-be realized collective institutions solved all questions and the answer to present problems was that they would not be around in the future.

Though theorists attributed great benefits to all of society from collective domestic institutions, in health propaganda, as elsewhere, only women were getting the message.[6] In plays, posters, and even in weeklong propaganda campaigns, reformers considered women the authorities within the home and the ones capable of substantial change.[7] Writers indicated that women were responsible for the home and for organizing the collective laundries, kitchens, and nurseries to free them from domestic slavery. The traditional connections of women, hearth, and home were consequently more deeply entrenched. As for other family members, although propaganda literature and posters urged husbands and children to lobby women, they did not deem men and children capable of changing the home themselves. In the play cited earlier, the father remained resistant to a new role for his wife even after the remarkable change in his home. The daughter's admonitions about clean hands indicated that the father still did not understand the new order and might infect the next generation through ignorance. In the propaganda literature on the home men remained passive or resistant, simply receiving change but not starting it. Children needed to be educated by Soviet institutions in order to see the path to a new life, and even then they remained dependent upon a compliant mother to institute lasting change.

For women responsibility for the home brought blame along with empowerment. The mother who chose not to accept writers' recommendations held back not just herself but her family and the entire Soviet experiment. Liza's red kerchief suggested that the household had become politically active; the mother attested that domestic changes had freed up time for political participation. Once the home was organized, political change resulted as the natural consequence of a rational domestic life. As activists from the *zhenotdel* and other groups argued, changing the home would alter the lives of all Soviet citizens. The emphasis on health brought a new dimension to discussions of the importance of the home to the Soviet state. Women could encourage entire neighborhoods to become more politically involved by choosing communal facilities, thereby improving individual health, their family's health, and the health of their entire community. While this play upheld a positive female model, other propaganda literature attacked negative models. Reformers consistently depicted women who did not maintain the new norms as backward, ignorant, and responsible for domestic and social problems. They lambasted husbands as uneducated, quarrelsome, or powerless and children as unruly and dangerous.

With blame came attempts at enforcement. Not content to leave women and families to arrive at these choices gradually, agents of the state targeted endangered families and sent in visiting nurses and doctors to investigate living conditions, urge change, and threaten those who did not comply. The state initiated change from above, but many of their most invasive propagandists arose from below. The good housewife was responsible for her home and was encouraged to nurture the rest of society by volunteering to organize a communal institution, investigate her neighbors, or get involved in delegate work. Apartment building health cells scrutinized their neighbors, as did volunteers from other groups. While hundreds of women joined inspectorates and health cells, lack of basic sanitary services ensured that even had they found a receptive audience, their recommendations could not be fulfilled by most households.

Inspectors figured heavily in health care initiatives in other countries; however, the pervasive and invasive nature of Soviet inspections distinguished them from global campaigns. Inspectors had limited power to help and also limited ability to reprimand the recalcitrant. Caught between their knowledge of the problems below and the pressures being exerted from above, the inspectors saw the worst of the city and were intimately aware of the problems faced by families living in dilapidated housing under overcrowded conditions.

The Bolsheviks believed that women's emancipation would arrive with the dissolution of capitalism.[8] Following the revolution, activists in the *zhenotdel*, the women's section of the party, led the fight. They agitated against restrictions on abortion, divorce, and women's sexual freedom and criticized the traditional distribution of power in the home—and even the home itself.[9] They argued for communal facilities to emancipate women from domestic chores and free them for political participation.[10] Building upon utopian, socialist traditions, Soviet planners of the 1920s wished to refashion domestic life by creating communal dining halls, nurseries, and laundries. Communal responsibility for housekeeping tasks was seen as an ideal way to fight domestic drudgery and make women politically active without sacrificing a comfortable life for the entire family.

The connection between domestic work and political consciousness was forged before the revolution, as was the link between environmental manipulation and political consciousness.[11] Socialists and utopians created plans to foster communal relationships and fight individualistic, competitive capitalism alongside the evil of women's oppression. For example, in *What Is to Be Done?* Nikolai Chernyshevskii praised communal living for fostering proper attitudes and values both immediately—as in Vera Pavlovna's sewing cooperative—and in the future, which she glimpsed in a dream. As a visitor to her cooperative noted, "Instead of poverty I saw contentment; instead of filth, not merely cleanliness but even some luxury in their rooms; instead of crudeness, considerable education."[12] The cooperative's idealized living conditions brought order, contentment, and refinement of life, home, and even person.

Although the Bolsheviks placed great stock on the ability of the material environment to modify behavior, others also looked to engineering homes to produce docile citizens. In Russia before the revolution, bourgeois factory owners attempted to control workers through curfews, fines, and barracks regulations. Factories maintained their own guards, in addition to supervisors, to surveil workers.[13] Elsewhere, reformers in France and Austria considered redesigning the homes of urban dwellers. The Red Belt of Paris was a planned community, and socialists in interwar Vienna saw living arrangements as a way to instill not only "orderliness but also decency and respectability."[14]

Soviet architects experimented with European models, like the communal house in France and the garden city in England. They analyzed communities in Germany, the United States, and Holland, and incorporated influences from the Russian arts and crafts movement. Drawing on these ideas, Soviet planners hoped to break down the barriers between nuclear families and encourage more efficient use of resources. Urban planners and architects envisioned joint bathhouses, laundries, and kitchens, where distinctions between individuals would break down.[15] In the novel *We*, Evgenii Zamiatin speculated about the consequence of such leveling in his glass-walled dystopia, where personal space and even the individual disappeared. Zamiatin's novel attested not just to the fears of some but to the saturation of society with these anxieties. Despite Zamiatin's dire predictions, most communes remained on the drawing boards. City planners preferred conventional apartment buildings, but the desire for utopian living inspired many in the population to try their hand. By 1921 865 communal living arrangements had been set up in Moscow, reflecting the outpouring of voluntary initiatives and enthusiasm for the concept.[16]

With so much social, political, and cultural import tied to the construction of the private home, it is no wonder that reformers sought to reeducate the public concerning the significance of the home. Hygienists added one more layer of meaning by stressing the health benefits of a properly maintained home and providing recommendations on all aspects of domestic care.[17] In *The Social Causes for Illness* (1928) Commissar of Health Semashko stated, "The home is one of the most important factors in the health or ill health of a person."[18] A. A. Ashikhmin's *Social Diseases in the Home* (1926) underscored the importance of the home to all of society: "The modern man, especially the city dweller, spends a significant portion of his life in the home. Leaving aside the fact that he sleeps here and prepares food here, he also often spends leisure time here and raises small children." Because of the amount of time spent in the house, Ashikhmin concluded, "it is understandable that health and welfare depend, to a very great extent, on the kind of home in which we spend time."[19] Semashko and Ashikhmin wrote about individual health, but in keeping with the tenets of social hygiene, the major reason for domestic health initiatives was the threat of the ill-kept individual to all of society. Semashko argued that life within the home directly influenced the spread of contagious disease. Citing statistics drawn from around the world, he linked unsanitary living conditions to high infant mortality and the spread of social diseases. The gravity with which Semashko regarded domestic health and its connection to disease drew upon and reflected ongoing, worldwide concern with urban health and societal strength.[20]

For Soviet officials the conflation of a healthy home and a healthy society transformed personal hygiene into a civic duty. In 1920 and 1921 they made it law, requiring Muscovites to maintain their housing in a sanitary condition.[21] A. V. Mol'kov, director of the Narkomzdrav Museum of Social Hygiene, explicitly made the connection between citizenship and sanitation when he wrote: "The maintenance of cleanliness within the home is the duty of every politically conscious citizen. It is important not just for [the citizen] himself but also for all of society."[22] Mol'kov's insistence on the civic nature of domestic maintenance served as the rallying cry for the early 1920s poster entitled "The Maintenance of Cleanliness within the Home Is the Duty of Every Politically Conscious Citizen" (figure 4.1). The poster consisted of three levels of information. The top picture showed an ordered, clean home. The middle picture featured a home that did not conform to a Soviet way of life. At the bottom a list detailed the changes that had been made, as reflected in the images. For Mol'kov a "good citizen" aimed for the well-maintained home of the top picture

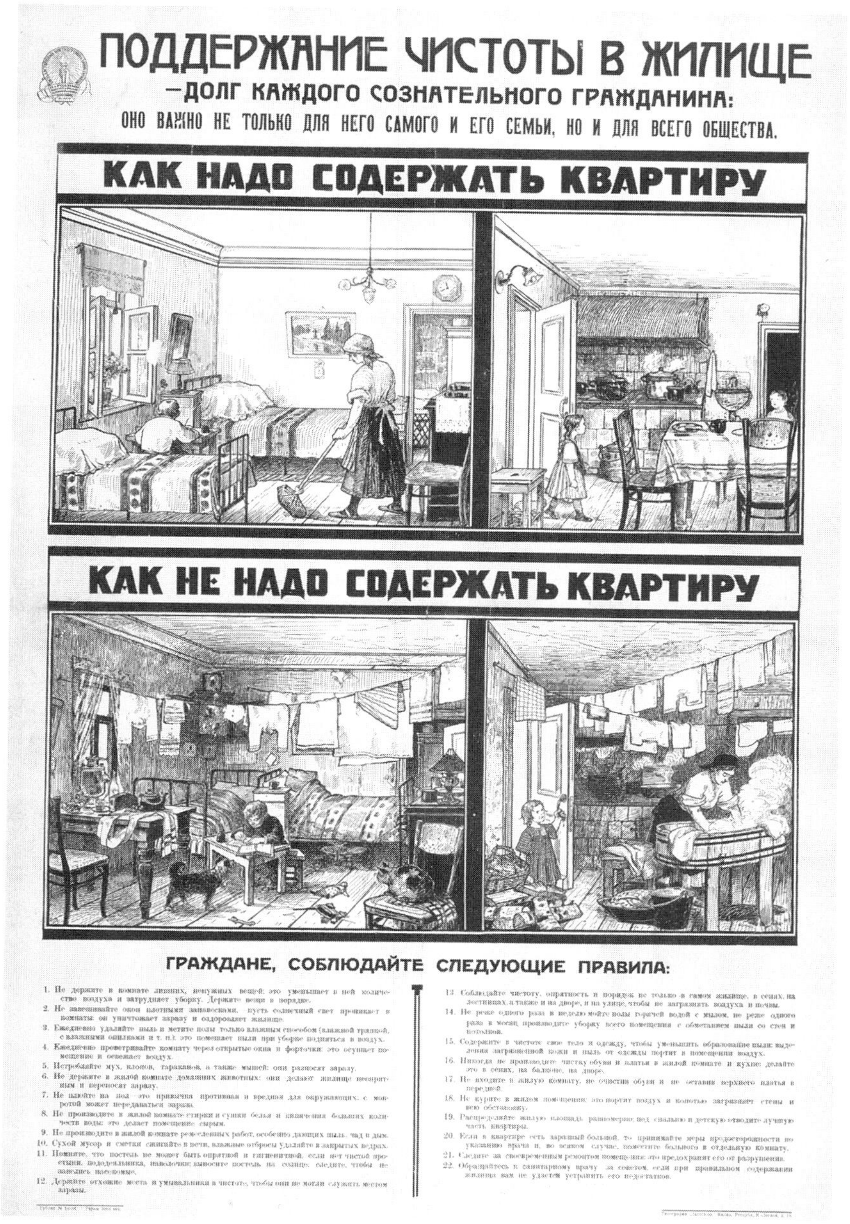

FIGURE 4.1. "The Maintenance of Cleanliness within the Home Is the Duty of Every Politically Conscious Citizen." State Institute of Social Hygiene. NKZ RSFSR, 1921–25. Pub. 5,000. Courtesy of the Russian State Library.

and thereby protected the welfare of the larger society. A healthy home became the basis for membership in society, its care serving the interests of society and government. Though Mol'kov referred to a universal citizen, it was clear that the target of the advice was a woman with children.

The poster delineated the benefits of the healthy home in scenes presented like heaven and hell in a style reminiscent of iconographic images and *lubok* woodcuts.[23] Whereas below laundry, domestic animals, and steam clouded the scene, above pristine spaces gleamed in a heaven of cleanliness. Light, both electric and natural, streamed through the top image, while steam and shadow billowed below in hell. Aside from the obvious difference of disorder/order, the poster conveyed the larger issue of hygienic choices for the home in terms of political awareness, technological advancement, and material comfort. In the top picture a woman damp-mopped her apartment, which, following Soviet norms, was decorated with clocks and images of nature instead of an icon corner and hanging clothing. Regimentation and technology replaced superstition and disorder. The window permitted fresh air and sunshine to enter—and, by extension, the future. It revealed the new, rationalized room, which now contained three rather than two children, implying that children thrived, or perhaps simply survived, in clean surroundings. Finally, electric lights, modern plumbing, and fire alarms surrounded the simmering pots on the stove, intimating a material prosperity to come. Since planners believed that maintaining a healthy home reaped such extensive benefits, it is little wonder that domestic chores were transformed into a civic responsibility.

As well as noting the necessity of a well-maintained home, poster art underscored the state's reliance upon women. The 1927 poster "Window" (figure 4.2), issued by the Moscow Department of Health, appeared to express concern for childhood safety. It cautioned that "with the onset of warm weather begins the tumbling of children from windows." It then catalogued the consequences of these problems for the rest of society: "In 1927 in Moscow there were 329 calls by the emergency service to help children suffering from falls from windows." The text emphasized not the injuries to the children—or even how many had died—but the number of times the state expended resources to respond to these problems. As the only adults featured in the poster, women were held responsible for the problem. The poster "Boiling Water," in the same series, similarly featured a woman as the sole caregiver in the home and emphasized the need to use state resources to care for improperly monitored children by observing how many times the government had to step in and treat them. In this poster wrestling children toppled a samovar in one scene, while in another an infant pulling at a tablecloth overturned a pot of boiling water. The fear

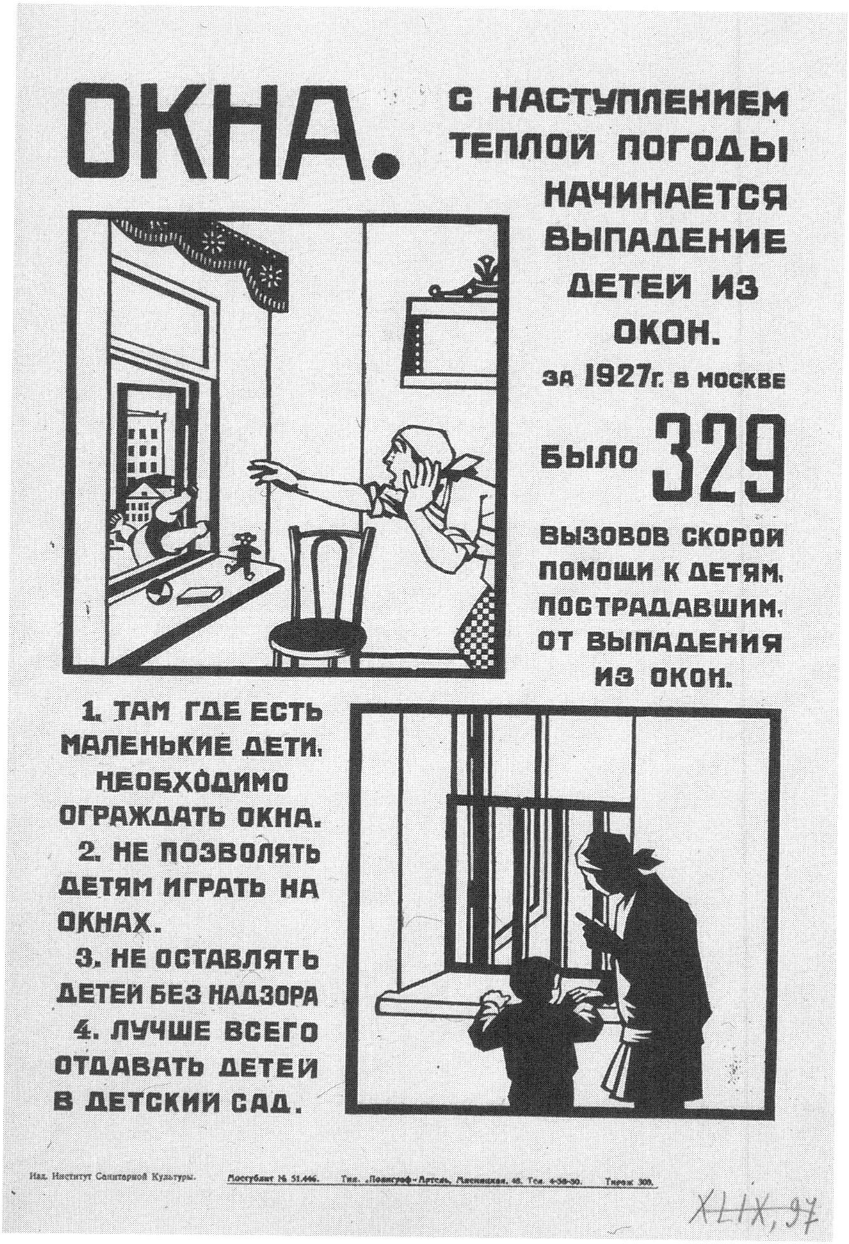
ОКНА.
С НАСТУПЛЕНИЕМ ТЕПЛОЙ ПОГОДЫ НАЧИНАЕТСЯ ВЫПАДЕНИЕ ДЕТЕЙ ИЗ ОКОН.
ЗА 1927г. В МОСКВЕ
БЫЛО 329
ВЫЗОВОВ СКОРОЙ ПОМОЩИ К ДЕТЯМ, ПОСТРАДАВШИМ, ОТ ВЫПАДЕНИЯ ИЗ ОКОН.
1. ТАМ ГДЕ ЕСТЬ МАЛЕНЬКИЕ ДЕТИ, НЕОБХОДИМО ОГРАЖДАТЬ ОКНА.
2. НЕ ПОЗВОЛЯТЬ ДЕТЯМ ИГРАТЬ НА ОКНАХ.
3. НЕ ОСТАВЛЯТЬ ДЕТЕЙ БЕЗ НАДЗОРА
4. ЛУЧШЕ ВСЕГО ОТДАВАТЬ ДЕТЕЙ В ДЕТСКИЙ САД.
Изд. Институт Санитарной Культуры.
Мосгублит № 51.446.
Тираж 300.
XLIX, 97

FIGURE 4.2. "Window." Institute of Sanitary Culture. Moscow: Mosgublit, 1927. Pub. 300. Courtesy of the Russian State Library.

mongering continued in the same series with "Stoves," which warned of improper ventilation. It presented an ominous picture of a stretcher being carried from a house, with a worried woman beside it. As with "Window," the image was stark and startling.[24]

Aside from shame and scare tactics, a prominent feature of hygiene recommendations was concern for air quality.[25] A. A. Ashikhmin's *Air in Our Homes* included question-and-answer sections with subheadings like "Air, Its Composition and Meaning," "Spoiled Air in Living Quarters," and "Dampness in the Home."[26] Reformers blamed bad air for a multitude of ills. Semashko cautioned that good air was "a necessary condition for the correct functioning of the breathing organs: clean air is the best remedy against lung ailments and against infectious diseases generally."[27] A. V. Mol'kov wrote: "The main characteristics of a healthy home are good air, freshness, proximity to nature, comfort, and spaciousness. Cleanliness is the sign of good air in a home . . . [as are] the absence of foreign adulterated gases and dust, [maintenance of] normal and uniform temperature, and the moderation of humidity."[28] While other issues continued to be important, air remained a primary consideration.

The belief in good air ushering in health was old and widespread. In the West and in Russia, the belief that miasmas (foul air) led to infection held sway throughout much of the nineteenth century, with remnants projecting into the twentieth century. From 1870 to 1900 the idea that germs caused disease was highly contested. Even Pasteur's and Lister's work exhibited some worry over foul air. Gradually bacteriology came to the fore throughout the world, including Russia. While hygiene and public health advocates initially rejected bacteriology, by the 1890s the two were being integrated.[29] Soviet conceptions of the healthy home retained a mixture of miasma and germ theory, as can be seen in recommendations on propaganda posters. For example, the simple companion posters "Air the Room Often" and "Close the Trash Bucket—Do Not Breathe in Infection," both dating from the late 1920s, implied that bad air could lead to ill health.[30] The previously cited poster entitled "The Maintenance of Cleanliness within the Home . . ." recommended the cleaning of areas surrounding the home (e.g., stairways, courtyards) "in order not to infect the air and earth" (figure 4.1).

Pamphlets went into even greater detail concerning the nature of good air. In the hierarchy of air presented in *Workers, Take Hold of Your Health!* country air occupied the top spot, followed by city air, and finally apartment (enclosed) air. The pamphlet further recommended that apartments be aired twice daily and throughout the night. It eschewed house plants because they spoiled the quality of the air by extracting essential oxygen at night.[31] Getting people to air out their homes was a struggle. Semashko railed against the superstition that kept people from opening their windows for fear of catching a cold. He pointed out that Swiss doctors put patients in front of open windows year round and argued that good ventilation could overcome even a poorly designed home.[32] Given the fact that so much was at stake, Soviet health organizations made ventilating transom windows a top priority of their work; when outlining their activities, they proudly featured the numbers of transom windows they had had installed.[33]

Dampness tainted the air, but dust stood out as the most dangerous contaminant. Dust was not an insubstantial concern but was pregnant with political, social, and cultural meaning. The removal of dust was integral to the creation of a utopia in the Soviet Union's obsessive ordering process, but the menace of dust floated across historical periods and international borders. As Mary Douglas argues, dust offends against order, and our discomfort with it predates the discovery of contagion.[34] From the nineteenth century onward, international experts identified dust as a probable cause of many illnesses and considered airing of the home an effective method for combating dust. In the United States the popular perception of the dangers of dust led to a surge in the manufacture of cleansing products and machines to aid in its removal.[35] German doctors linked specific types of dust to cancer. The connection of dust to tuberculosis led to the implementation of wet sweeping and street sprinklers in Canada, as well as to U.S. campaigns to wipe feet, avoid long skirts, and eradicate flies.[36] Soviet hygienists aligned themselves with international opinion on dust. One Soviet pamphlet cautioned that tuberculosis floated in the air and could settle on anything; the homemaker was advised to clean bedding and clothing frequently.[37] Calling the inhalation of dust "one of the most dangerous occurrences," another reformer worried over "the air thickly saturated with dust, which is found in work and educational premises."[38] Still another pamphlet remarked: "Ventilation cleans and freshens the air, aids in the removal of dust, and decreases humidity."[39]

To minimize dust, reformers advised simplicity in home decor.[40] The first recommendation on the poster "The Maintenance of Cleanliness within the Home. . ." was "Do not keep superfluous, unnecessary items in the home: it decreases the amount of air in it and hampers cleaning. Keep articles in order" (figure 4.1). Furniture was to be kept to a minimum, preferably spartan in appearance. Wooden beds, which hid bugs, were to be exchanged for iron beds. Soft, overstuffed items, associated with bourgeois luxury, were generally condemned as unhygienic because they attracted dust, in addition to being poor political choices.[41] The emphasis on simplicity over collections of knickknacks coincided with political calls for ascetic behavior. In 1928–29 this distaste surfaced in a Komsomol campaign that urged "Down with Domestic Trash" and targeted figurines, statuettes, and other physical symbols of petit-bourgeois culture.[42] In another bit of political serendipity, reformers singled out the icon corner in the house as attracting dust. Even ideal homes, however, were not completely devoid of decoration. Pictures of nature or portraits of politically approved, charismatic personalities repelled dust—or so one was led to believe (figure 4.1; plate 3).

To keep the dust of the city from invading the home, elaborate cleaning rituals were established for entering the home and the entryway space itself.[43] In the pamphlet *Take Hold of Your Health!* an entire regimen described "the cleaning of dust from shoes before entering the lodging (especially in relation to unfortunate felt boots), the cleaning of clothing not within the living area, the washing of the floor using a 'damp' method (damp sawdust, wet twigs, a brush wrapped in a damp towel), and frequent dusting with a similarly wet towel of the items in the room."[44] Recommendations for cleanliness did not stop at the door. Writers counseled the cleaning of stairways, courtyards, and common areas. A typical cleaning regimen included sweeping stairways, windows, hall lamps, and disposing of animal waste.[45] Instructions even commented on airing these transitional spaces: "The entrance doors of the stairs must be supplied with springy closing devices so that in the wintertime staircases will not be exposed inadvertently to the chill air."[46] Prescriptions led to some action. The apartment dwellers in one Moscow suburb chose lots to see who would wash the stairwell every other day.[47]

Spitting and smoking also compromised air quality. Smoking hurt everyone in the home by dirtying the air and walls.[48] Reformers maintained that when spittle containing the tuberculosis bacillus dried, it could be carried aloft and infect others.[49] The late 1920s poster "Comrades! Do Not Spit on the Floor" (figure 4.3) admonished the spitter while simultaneously suggesting he use a spittoon. A simple picture of the necessary bucket ensured that reading the poster was not necessary for comprehension. Local health authorities provided spittoons to residences, clubs, and factories and reported this as part of their work.[50] Manuals advised people to avoid expectoration, coughing, and sneezing; if they could not, the mouth and nose should be covered, preferably with a handkerchief.[51] In the West similar rules regarding spittle filled public health campaigns. Canadian activists fighting tuberculosis condemned spitting and kissing as responsible for spreading the disease and promoted anti-spitting laws.[52] The United States also passed anti-spitting laws in the 1890s.[53] Other beliefs may have guided health advocates in their admonitions against spitting.

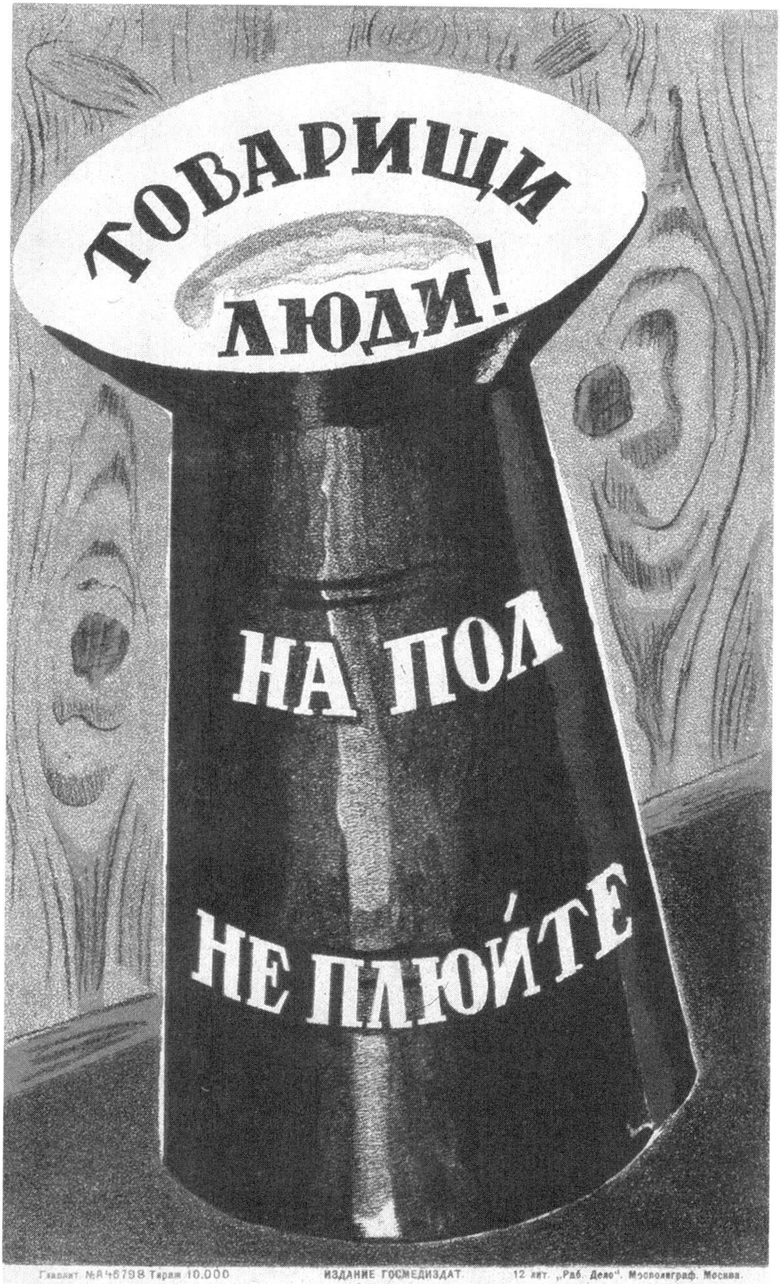

FIGURE 4.3. "Comrades! Do Not Spit on the Floor." Moscow: Gosmedizdat, 1926–29. Pub. 10,000. Courtesy of the Russian State Library.

Many demonized the habit for being antisocial and vulgar as well as dangerous.[54] In any case, laws and admonitions were deemed ineffective. In the United States the police only issued warnings, fearing that people would not tolerate prosecution for such a minor offense.[55] Clearly, public attitudes did not meld with health advisories.

While spitting abetted tuberculosis, reformers in Russia and abroad hailed sunlight as the friend of health. The sun provided a natural disinfectant, a deterrent to disease, and was particularly lauded in the fight against tuberculosis.[56] *Take Hold of Your Health!* praised the sun as the greatest weapon in the fight against infection and declared that tuberculin houses contained more dark or shady rooms since in well-lit rooms only thirteen out of every ten thousand people died of tuberculosis, whereas in dark rooms eighty-two died.[57] Writers emphasized the bacteriological benefits of sunlight and reinforced calls for open windows by noting that windowpanes blocked the qualities of sunlight, which killed microbes.[58] While reformers preferred sunlight, they championed anything that might brighten the environment. Electrification and whitewashing were similarly seen as important in fighting disease.[59]

Damp air was believed to be as hazardous to a healthy house as dusty, dark rooms. To combat it, pamphlets and posters recommended that laundry be done outside the house to avoid extra moisture. The poster entitled "The Maintenance of Cleanliness within the Home . . ." vividly showed clouds of steam resulting from doing wash indoors and advised that clothing should only be cleaned in the courtyard or on the balcony to avoid fouling the air of the apartment (figure 4.1). Because communal laundries did not exist in sufficient numbers to farm out this task, women who wished to follow hygienists' recommendations were left with the choice of either doing laundry outside—which was nearly impossible during certain times of year—or founding a communal laundry themselves.

Although dust, dark, and damp all contributed to problems in the home, the kitchen held special risks. Collective eating facilities were few in number and often served food of inferior quality at inflated prices, so most workers ate at home. Of particular concern to health care advocates was the cleanliness of utensils, plates, and napkins since they believed these objects to be vectors of syphilis infection.[60] Writers noted that kitchen trash served as a breeding ground for disease. Cockroaches needed to be similarly discouraged, despite the folk belief that black ones brought good luck. Flies could foul an entire house by flitting from filthy to clean surfaces and spreading disease in their wake. To keep cockroaches from invading and flies from breeding, trash had to be kept in a sealed receptacle and stored in a dark place; it also had to be emptied every week. Even the dispensation of trash outside the home aroused concern. Hygienists cautioned that the trash heap had to be at some distance from the dwelling.[61]

Bathroom strictures only appeared in a few pamphlets and posters. This may have reflected the dearth of facilities and was also a way of avoiding discussion of the utterly filthy nature of the toilets then available. Still, one text advised paying attention to the bathroom "for the sake of one's own health and the health of those around you." Pioneers were advised sit on the toilet only if clean; otherwise the user should assume the posture of an "eagle" (*sadit'sia orlom*—which presumably meant a crouching posture) and then carefully use the bathroom.[62] The pamphlet *Infectious Disease and Life* recommended "tidiness" in bathroom use, as well as utilizing toilet paper and hand washing.[63] A helpful late 1920s poster even showed how to operate the toilet under the slogan, "Flush after Every Use!" (figure 4.4).

A flushable toilet was a rarity. Reformers recommended wet cleaning of floors, surfaces, and common areas, but they never discussed from where the water was to come. Women required water for the laundering of linens and clothing, the washing of dinnerware for each family member, as well as the two daily personal washings.[64] All of the cleaning surely led to an almost unbearable washload. Nowhere in all of these recommendations for increased water use did reformers suggest that these needs would add to women's chores—or to children's or husbands' tasks—indicating that writers and activists lived under far different conditions than the average worker or simply did not consider the difficulties.

Not only did reformers ignore the problems of water use, they also neglected to suggest changes in the way chores were distributed in the home, preferring to focus their attention on the future rather than on an unpleasant present. In the streamlined, efficient homes of the future, women still were solely responsible for domestic tasks. Even in communal and utopian groups, tasks were often sex-segregated based on traditional divisions of labor. Still, reformers aimed to improve the status of women. By relocating many domestic tasks outside the house, hygienists hoped to free women for the more important pursuit of political activism. Elizabeth Wood argues that this focus upon women was based on two points: the commitment to social reform and a perception of women's backwardness. These two points were seen as sufficient reason for invading the home.[65]

While party discussions might have become heated on the subject of the harm done by untutored women to the cause of revolution, hygienic propaganda presented women as both a positive and a negative force. The poster "Women

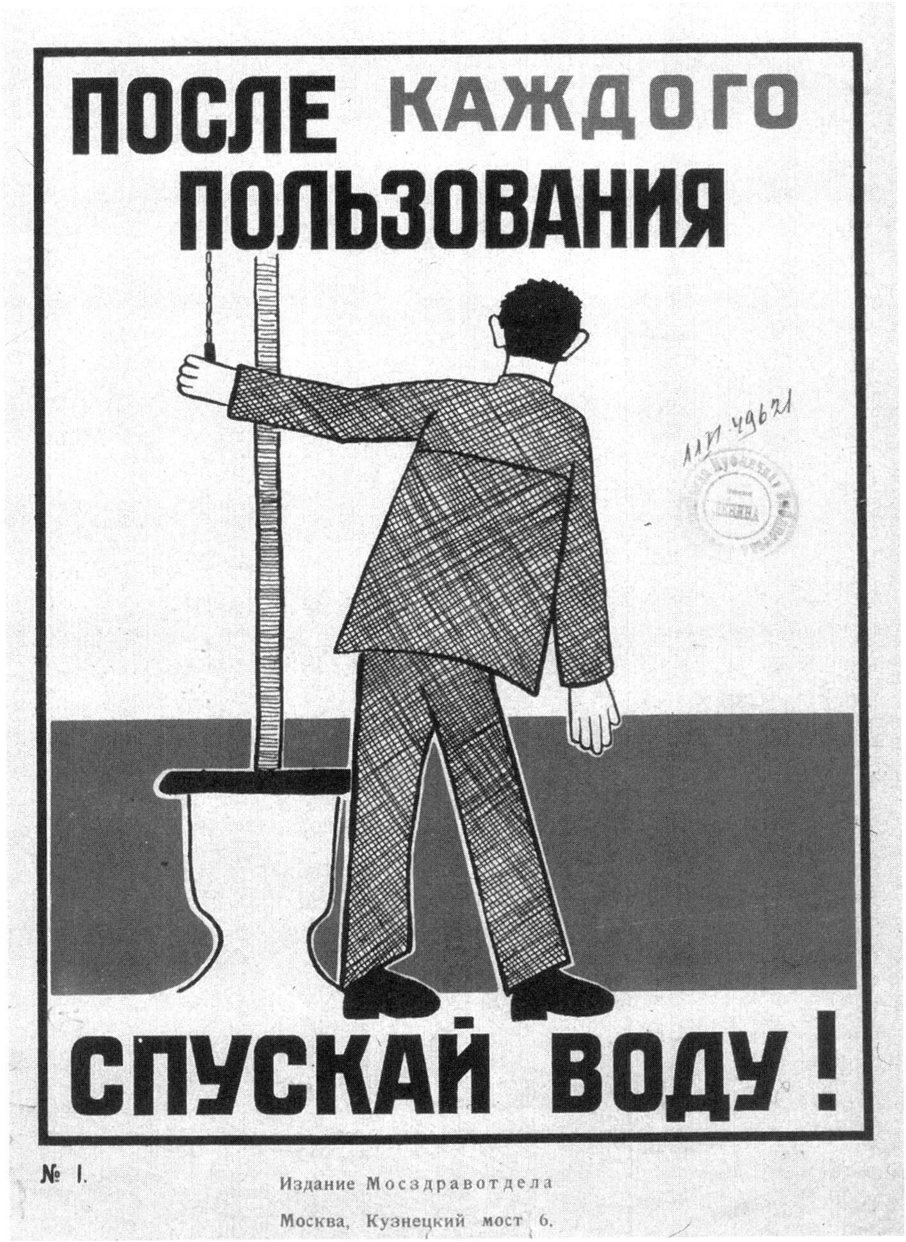

FIGURE 4.4. "Flush after Every Use!" Moscow: MOZ, 1926–29. Pub. 10,000. Courtesy of the Russian State Library.

Workers Build Cooperation" from the early 1920s showed woman as the catalyst for the creation of new life and placed the responsibility for developing collective nurseries and other institutions on women alone (plate 3). At the bottom of the poster a female figure in a circle of action connected left and right panels showing old and new urban settings. Under the watchful eye of Lenin's portrait hanging on the wall, the woman in the circle struggled with geometry. Presented in a pivotal position, her mathematical struggle bridged the gap between irrational past and calculated future, making her a gateway to a new life. In the panels on either side, her individual actions pulled the rest of society from squalid homes to communal nurseries, from street bartering to the cooperative, and from the barroom to the classroom. In the upper left a woman in bright red clothing with a kerchief secured behind her neck (a style that denoted political activism in poster iconography) guided the reader from the sphere of individual activity below to communal activity above, while pointing to the means of transformation (individual development) and its goal (societal development).[66] A gleaming sunburst, shining cooperative, belching smokestacks, and even a buzzing airplane connected women's activities to political activism, industrial productivity, and even pioneering technology. The scope of women's actions seemed empowering.

The size of the guide hinted at the task's difficulty. It must have been an extraordinary, larger-than-life woman who could achieve all this—work, home, and social activism—but, according to the propaganda, these powerful women struggled together in large numbers. In her 1926 pamphlet *The Path to Social Work* Liza Kagan reported that in the mid-1920s nearly ten thousand housewife delegates volunteered and approximately seventy thousand participated in elections. Undoubtedly many more claimed participation than were actually involved, and even in volunteer work women followed traditionally feminine pursuits.[67] Early on Lenin had viewed women as an essential component of the hygiene campaigns. In 1919 in meetings with Semashko he stressed the need to get women involved in cleanliness commissions because of their better grasp of the issues.[68] On the tenth anniversary of the revolution, Semashko acknowledged women's volunteer work and noted that women had made great contributions in the fight for better health.[69] Perhaps to acknowledge those who were working or to encourage women to undertake greater action, the health magazine *To a New Life!* regularly featured short biographies of female delegates and inspectors who had dramatically changed not only their own lives but had also bettered society.[70] One such biography glorified delegate Tsarkova of the Krasnaia Presnia district of Moscow. A housewife, she worked in two small bureaucratic departments, organized other housewives into health cells, lectured on sanitary enlightenment, helped several workers to move, and represented others at trial. At home she was the model of Soviet domesticity, raising five children. To canonize this saint of Sovietized womanhood, the article pointed out that she was now learning to read.[71]

It is not surprising that propagandists pointed out connections between self-improvement and progress, but in biographical statements women themselves credited their delegate and social work with changing their lives. Their descriptions of their sacrifices and diligence contained a call to arms to others. These transformations, which were highly formalized in both their language and imagery, turned the private home into a public display.[72] In a book devoted to the female delegate, one woman insisted that political work had changed her: "Before, I rarely cleaned the apartment. Everything was put off. There were a lot of troubles with the children and simply no time. I just made it to the holidays and the bustle began. But now, when I hear lectures at the delegate meeting on the dangers to people of filth, which illnesses multiply, and how you should clean, things have completely changed for me. I've gotten used to shaking out the door mat, sweeping with a damp broom, dusting everyday, etc. Now you would not know the apartment. It is not neglected. It is easy to clean daily."[73] Oddly enough, taking on greater work outside the home had allowed this woman to do more work within its confines. Another woman attributed increased marital harmony to her attendance at delegate meetings: "I stopped scolding my husband. . . . Now I go with my husband to the club or to some kind of lecture, and together we follow the advice and our lives have completely turned around."[74]

According to inspirational tales, relations between mother and child improved with delegate work. One mother-delegate admitted that before becoming active she quarreled with her children and even beat them, confessing: "It's well known that a mother loves her children, but I just did not have enough patience with them."[75] Becoming a delegate enabled her to improve her relationship with her children. She discovered that beating her children could affect their character development, and she reported that once she had sent the oldest child to camp, she found greater strength.[76] Delegate work bolstered her ability to express what she considered her natural feelings, enhanced her family's happiness, and ensured her child's future.[77] The woman claimed an increase in motherly affection after handing over one child to Soviet institutions. Nevertheless, the article underscored the idea that delegate work was only one aspect of an entire revolutionary life.

Often these laudatory tales included a villain. In fawning biographies, cautionary tales, and agitational plays, women overcame male prejudice and bullying, along with poor material circumstances and overwork, and maintained active participation in social work. The biography "*Vydvizhenka* to Work" noted that even though Filipenko's husband grumbled, she continued her party and health inspector work in addition to an eight-hour day and raising three kids.[78] In Andreev's play *Trial of the Old Life* (1926), a politically aware wife divorced her abusive husband and became a different, better person.[79] In another play by Andreev the wife gradually had her consciousness raised thanks to the advice of a young, forward-looking male worker. With the support of her Octobrist son, she divorced her primitive husband, who failed to understand that "his wife has a right to a social life and work."[80]

In these tales women collapsed in the face of party logic, almost always being saved by a male activist, but men were not educable like women. The husband who refused enlightenment was abandoned instead of being forced to reform. Men attacked women who were already radicalized, and other depictions blamed men for women's backwardness in political matters. One 1921 article contended that ignorant men kept women in the dark. It related the story of a politically active woman whose husband beat her for catting around, though in truth she was attending meetings. The author commented, "It is clear we do not need to fight political unconsciousness just among women."[81] Men of authority did not escape blame for keeping women down in fiction or in reality. In a letter to the newspaper *Communist Labor* two women wrote of their efforts to bring a militia man to account for not intervening with a man who was beating his wife.[82]

Battering, backward husbands constituted sufficient reason for divorce in propaganda literature and plays. In I. V. Rebelskii's play *The Trial of a Husband Who Beat His Wife While in a Drunken State* (1926), the drunkard Vasilii Petrovich abused his wife because he said it was his right, especially after she became politically aware and consequently not as subservient. Friends convinced his wife to sue. She admitted to being reluctant at first because she did not want other women to think that *zhenotdel* membership automatically meant divorce, but she eventually filed and won.[83] Kollontai's heroine in *For Love of Worker Bees* (1923) similarly left a politically backward spouse. The belief that female political activism automatically led to estrangement found expression elsewhere. The general conception that political women were independent of men hearkened back to images of saintly women who had renounced the world and their femininity for God.[84] Lenin's wife Nadezhda Krupskaia related her experience in a factory, where a female activist told a group of workers that once they entered the party, they must renounce their husbands and children. Krupskaia emphasized that this was not true and said that instead women must make fighters of their husbands.[85] What was to be done with a husband who refused his wife's counsel was left unspoken.

While Krupskaia disputed the idea that political activism meant that women must abandon their families, a definite distaste for the confines of the family emerged from utopian tradition and Bolshevik distrust of isolating, noncommunal relations.[86] They spurned domestic concerns and forced women out of the house, away from the family, and into a more masculine public sphere. As theorists worked to construct a model of a female comrade that was more and more masculine, their propaganda presented an increasingly hostile relationship between husband and wife. In stories about the domestic sphere, this emerged as a husband who had nothing constructive to offer in the running of the home. Health care propagandists downplayed any positive influence of men in the domestic sphere. Even men who did not beat their wives fell short of helping them. Although men passively received the benefits from the women in their lives and were educated by them as to proper deportment, hygienists did not call men to task for their passivity. Before the revolution Krupskaia had suggested that men help with housework until children could be trained to perform this service, suggesting that any need for them to help out would be temporary.[87] After the revolution such suggestions were absent. Criticisms targeted men's inability to accept change, not their failure to promote it. Reformers left almost completely unquestioned women's responsibility for transforming the home.[88] Criticism that focused on men for not helping out was infrequent. *The Bourgeois Woman,* a late 1920s play performed in Leningrad, attacked the prison of the home, which made it hard for recently married, young female activists to do political work.[89] Generally appeals were few.

The following passage from the pamphlet *The Female Worker and the New Life* (1927) stood out in its recognition of woman's double burden of work and family, as well as in its many small details of domestic drudgery that were neglected in theorists' depictions of utopia:

> Look closely at how life is in the majority of even our working families. The husband, returning from work, mainly relaxes at home or elsewhere, but the wife, even if she has worked her eight hours at the factory, hurries home quickly in order to serve the family. Who cares for the children and cleans up after them? Who must set the table and clean up after the "master" has eaten? Who makes sure that his shirt is clean, washes the whites, sews on buttons, darns socks? Who makes lunch? All of these obligations fall upon the wife even though she has worked at the bench the same eight hours alongside her husband. And only infrequently does it occur to anyone that this is incorrect, that a man must also

> help a woman in the household while there are still an insufficient number of establishments to assume these cares from women.[90]

It is noteworthy that the writer likened the husband to a "master," calling to mind images of slavery, serfdom, and, of course, defunct capitalism. The tensions between women's traditional role as wives to serve their husbands and their new, revolutionary duties to serve society remained unresolved.[91] This inattention reflected the denigration of these activities as unimportant and undesirable. Not surprisingly, in posters men were missing from the home. They consistently depicted women as responsible for tasks around the house, with men only appearing as helpers in outdoor tasks, such as window washing, chopping wood, or cleaning courtyards. This connection of men and women to exterior and interior spaces, respectively, linked women to the domestic and men to the public sphere. For example, in the companion posters "Close the Trash Bucket—Do Not Breathe in Infection" and "Air the Room Often," only two men appeared in the six tasks highlighted. One chopped wood in the courtyard and the other, a young boy, washed windows while a woman mopped the floor in the foreground.[92] Young boys, themselves in a liminal state, were shown doing domestic tasks within the confines of the home. Adult men did not engage in domestic work.

With sole responsibility for the home, women wielded considerable power. In recognition of women's domestic power, if a politically aware man wanted a better home, he could not achieve it alone. Zetkin noted that male activists who were "brave eagles" would often become "cowardly geese" if a recalcitrant woman awaited them at home.[93] Her comments intimated that women held more power in the home than men and that they could override men's wills. According to propaganda, although women pointed the way to a new life, unenlightened women had the power to hold back husbands, children, and society. The cover of the 1926 book *Workers Hold on to Your Health* presented this concept in a visual allegory (figure 4.5). A barefoot, politically backward woman (with a kerchief tied under her chin) created a barrier between the revolutionary, leather-clad man and the future and prosperity symbolized by the child and smokestacks in the distance. The wife blocked man's power in the home. In a petitioner's gesture, the male worker passed to the woman a paper captioned "Hygiene." For the man to improve the health of the next generation (the child) and achieve prosperity (the smokestacks), he had to get past the woman. The man introduced the information to the woman, thereby reasserting the paternalistic relationship of teacher and pupil, but it was still the woman who had to be convinced to make the effort.

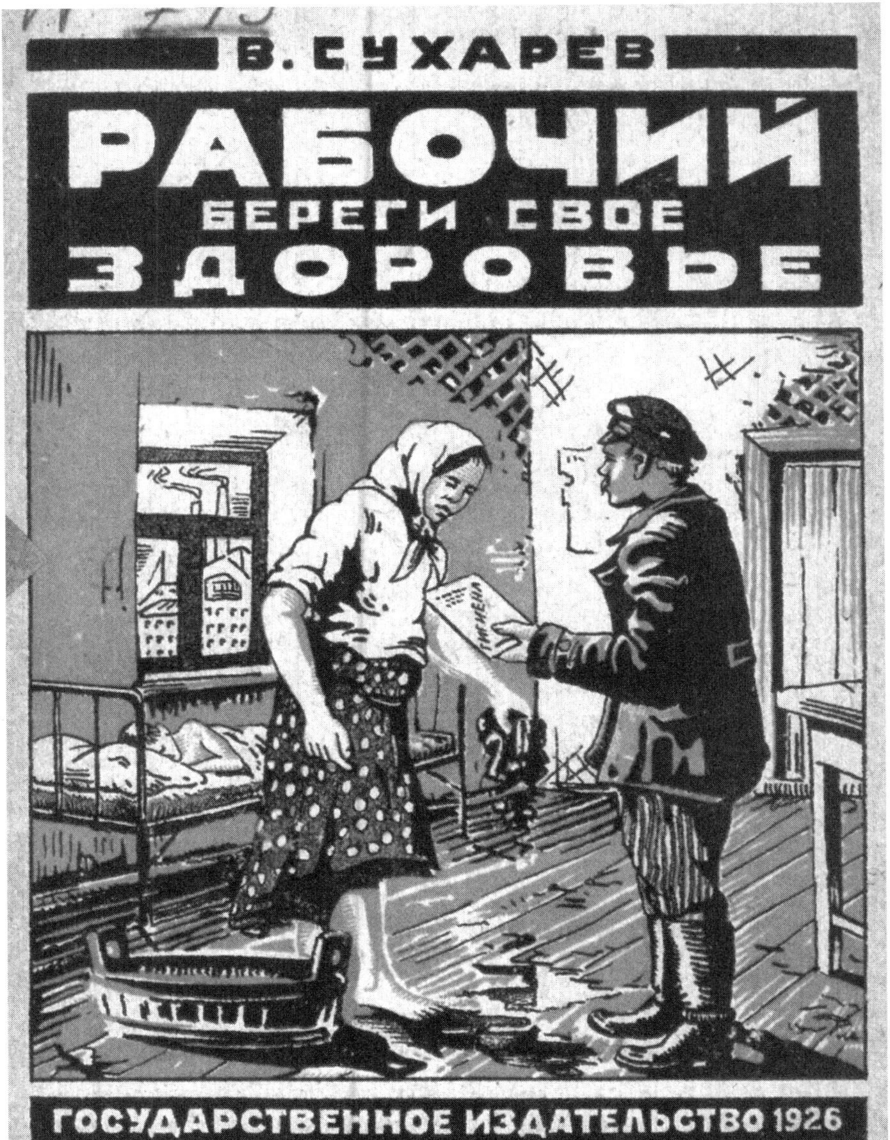

FIGURE 4.5. Cover, B. Sukharev, *Workers Hold on to Your Health*. Moscow: Gosizdat, 1926. Courtesy of the Russian State Library.

In a common theme, women held up change until their husbands resorted to the courts as a way to force them to accept enlightenment with the help of the state. In the play *The Trial of a Housewife* (1927), Vlasova, the wife of a communist, refused to go to the cooperative or allow her children to become Pioneers. She did not attend club meetings or open windows around the house.[94] The husband finally resorted to Soviet justice since he had no power over his wife or control of his home. In contrast to women's experience with politically backward spouses, this husband did not divorce his wife but instead sought her advancement, perhaps acknowledging women were irreplaceable to the home and children. Divorce would have meant abandoning the next generation to ignorance since children commonly stayed with their mothers. The pressure to change wives but abandon husbands implied that only men could assume power over other men, whereas women could be brought to a state of social enlightenment by men, women, or even by their children.

While husbands had little influence over the running of the home, children produced both good and ill effects. Without exception children unexposed to Soviet institutions ravaged the health of a home. These children lived in a Hobbesian state of nature—nasty, brutish, and short. Their poor conduct held women back. In most cases, placing children in Soviet day institutions resulted in an ordered home. In a 1927 article documenting nurse inspectors' work, after one nurse placed the children of five patients into Soviet care (kindergartens, Pioneers, and nurseries), the conditions of the homes and patients improved.[95] For the home to be ordered, healthful, and peaceful, children had to undergo Soviet education. Once children left the home, women were free to pursue the political participation deemed so important by social reformers. Most radically, a female activist speaking before the Moscow soviet explained that sanitary reformers urged women to place their children in institutions so that the women could increase their volunteer work.[96] The happy Soviet home was, it seems, an empty one.

Theorists promised women that Soviet education would make their children agree to help around the house. In the Pioneers children purportedly learned how to order their personal lives and clean up after themselves. The 1925 pamphlet *Pioneer's Hygiene* recommended not just personal hygiene but also explained how Pioneers should maintain their rooms within their homes. The writer assumed a single-occupancy room for the Pioneers, which they needed to care for conscientiously by wiping their feet before entering the house, ventilating and lighting their bedrooms, dusting thoroughly, and washing the floor.[97] Another writer widened the arena by suggesting that the Pioneer would be so busy transforming the home that a monthly schedule might become necessary:

eliminating clutter during the first week; dusting the second; general cleaning the third; and laundering clothes and linens the fourth.[98] If this schedule were carried out, all tasks excepting cooking would become the child's responsibility. Few went this far.

According to the propagandists' biased presentation, women inexplicably resisted enrolling their children in the Pioneers despite the benefits membership brought to the home. Propaganda attempted to show the major positive changes Pioneers could effect as a way of urging women to enroll their children. In the pamphlet *The Path to Social Work* (1926) Kagan retold the story of one exhausted housewife who only saw her children when they wanted to eat. She finally acceded to her husband's urgings and allowed the children to join the Pioneers. Within two weeks the housewife insisted they were different children; they did their homework, the wash, and even asked to help around the house.[99] In the short story "Why Varia Gave her Children Over to the Pioneers," the title character initially opposed her children's call to join the Pioneers but finally relented, confessing that "I am their mother and not their enemy." The power of the Pioneers quickly manifested itself: "Varina's children have attended the troop for four months, and in reality Varia's life has eased." The children attended school while she worked, and they were kept occupied in the evening learning positive behavior: "Everyone picks up after himself or herself and wants to help Varia clean. Fights and screams have lessened."[100] In both the reported case and the fictional representation, placing children into Soviet care improved the home. The children became obedient and even helpful. Domestic order reigned because of Soviet power.

Despite the assurances of propagandists, the Pioneers' presence was not always the calming palliative presented to reluctant mothers. Meetings, troops, and literature encouraged Pioneers to attack poor conditions in the home on multiple fronts. Triumphant tales were told of those who had created change. A 1927 article entitled "Fighters for a New Life" argued that "Pioneers do not want to be shut up in the narrow framework of individual health." Instead, they wished to transmit Soviet ideas to the family and society, to "take up the fight against smoking and alcoholism or for cleanliness and fresh air in the home."[101] Far from making their own beds or sweeping the floor, Pioneers were urged to take a more combative stance in the transformation of their homes. Activists encouraged children to confront the parents of their fellows as well. At a conference of school health cells, one young woman praised such activism: "We compel our parents not to fear fresh air. We fight smoking in the school and in the home. . . . We ask for ourselves our own plates, our own beds." She went on to speak with pride of the work of the collective on behalf of one of their fellows whose father drank: "We told the father that he was not just harming his own health but that he was drinking up the milk money of our comrade. And the father was ashamed."[102] Children forced others into compliance by promoting Soviet norms, becoming the shock troops of revolutionary life.

Children did not just target drunken fathers. Rather than helping their mothers, propagandists urged children to confront them and other female figures in the home. A 1925 short story entitled "Who's Right?" depicted a child bringing change to the home over the objections of the mother. At issue in the story was the quality of air within the home. The mother attempted to prevent the son from opening the window, but he finally prevailed.[103] Lenin himself noted the ways in which children could change the habits of those within the home: "Children learn in school how to brush their teeth and wash their hands. They inspect their own clothes and they ask their mothers and sisters that their own clothes be examined and, as much as possible, put in order."[104] Here Lenin suggested that children instruct and agitate. Tellingly, it was mothers and sisters who received instruction, not fathers and brothers. This comment by Lenin hinted at the deep ambivalence toward women's liberation.

A. Zheleznyi argued in 1925 that agitation for change could increase tensions in the home: "Of course, such a big job must attract all the forces of the home up to the old grandmother, who perhaps does not take all this innovation to heart." But these old authorities were not to be heeded; their excuses proved inadequate or hypocritical. As he explained, "Often our mothers complain of the impossible clutter, but at the same time the corners are crammed up with all kinds of odds and ends, old galoshes, teapots, samovar tubes, and so on. This rubbish typically sits from Easter to Easter. Mice nest there, and cats use it as a bathroom. You must permanently remove these hotbeds of dust—soft curtains, rugs, photos, and icons from the walls. In general you must minimize those places above which dust may settle."[105] The child was forcibly to reorder the home and, while doing this, to attack symptoms of bourgeois complacency, like curtains, and evidence of counterrevolutionary mind-sets, like religious icons. They introduced a strict order and regimentation, which allowed no place for dust to settle on the flotsam of the old order. In a 1925 cartoon published in *To a New Life!*, the relationship of mother and child was depicted as even more hostile. The crude line drawing showed a young male Pioneer attacking his mother with a water hose. The caption noted that he was doing this in the name of "wet cleaning" (figure 4.6). While outwardly humorous, the message was clear: women needed to be cleaned up—by force, if necessary.

While propaganda urged children to change their homes, the Department of Health did not rely solely on their help. Other groups were formed and

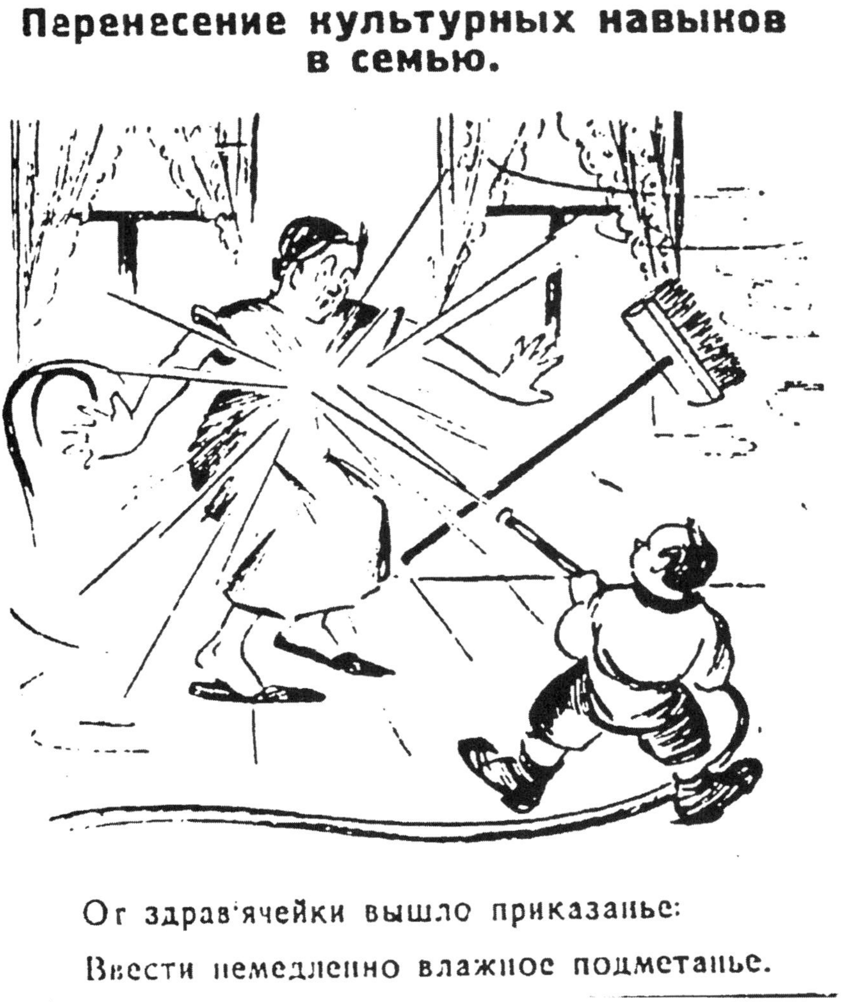
Перенесение культурных навыков в семью.
От здрав'ячейки вышло приказанье:
Ввести немедленно влажное подметанье.

FIGURE 4.6. "Play Corner." *ZNB* 13 (October 1925): 21. Courtesy of the Russian State Library.

instructed to go forth and spread propaganda far and wide. As part of the effort to encourage "self-help," authorities pushed for health cells in apartments and houses, arguing that "in cities and villages every large property or group of small properties must have its own health cell."[106] The ideal health cell was chosen at a meeting of the inhabitants. Following their election, cell members were assigned several major tasks: to assist the dispensary; help monitor investigations; urge better construction; conduct sanitary enlightenment work; provide help for mothers, children, the chronically ill, and the psychologically disturbed; and investigate workers on disability to ensure that they were making proper use of their leisure time. The cells first tackled tuberculosis but expanded soon after 1922 to include venereal disease, sanitation, obstetrics, and so on. Ia. Iu. Kats, the foremost theorist of the dispensary and health cell, recommended that cell members be drawn from both the proletariat and intelligentsia and that they resemble professional organizations. To support the Moscow dispensaries, in 1925 389 health cells were assigned to factories, 8,516 to housing, and 300 to anti-tuberculosis work. With an average of three to five people per cell, this meant that nearly thirty thousand workers conducted sanitary enlightenment and organized children's services.[107] According to a Moscow Department of Health report, "The inclusion of so many workers in the construction of health care significantly lifted the consciousness of the masses, which helped the organs of the Moscow Department of Health in the fight against infectious diseases."[108] These estimates, however, inflated participation since many cells only existed on paper. A 1927 investigation reported six thousand health cells with twenty thousand participants, yet the same report also suggested that many were fictitious.[109]

In these health cells Muscovites supposedly came together under their own initiative to improve their factories and homes and ultimately the city. Apartment dwellers, workers, and even schoolchildren organized cells. Health cells engaged in a great deal of labor-intensive contact with the population: "Their work consists of distributing educational pamphlets, carrying out public health campaigns, ferreting out the sick and bringing them to physicians, etc."[110] In practice, health cells varied greatly in their abilities and powers. One health cell described its duties as follows: it had weekly meetings with the sanitary doctor and the nurse-investigator and followed experts' instructions while enforcing "individual social-prophylactic measures" in worker homes through inspections. The listing of two months' worth of accomplishments showed the mundane nature of its goals, the modest changes it had achieved, and a hint of how far it still had to go. The health cell boasted it had performed 114 exterminations, "tidied" up 41 apartments, aired 14, installed 3 transom windows, acquired individual towels in 4, added trash cans in 2, moved clothes washing outside in 2, and set up spittoons in 4. Perhaps most impressive, in four extreme cases the health cell helped families move to different apartments.[111] The meager accomplishments reflected the very poor circumstances where simply opening windows and obtaining trash cans became a political act worthy of note.

A more extensive view of health cell work can be culled from the forms used in the Moscow Department of Health's 1924 group competition. The department asked the cells to provide information on the material circumstances of their building, together with its social breakdown and density, what they had remodeled, and their role in the fight against infectious disease and social problems—specifically tuberculosis, sexually transmitted diseases, and alcoholism. In addition, cells provided information on their relationship to the sanitary bureau, the Committee for the Sanitation of Labor and Life, and the dispensary. Finally, they explained how they helped tenants with children; created green spaces, playgrounds, and cafeterias; and organized sanitary enlightenment activities and general meetings of the tenants.

Of the roughly seventy respondents to the competition, many returned nearly blank forms, having only formed a few months earlier, perhaps in response to the competition. Some, however, filled out their forms exhaustively and mentioned activities that they hoped would set their cell apart. The health cell of 3/24 Meshchanskaia highlighted its efforts to keep the building clean by disinfecting it regularly, keeping the yard tidy, sweeping the stairs on a daily basis, and doing a weekly wash. It also organized summer gymnastics for the children, built a sandbox, installed transoms in all rooms, lectured on sanitary hygiene, organized excursions to a health museum, and put up posters in its own red corner. All this was accomplished by just three people—a chemist, a worker, and an unemployed colleague.[112]

Other cells reported extensive activities in different areas. At 9 Malaia Spasskaia the cell's two workers and one office worker inspected all thirty-eight apartments on a monthly basis to ascertain "how accurately the tenants of the building fulfilled the laws of sanitary housekeeping." They brought violators before the building's tenants' council, which could fine problem tenants.[113] Another cell conducted monthly inspections and prodded people to open their transoms every day, take their trash out more frequently, keep the bathroom moisture-free, and clean their homes using a "damp" method.[114] In some cases, such as alcoholism, the cell might recommend treatment; in extreme cases the cell evicted the alcoholic.[115] This, however, was the exception rather than the rule. Generally health cells wielded no administrative power, instead focusing on education.[116]

In the records of the competition, few cells admitted to a complete lack of sanitary enlightenment work, though they varied in the amount of work attempted. One of the more active cells, the group at 14/30 Matrosskaia tishina, with a total of 908 people under its purview, organized a sanitary agitational trial, an excursion to a health museum, an agitational play on venereal disease, and propaganda installations, including a health corner and a wall newspaper.[117] Other, less active groups admitted only to an occasional letter or tenants' meeting while still maintaining that they influenced their building. One cell admitted that though it had not organized any lectures, it did "conduct discussions at convenient opportunities with every tenant" in the apartment building.[118] If these guerilla lectures did occur, and were not just a way of padding the form, residents of this building undoubtedly looked up and down the corridor before leaving their apartments.

Given their involvement in the spread of sanitary information, organizers felt it essential that cells "grasp and master the elements of sanitary culture." For this purpose they recommended "systematic lectures, excursions, and the consistent instruction of the health cell in its work alongside specialists."[119] In addition to instructions on proper hygiene, officials bombarded cells with lessons on how properly to advise those under their care. An article addressed to members of tuberculosis cells stressed that they had to do more than just forbid certain behaviors. They had to explain why these behaviors endangered others and why new hygienic norms helped. The social consequences of disease also needed to be pointed out: "We need to show why it is dangerous to drink spirits and how it affects the health of the most ill, the economy, and consequently the family." Finally, disease had to be blamed on not following instructions: "We need to know that we fall ill with tuberculosis not just thanks to poor conditions but also thanks to our ignorance."[120] Citizens' ignorance was probably not the only problem. With little time for reading or training, and relatively little supervision, cell members very likely peppered their medical advice with their own homespun theories and moral lessons.

Letters to the magazine *To a New Life!* suggest that Muscovites counted on their health cells to be effective since readers held the cells responsible for poor conditions in apartment buildings and dormitories. Of course, if the magazine printed letters from readers who held the health cell culpable for their problems, the editors obviously wished the public to consider cells responsible agents. This conveniently displaced responsibility for poor living conditions from the state onto volunteer organizations. Although a 1926 letter of complaint about the 53 Smolenskii Boulevard student dormitory criticized students for throwing garbage out their windows and destroying their newly remodeled building, it concluded that ultimate responsibility for the mess lay with the health cell.[121] In one 1926 complaint about the awful conditions of another dormitory, the writer claimed that the lack of a health cell was the only reason that trash was not emptied and conditions were filthy.[122]

More often letters in the press praised health cells in an apparent quest to encourage good works through positive examples. One letter extolled the health cell at 18 Staromonetnyi Passage.[123] Another congratulated the cell at a student dormitory, which improved a filthy kitchen by constructing a laundry room for the boiling of linens.[124] Worker O praised the health cell of his factory, which had done far more than the Commission for the Sanitation of Labor and Life, because, the worker felt, it went beyond instructions and circulars and remained closely tied to the dispensary, ambulatory, and nursery.[125] Indeed, writers admired some cells for going above and beyond the call of duty. A letter commended the health cell of 2½ Polianka because the cell did its work and also constructed a Lenin corner for political and cultural enlightenment.[126]

The grassroots nature of the health cell closely resembled education programs aimed at the working class and urban dwellers in the West. In the United States a movement emerged at the turn of the century whose purpose was to educate tenement dwellers in cleaning techniques and decorating norms. Best exemplified by Lillian Wald's Henry Street Settlement, it led to many other "model apartments" and schools set up by well-meaning yet condescending, volunteers. In 1914 the U.S. Congress became involved by creating a pool of matching funds to help states and counties hire people to enter homes in order to teach about domestic organization.[127]

Alongside the health cell existed the dispensary, the more formal institution of Soviet health care and prophylaxis. In addition to treating sick workers, inspecting homes, and providing sanitary education, in 1926 alone the dispensary collected information about workers at the factory and through questionnaires in 64,075 cases.[128] Working under dispensary orders, nurses and doctors carried out targeted home inspections, which was another form of domestic control. The dispensary doctor ordered investigations "where the character of the disease requires an explanation of the standard of living and its influence."[129] The doctor noted the results in the patient's sanitary journal. Since most everything qualified as a "lifestyle" illness, home inspection marked a logical progression. According to a 1926 assessment by V. A. Obukh, the head of the Moscow Department of Health, the Moscow dispensaries examined 120,000 people and carried out 32,000 home inspections, of which doctors undertook 12,000 and nurses 20,000.[130] In addition to these inspections, the doctors within the house call group (*pomoshch' na domu*), established in 1925, visited those too ill to make it to the dispensary. Organizers boasted that this type of care, unique to Soviet practice, brought "sanitary culture into the lives of workers."[131]

Those involved in the dispensary system felt that the home inspection constituted an essential part of treatment because of the details it provided about workers' lives. According to Obukh, "When the doctor knows the condition of the worker's life and labor, the doctor can give advice, pursue sanitary and san-technical measures (through responsible organizations), and prevent harmful consequences from abnormal conditions of labor and lifestyle."[132] Health care advocates hoped that by observing and instructing sick workers, they could turn them away from habits that made them ill. The inspector "must closely and ably observe the personal and intimate life of the patient to diagnose and remove that which pushes him toward this or that poison."[133]

The idea of the nurse-inspector sprang from the nineteenth-century tradition of charitable work and Enlightenment faith in the power of education to transform peoples and societies. European and American health care systems instituted similar inspections. In 1887 Scotland led the way, attaching "Samaritans" to the dispensary to assist with social problems. Vienna's socialist government employed inspectors to make sure people cleaned their apartments and kept up communal areas. By 1932 municipal clinics in Vienna had performed 91,000 home visits. In the United States, many visiting-nurse groups worked in major urban areas like Boston, Philadelphia, and New York City. Around 1900 Boston added nurse investigations to its health institutions. The visiting nurse idea spread rapidly and by 1908 the United States had ninety-eight dispensaries with visiting nurses who numbered over 3,000 by 1912.[134]

Nurse inspectors played important roles in the dispensary system, helping to control patients and imposing healthful regimens. Organizers in New York City found the nurse's role vital since she demonstrated how to change circumstances rather than just handing out circulars. This proved important when dealing with the (often illiterate) lower classes. This emphasis on their lack of education seemed ironic given the fact that inspectors seldom received any special training for their work. Inspectors were not, however, just a force from above. Inspectors in the West used their knowledge of worker housing to agitate for change.[135] Soviet nurse inspectors reflected this conflict between above and below in their reports. One Moscow nurse noted that she could not find anything in common with the mother of two children she was visiting because the uncultured woman never attended the theater and was illiterate. Instead she found common cause with the husband, but she attacked him as well for his tendency to drink. While she was quick to criticize poor health choices, she also took care to describe the poorly designed lodgings. Construction was so inadequate that even though the transom was not open, a breeze came from the walls, window, and floor. The nurse was instrumental in moving the family to a house-commune.[136]

Nurse commentaries on family problems extended to use of leisure time and political activity. Sympathetic understanding often colored criticism. In one inspection report the nurse commented that the family did not engage in cultural pursuits because they had no time. She did, however, take time to criticize the young son who had no political interests, did little reading, and spent no time at the club. The pitiable condition of the home, which had neither water nor a sewer, merited particular ire on the part of the inspector as she described the arduous ritual of hauling water from a communal pump on the street. The full range of concerns of the nurse-inspector emerged in the additional commentary regarding the pleasing number of flowers and plants in the room, as well as her description of the clock, pictures, and icon corner in the main room.[137]

Other groups also became involved in inspections. In 1926 official government building inspectors, citizens connected to the Committee for the Sanitation of Labor and Life, members of the *zhenotdel*, and some schoolteachers conducted inspections in the Chistie prudy neighborhood of Moscow, looking at the homes of 342 families totaling some 1,235 members.[138] In the Khamovnicheskii district *zhenotdel* members joined with the Department for the Protection of Motherhood and Infancy to carry out 4,620 investigations and even went to court to improve the living conditions of some women.[139] These organizations carried out 200,000 visits in 1924–25. By 1926 inspections reached an estimated 500,000 Muscovites, representing approximately a quarter of the city's inhabitants.[140] Later histories noted the 1920s push for even more women to serve as visiting nurses.[141] Though inspections were not universal as the Soviets claimed, they far exceeded in number those of other countries.[142]

In theory Soviet inspectors diagnosed problems and prescribed antidotes. During their visits, however, they surely recognized the impossibility of substantial improvement no matter how much the wife dusted. As the Western observer Fannina W. Halle commented, "Nowhere, perhaps, do the contrasts between the new and the old appear so crude, so glaring, as in the Soviet Russian house and home."[143] For Frenchman Henri Béraud, who visited in 1925, the revolution had left Moscow in an abysmal state. He lamented: "The real misery of Sovietism is not in the street but in housing. . . . In Moscow you smoke as much as you possibly can so as not to be conscious of the room." The floors, covered with loose flooring and pebbles, "crunch like the paths of a Casino." The overcrowding led people "to hate each other like the chained galley slaves of former days." Béraud bemoaned the fates of families squeezed into a kitchen or entryway and the general lack of sanitation. Tenants lived under horrific circumstances: "Lids of old boxes replace broken windows. Some of the more particular tenants have made doorways with smelly bags of pitch. Everyone lives immured in a sort of surly terror." He concluded that Moscow was "a mixture of barrack, monastery, and prison."[144]

The living condition in Moscow in the 1920s was disagreeable, but that was nothing new to most working-class inhabitants.[145] Nineteenth-century Moscow experienced rapid and drastic urbanization, making it one of the world's ten largest cities and twice as densely populated as most European capitals.[146] Prerevolutionary worker housing in Moscow had been in poorly ventilated, badly lit, minimally maintained barracks. Despite the lack of amenities and the overcrowding, Moscow workers jammed into whatever accommodations they could find.[147] Whereas the effects of war, domestic turmoil, and hunger drastically reduced the population of Moscow between 1917 and 1920, the introduction of NEP in 1921 swelled the city. Moscow's population in 1920 was just a little over 1,000,000; by 1926 it reached 2,026,000; and by 1933 it swelled to 3,663,000.[148] As the population multiplied, the housing was in worse repair than before the revolution. Neglect marked the civil war years as rent controls and restrictions against evictions led landlords to hold up repairs.[149] As one traveler reported in 1921, "In neither of the capitals has it been possible to replace the innumerable broken window-panes or to replace burst pipes; with the result that the condition of the housing in all quarters of the town and in the dwellings of all classes of the population beggars description."[150]

In August 1918, before the rapid influx of people began, the government recognized that there was a housing crisis and began resettling workers in the houses of the rich. After October Lenin drew up a plan allocating space to people on the basis of square meters rather than rooms. This often resulted in odd configurations, with the former inhabitants squeezed into one or two rooms. Between 1918 and 1924 half a million workers relocated as part of this revolutionary redistribution. For many workers these subdivided apartments proved uncomfortable, hard to heat, and difficult to live in with the former owner's oppressive presence still felt. At first the reclamation of bourgeois houses eased housing problems, but foraging, deterioration, and overcrowding conspired to make many of these lodgings virtually uninhabitable soon after their repartition. The houses that remained proved inadequate, and by 1922 there was a severe shortage. When housing did become available, it was assigned in theory based on health considerations. The homeless and tubercular came first, followed by cellar dwellers and those in unfit housing. Some workers attempted to manipulate their environments through communal arrangements and by forming cultural organizations.[151]

Even with progress, there were still problems. Moscow contained 26,586 properties in 1925, with roughly sixty inhabitants per dwelling. The average property was divided into eight apartments, leaving roughly eight people per apartment.[152] Of these dwellings, teeming with humanity, 35 percent had running water, 62 percent had sewers, and just over 11 percent enjoyed central heating.[153] While city services expanded and contributed to a decrease in health problems, they remained far from adequate.[154] Health care advocates devoted increased attention to sewers and water services and contrasted Soviet death rates with those of economically advantaged countries with more sanitary cities, especially Germany, England, and France.[155] These conditions undoubtedly complicated the mission of Narkomzdrav. As one observer reported, "It is self-evident that in these barracks-like conditions any kind of home-life is unthinkable, and all hygiene suffers, whilst immorality flourishes."[156]

While conditions were poor, these descriptions also served as feints to cover the inadequacy and ineffectiveness of their own prophylactic efforts. Inspectors' reports generally focused upon the lack of beds, the filthy rooms, and the inadequate construction, ignoring the obvious complications for home care in their propaganda.[157] Instead, they assumed water, sewer, gas, and even electrical services as givens. Posters routinely featured apartments with running water (figures 4.1, 4.4, 4.7, 4.8). In two telling illustrations, the faucets literally hang in midair, taking on a fantastic quality (figures 4.7, 4.8).[158] While posters frequently showed running water, the images in the posters "8 Hours for Leisure—8 Hours for Sleep—8 Hours for Work" (plate 4) and "Get into the Cultured Habit" (figure 6.1) probably coincided with reality by depicting running water only in the communal baths and a simple bucket for home washing.

Muscovites without running water lugged water from pumps and wells in courtyards or even from rivers and ponds. In the winter they had to chop through ice. To add to the labor, water was often of questionable quality and needed to be boiled.[159] They drew the water and carried it home, sometimes up multiple flights of filthy, treacherous stairs.[160] Having to carry water for even a short distance greatly increased the time women spent on laundry. For example, if a woman did four loads of wash a week on average, that meant carrying about eight gallons for each of two to three washtubs. A bucket holding three or four gallons of water weighed about twenty-five pounds.[161] After hauling the water from the pump, women next had to heat it. If they could have afforded it, Muscovites might have hired others to do their washing, but laundry services in the capital were expensive. Perhaps exaggerating a bit, in his memoir

Béraud commented that washing was "the luxury of millionaires," and that laundry was done by Chinese immigrants at such exorbitant prices that a clean shirt cost the same as a new one in Paris.[162]

Given the expense of time and/or money, most citizens probably did without laundered clothes, bathed bodies, or clean linens. Those who did have water and sewers had to be taught their proper use. Such slogans on posters as "Flush after Every Use!" (figure 4.4) suggested that plumbing was not always well understood. This would lead to further problems for the apartments since tenants who did not correctly care for plumbing would flush all manner of waste down the pipes. Upkeep was difficult, and burst pipes destroyed even more of the limited housing.[163] Worse problems prevailed in the countryside. Conditions in villages exposed the lack of penetration to the periphery of new norms. According to a 1928 survey of fifteen hundred Ukrainian rural homes, only 62 percent could be considered "clean." Nearly 75 percent of those inspected had insects of some kind.[164]

Providing food for the family also proved more difficult than activists admitted. Gathering ingredients for cooking in an environment of scarcity remained costly in terms of time and money. Once they returned home, many women did not have private or communal kitchens; they either shared a general-purpose room with others from their floor or used a small primus stove in the apartment with room for a single pot. If a separate kitchen did exist, it often served as

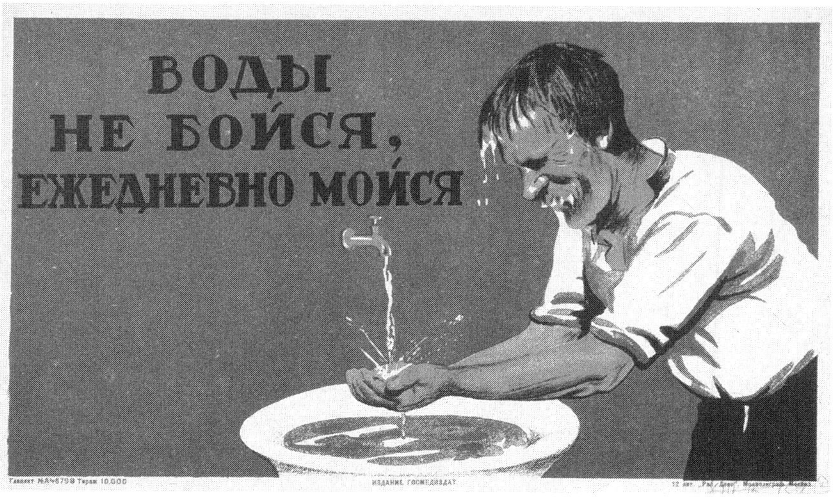

FIGURE 4.7. "Don't Be Afraid of Water. Wash Daily!" Moscow: Gosmedizdat, 1926–29. Pub. 10,000. Courtesy of the Russian State Library.

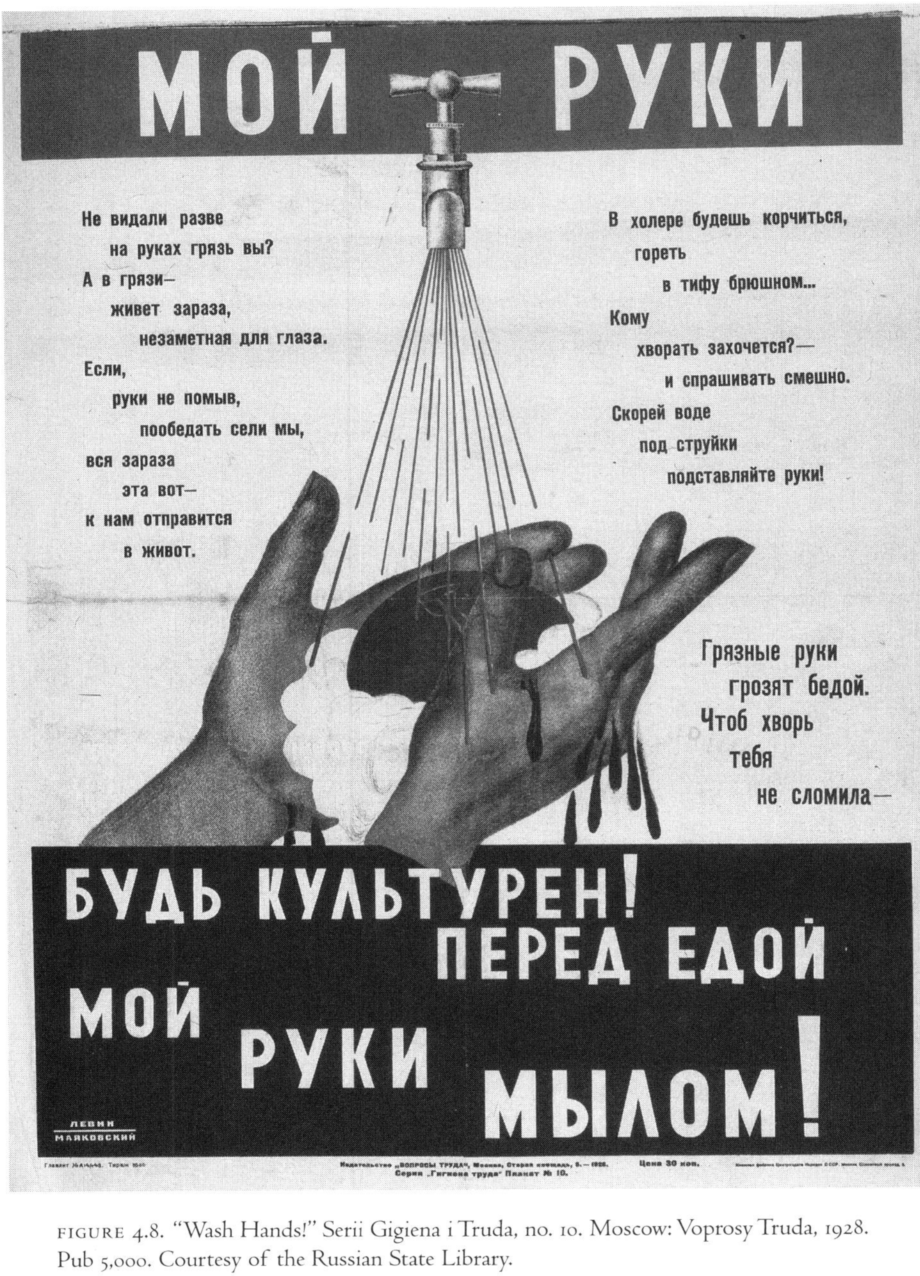
МОЙ РУКИ
Не видали разве
на руках грязь вы?
А в грязи—
живет зараза,
незаметная для глаза.
Если,
руки не помыв,
пообедать сели мы,
вся зараза
эта вот—
к нам отправится
в живот.
В холере будешь корчиться,
гореть
в тифу брюшном...
Кому
хворать захочется?—
и спрашивать смешно.
Скорей воде
под струйки
подставляйте руки!
Грязные руки
грозят бедой.
Чтоб хворь
тебя
не сломила—
БУДЬ КУЛЬТУРЕН! ПЕРЕД ЕДОЙ
МОЙ РУКИ МЫЛОМ!
ЛЕВИН
МАЯКОВСКИЙ
Цена 30 коп.
Серия „Гигиена труда" Плакат № 10.

FIGURE 4.8. "Wash Hands!" Serii Gigiena i Truda, no. 10. Moscow: Voprosy Truda, 1928. Pub 5,000. Courtesy of the Russian State Library.

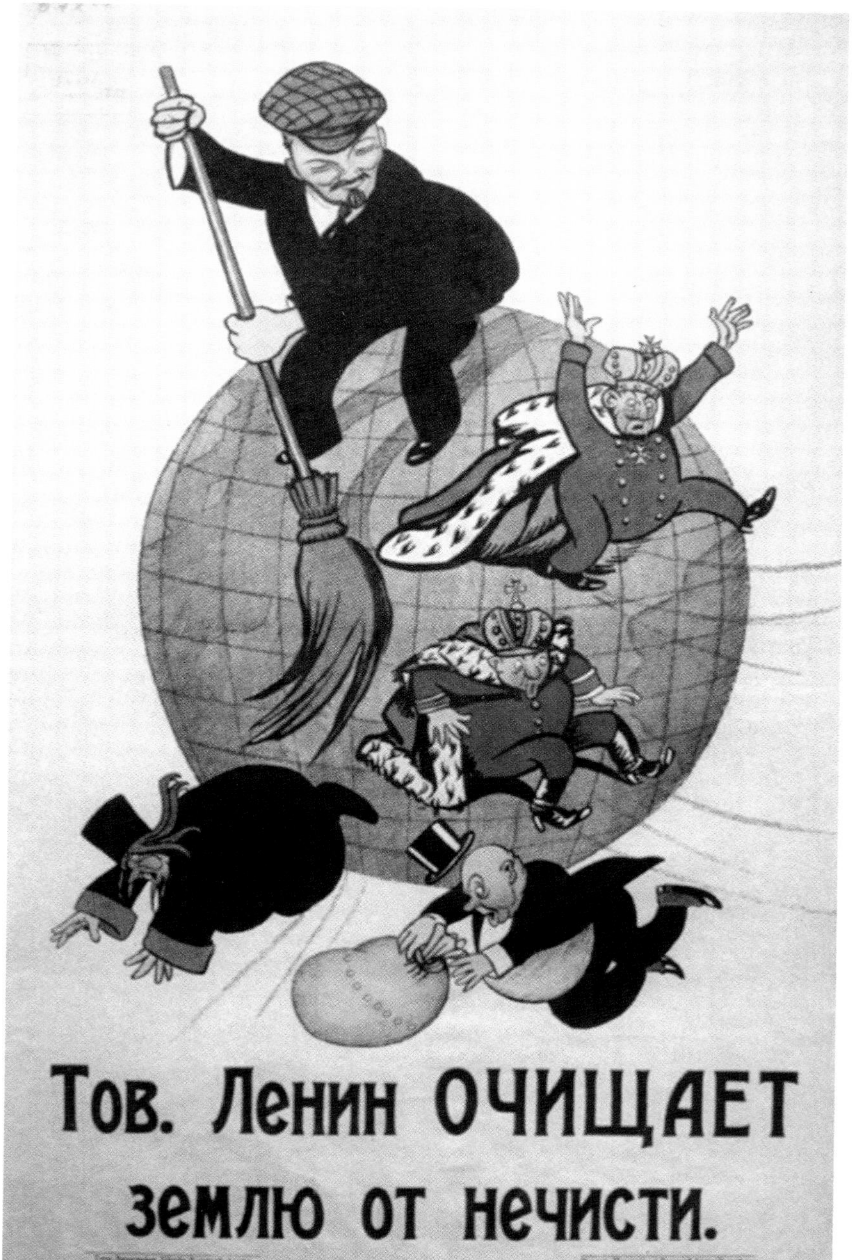

PLATE 1. "Comrade Lenin Sweeps Clean the Earth of the Unclean." Courtesy of Stephen White.

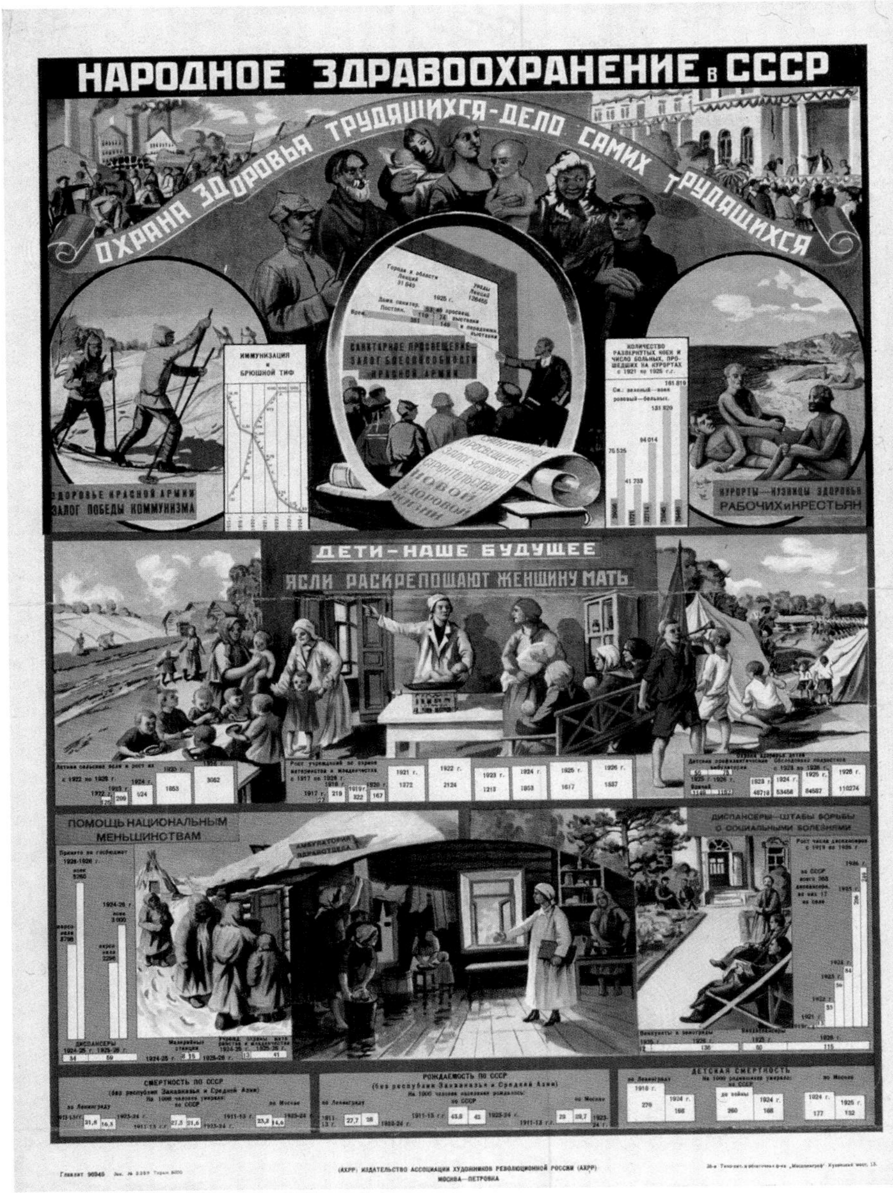

PLATE 2. "People's Health Care in the USSR." Moscow: Association of Artists of Revolutionary Russia, 1926–29. Pub. 5,000. Courtesy of the Russian State Library.

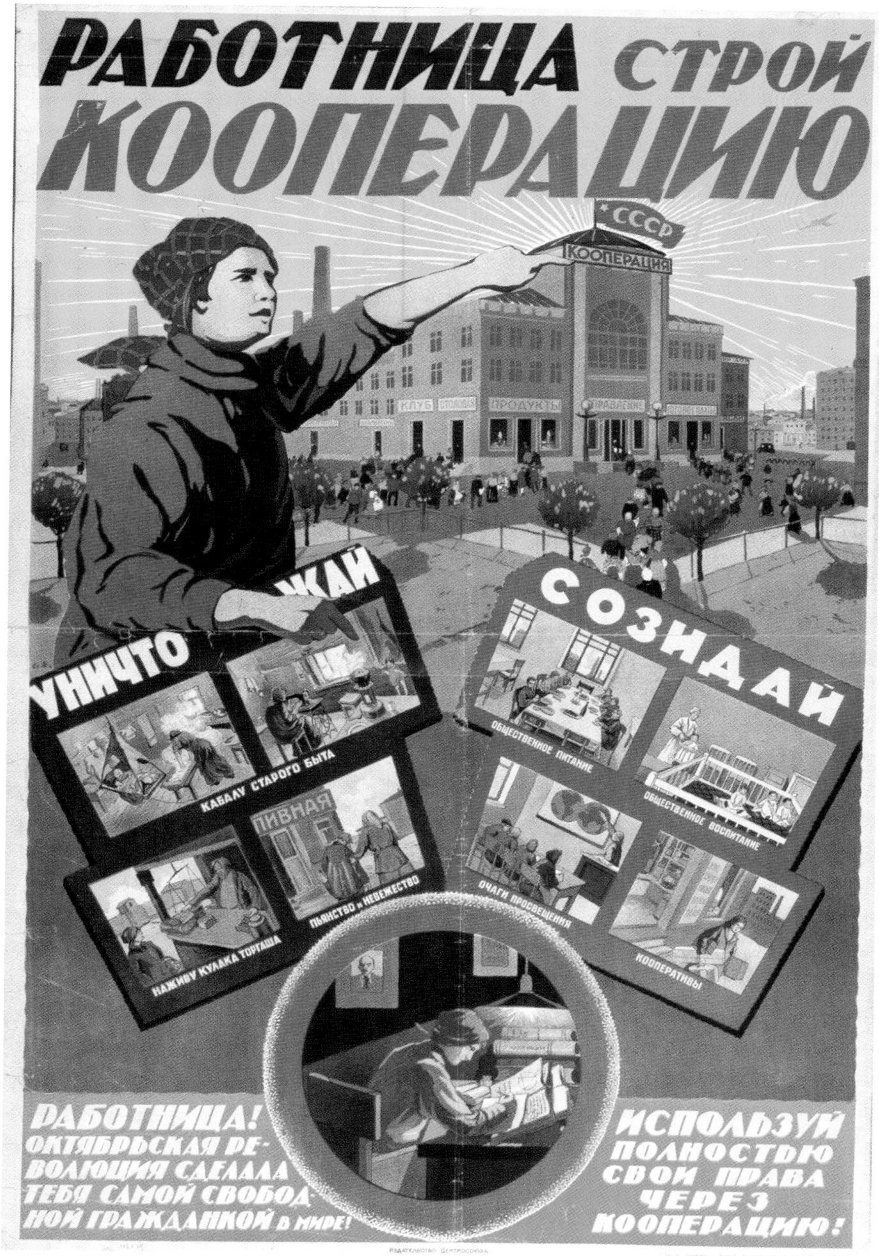

PLATE 3. "Women Workers Build Cooperation." 1921–25. Pub 20,000. Courtesy of the Russian State Library.

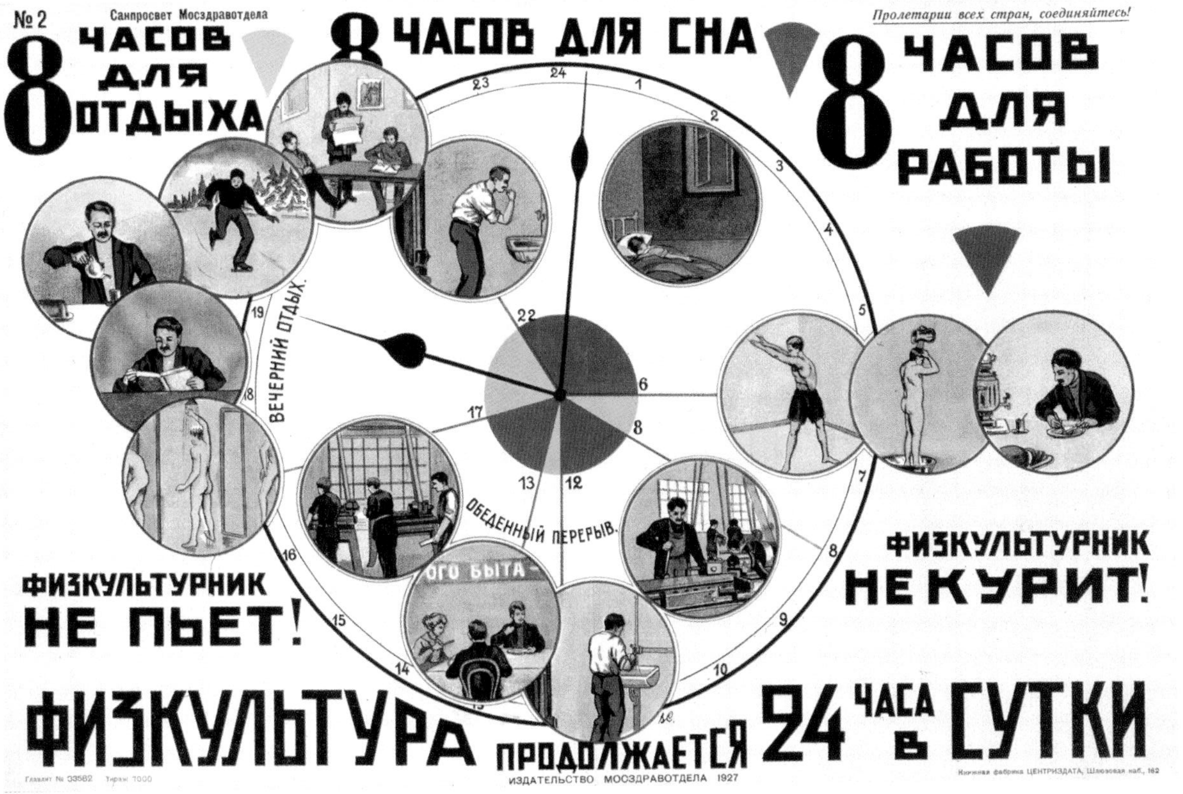

PLATE 4. "8 Hours for Leisure—8 Hours for Sleep—8 Hours for Work." Moscow: MOZ, 1927. Pub. 7,000. Courtesy of the Russian State Library.

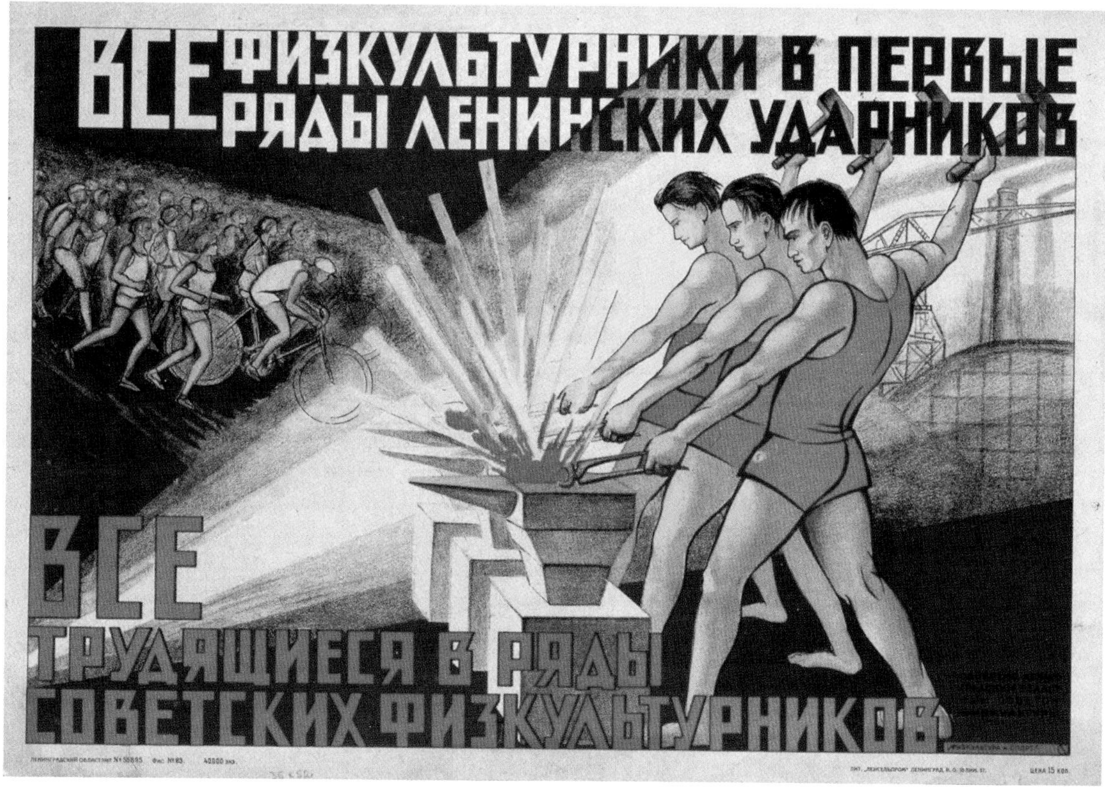

PLATE 5. "All Athletes to the Front Lines of the Lenin Workers!" Leningrad: Lenselprom, 1921–25. Pub. 40,000. Courtesy of the Russian State Library.

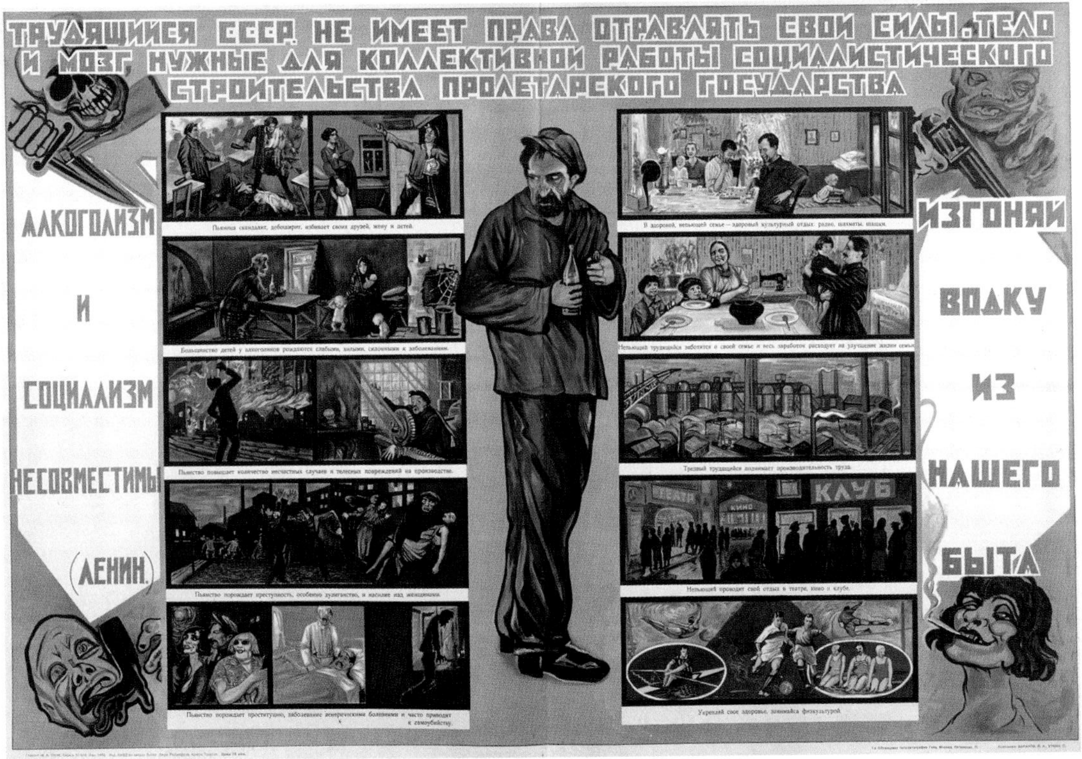

PLATE 6. "The Workers of the USSR Do Not Have the Right to Poison Their Strength, Body, and Mind, Which Are Needed for the Collective Work of the Socialist Construction of the Proletarian State." Moscow: NKVD, 1922. Pub. 20,000. Courtesy of the Russian State Library.

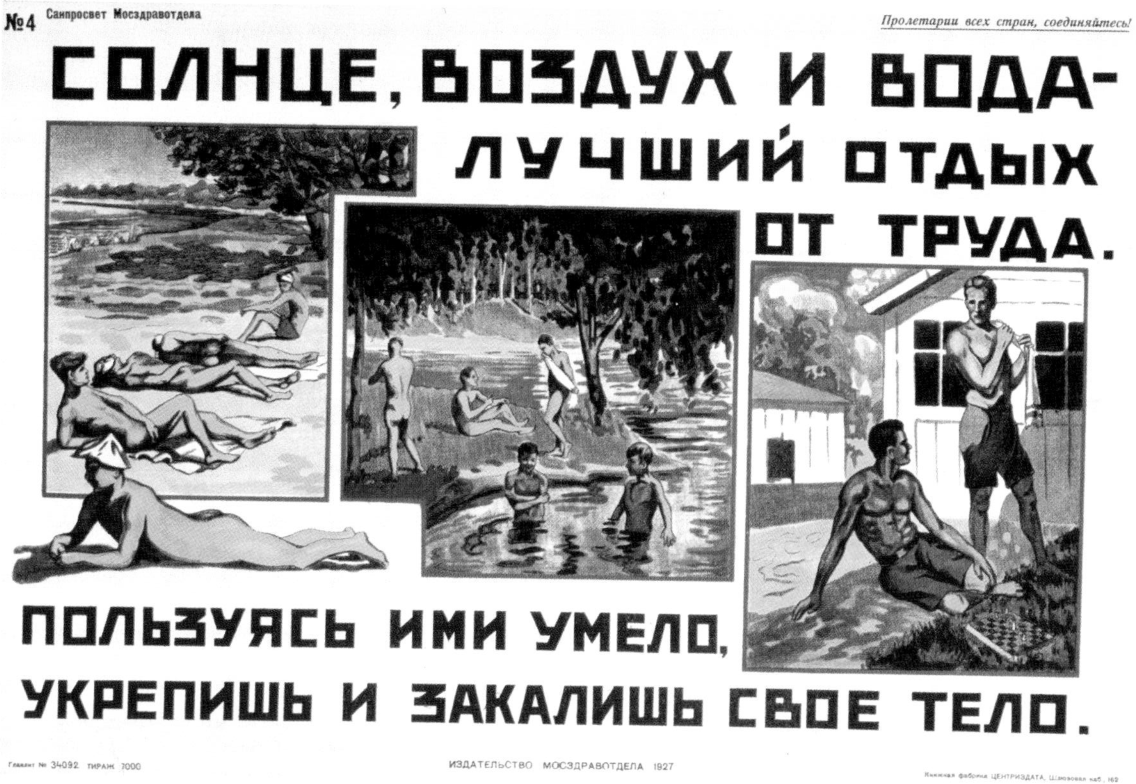
№4 Санпросвет Мосздравотдела
Пролетарии всех стран, соединяйтесь!
СОЛНЦЕ, ВОЗДУХ И ВОДА-
ЛУЧШИЙ ОТДЫХ
ОТ ТРУДА.
ПОЛЬЗУЯСЬ ИМИ УМЕЛО,
УКРЕПИШЬ И ЗАКАЛИШЬ СВОЕ ТЕЛО.
Главлит № 34092 тираж 7000
ИЗДАТЕЛЬСТВО МОСЗДРАВОТДЕЛА 1927
Книжная фабрика ЦЕНТРИЗДАТА, Шлюзовая наб., 162

PLATE 7. "Sun, Air, and Water—The Best Rest from Labor." Moscow: MOZ, 1927. Pub. 7,000. Courtesy of the Russian State Library.

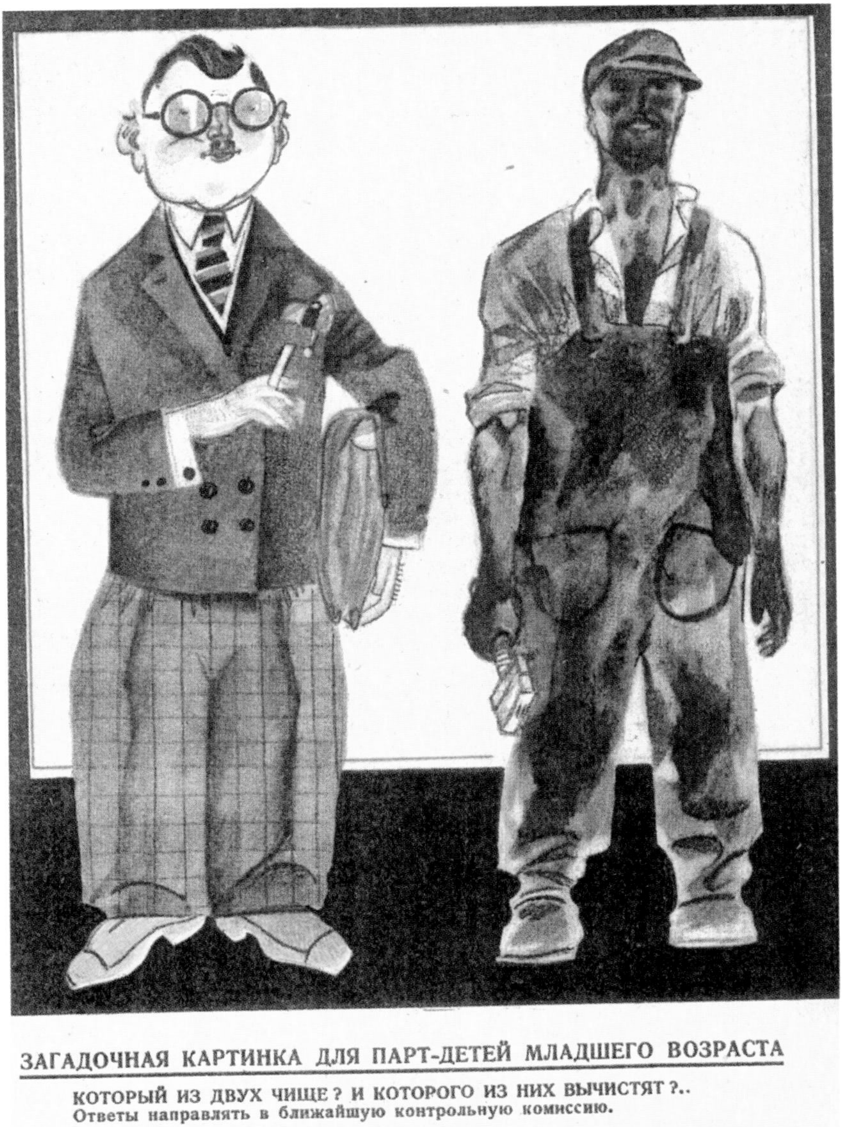
ЗАГАДОЧНАЯ КАРТИНКА ДЛЯ ПАРТ-ДЕТЕЙ МЛАДШЕГО ВОЗРАСТА
КОТОРЫЙ ИЗ ДВУХ ЧИЩЕ? И КОТОРОГО ИЗ НИХ ВЫЧИСТЯТ?..
Ответы направлять в ближайшую контрольную комиссию.

PLATE 8. "Puzzle Picture for Party Children of a Young Age." *Krokodil* 7 (February 1929): 7. Courtesy of the Russian State Library.

housing for yet another family. Under such conditions, the average diet remained limited in both quantity and variety.[165]

Reformers occasionally acknowledged these problems. For example, they pointed to inferior construction and overcrowding as the reason for poor health. One 1927 pamphlet observed, "It has already long been noticed that from a sanitary point of view poorly constructed houses (close, dirty, deprived of light and air) are the centers of this or that disease. Epidemics of typhus . . . diphtheria, scarlet fever, and so on, often emerge from uncomfortable living spaces."[166] Hygienists blamed overcrowded conditions for everything from infant mortality to the breakdown in morals. They argued that in the United States, France, and Britain less crowding led to lower infant death rates.[167] Semashko cited statistics dating from 1899 claiming that Viennese workers "in poor, crowded apartments" died at five times the rate of others.[168] To remedy this problem, he stipulated that the minimum requirements for health were fifty-five cubic meters of well-lit space per person and about one cubic meter of window for every three to five cubic meters of space.[169] Of course, declaring a minimum and enforcing it were two different things. In 1926 in Moscow the average person lived in a little under one cubic meter of space.[170]

The hygienists' grasp of reality was tenuous. In such packed spaces, individual beds were obviously impossible, but this did not keep reformers from commenting upon their necessity. The 1923 all-union health survey counted individual beds as one important criterion. It found that 31.6 percent of urban worker youth did not sleep in an individual bed.[171] Reformers blamed overcrowding for a slew of health problems. The author of *Scabies and the Fight against Them* (1926) directly indicted the practice of sharing beds for this hygienic danger: "In the cities, in view of their current overcrowding, people live closely and often also filthily. Sometimes several people use the exact same bed, not changing the bedding after their use. There are families in the city that have maintained the habit of sleeping together. . . . The unemployed, staying in boarding houses, and the newly arrived—for example, seasonal workers—live in 'eternally dirty due to overcrowding,' poorly cleaned locations."[172] The writer worried about the proximity of bodies almost as much as filth. Others expressed the same concern. While the state hailed communalism as a sign of Soviet mentality, this did not extend to the sharing of beds. According to hygienists, the crowding of many into one bed endangered children's development because it prematurely awakened the sexual instinct. Perhaps as much to discourage the family sharing the same bed as to save infant lives, pamphlets aimed at expectant mothers warned that infection or accidental suffocation of the infant resulted from shared beds.[173]

Health care activists blamed overcrowded conditions for other social ills, such as alcoholism. They contended that the unpleasant situation in the home led people to participate in unhealthy leisure activities. One writer commented:

> Upon returning home from service or work, every person wishes to relax in a clean, comfortable, quiet home. It is not a whim but a natural, essential requirement. Nothing gives such complete rest as quiet, comfort, and cleanliness in the home. But can this be achieved in crowded, overfilled, filthy homes where there is no place to escape from the noise or other people? Crowding, noise, and turmoil not only do not permit rest and relaxation but, on the contrary, further irritate the worker's nerves. He would involuntarily wish to leave such conditions and run from them to the nearest pub.[174]

Emphasizing at every turn the noise and overcrowding, the writer provided a much more likely depiction of the average home than those contained in domestic advice literature. The passage critiqued urban life generally. The city dweller can go nowhere to escape urban pressure. The writer concluded that these conditions led to a breakdown of the family, caused adults to drink, and introduced children to alcohol as they watched the example of their elders.[175]

Overcrowding did more than harm individual health; it also threatened the dynamism of society. Doctor Ashikhmin held that one of the greatest problems resulting from overcrowding was that "it made it necessary for people to always be under the gaze of others, often complete strangers unwillingly sharing the apartment." This situation threatened to wear down the individual and destroy the moral order. He cautioned: "It leads to the dulling of that natural sense of bashfulness and people become accustomed to speaking crudely concerning many things about which it is not fitting to speak. Children begin to look prematurely upon sexual relations, and the example of adults affects them and corrupts them. To this it is still necessary to add that in a crowded home children of both sexes sleep together, and with the example of elders around them, this prematurely awakens the sexual instinct in children. Joint living and sleeping of people of different sexes not only leads to premature awakening of sexual feelings but also leads to sexual dissipation and to a chaotic sexual life."[176]

For Ashikhmin humans in close proximity inevitably lapsed into carnal feelings, which led to a corruption of modesty and a sexually dissolute lifestyle. While other authors expressed concern over filth, much of their anxiety about shared beds and crowded apartments sprang from a concern over sexual misconduct. As Olga Matich argues, the avant-garde much preferred the bed of nails of Rakhmetov to the double bed, with its symbolism of bourgeois, sexual, noncommunal life.[177] While reformers deplored the filth that accompanied overcrowding, they took full advantage of the window overcrowded conditions provided into the private lives of citizens and encouraged others to use this vantage point to inform on their fellows. The "gaze of others" could open a window on the proletariat.

Following the revolution, theorists anticipated that collective institutions would liberate women from domestic labor, vilified as the source of women's subjugation and a cause and symbol of their ignorance. Reformers hoped that domestic responsibilities would shift to the social sector and that the domestic arena would be transformed. This disregard for the enormity of the task of relocating and reallocating domestic labor crept into and mirrored popular sentiment. The public regarded it as not just the lowest form of labor but also of little significance generally.[178] One couplet underscored the insubstantial nature of domestic work by implying that it took no time at all: "8 hours of work / 8 hours of rest / Finish the chores / Sleep the 8 left."[179] Even in plays and stories devoted to refashioning the home, the multiple tasks necessary for maintaining a clean home remained obscure, as if they were self-evident and unworthy of serious study. In Zamiatin's *We* the mechanisms by which this exquisitely ordered society kept itself clean were left in the shadows. Perhaps most damning, in a diatribe addressed to Zetkin, Lenin attributed women's backwardness to the domestic scene, insisting that "the home life of the woman is a daily sacrifice to a thousand unimportant trivialities."[180]

Though they minimized the problem of maintaining the home, hygienists paid serious attention to it as the basis of a healthy society. Semashko summed up the recommendations for maintaining the home: "Choose a spacious, sunny, and dry place; do not encourage humidity (do not spill water or do wash in the apartment); open the window and transom more often; and heat well. The most important thing is to keep it clean."[181] He and his colleagues were not merely commenting on laundry and windows. In their recommendations they made assumptions concerning the proper role of men, women, and children. Health care reformers targeted women as the source of problems in the home, but they also viewed them as the only ones with the power to effect change. Husbands and children had to persuade mothers, whereas wives applied their knowledge and overcame sexist, abusive husbands in order to propel their homes into the future. According to propaganda and even contemporary observations, men held little power when it came to their domestic lives.

While nurses and doctors inspected and recommended ways to maintain a more healthful home, the lifestyle they advocated would push women into unhealthy cycles of overwork and stress, with less time than men for political activism, leisure, and sleep. Many women absented themselves from the question entirely, leaving it to others to answer by hiring domestic servants.[182] For those left to do the work themselves, time studies documented the burdens on women. One study noted that in 1923, 80 percent of women workers were also housewives. Moreover, although they worked alongside men, they lived divergent lives. A man's working day lasted 13:02 hours, while a woman worked 14:55 hours. Their leisure and sleep times were also disparate. Men had 3:23 hours of leisure and slept 8:14 hours, while women had 2:42 hours of leisure, with 7:23 hours of sleep.[183] According to studies done in the 1930s, women's household duties only increased. Women workers spent an average of five hours a day on chores and child care, whereas men spent only two.[184]

In the rhetoric of domestic health, contradictions were omnipresent. Certain reports explored the horrendous difficulties, while others railed against women's backwardness as the real reason for these problems. Undoubtedly, the lack of running water, electricity, sewage lines, laundries, or convenient shopping greatly complicated domestic tasks. If followed, new hygienic norms for housework would have greatly overburdened women, but Semashko and other officials considered more sanitary homes essential. A clean house became a hallmark of citizenship, and since the government targeted women as the parties responsible for the home, it became integral to the definition of Soviet womanhood. As guardians of the home, women's individual efforts at domestic hygiene and economy could point the way to the new world. In posters women's actions led to a bright future of cooperative living, order, and political consciousness. In those areas deemed least important in Soviet life women were all-powerful.

While activists touted nurseries, Pioneer groups, and *zhenotdel* membership as cure-alls, in reality these barely instituted programs could not begin to address the insurmountable problems women faced within the home. Although health care advocates recognized the lack of facilities as a problem, they did not tolerate this as an excuse for women's social and political apathy.[185] Since communal facilities remained insignificant in the face of increased demand, the state called on women to muster their own resources to meet their household needs. While Lenin wished every cook to learn how to run the state, it was clear that for the present she would have to continue to attend to the pots and pans.[186]

5 The Family

Maternity, Birth, and Parenthood

In the eyes of the young mother entering the consultation room, everything looked bright and clean, so different from her own home. Doctors and nurses wore spotless white gowns, as did the medical personnel featured on the posters affixed to the walls. Two other mothers awaiting medical attention chided the newcomer for bundling her baby and cradling it to still its cries. A third woman called the mother's attention to her maternal lapses by pointing to the didactic posters, as if to say, "Heed the expert advice!"

Just a few months earlier the attitudes of the waiting women had been quite the opposite. While the consultation room sparkled just as brightly, the chorus of women behaved differently. The women had accused the consultation of all sorts of corruptions and perversions. They bundled their children and distrusted the nurse, who they doubted had children of her own but who seemed quite willing to tell them how to raise theirs. One woman suspected they were weighing the children for some nefarious purpose. Another mother even asked worriedly about the "confiscation" that was being planned.

Anna J. Haines, the enthusiastic American nurse who recounted these dramatic scenes, depicted them as a triumph of Soviet public health.[1] Suspicion and distrust, she claimed, had been transformed into a devotion to the new system, which led these once reluctant mothers not only to follow but also to proselytize the consultation and its techniques for rearing children, yet the mother who had confused the consultation with the well-known grain confiscations had a better sense of the reality of maternal health campaigns. In many ways the consultation, set up by the Department for the Protection of Motherhood and Infancy (Otdel okhrany materinstva i mladenchestva), a subdepartment of Narkomzdrav, hoped to rob women of authority in matters of child rearing and replace mothers and fathers with the consultation nurse and the male doctor, representatives of the new scientific Soviet lifestyle.

The campaign to medicalize motherhood and professionalize child care with new norms, authorities, and institutions was not unique to the Soviet state, nor were its techniques radically different from efforts in other countries. Soviet natalist propaganda and policies bridged pre- and postrevolutionary thought, blurred the boundaries between public and private, and mirrored the methods of capitalist population policies.[2] Although Soviet methods reflected those of other world powers and prerevolutionary reformers, the application of these programs differed because of Soviet concepts of citizens' duties and state imperatives. While Narkomzdrav did not succeed completely in taking over child rearing from women or infiltrating every home with advice through the consultation, birth home for infants, and other new institutions, it did apply techniques to manage motherhood more thoroughly than any other country at the time.

The Soviet consultation—with its attendant propaganda, visiting nurses, and vacation houses—attempted to spread new methods of child rearing among women. In place of the mother's intuition, the midwife, folk methods, or the father, officials substituted science, interpreted by doctors, as the ultimate authority. The male doctor, aided by his handmaiden the consultation nurse, chipped away at the standing of the midwife, denied that motherhood was a natural ability of women, challenged traditional methods of healing, and assumed the father's place in the home.

By injecting a physician into the parent-child relationship, health specialists tried to depersonalize and discipline parenting and thereby weaken the authority of mothers and fathers. Once hygiene was trumpeted as the deciding factor in a child's health and happiness, the good mother ensured her child's physical and mental well-being by following the instructions of the experts. Essentially, good mothering became a skill to be acquired, and any woman could perfect this skill by following the doctor-recommended regimen, and therefore any authority she could derive from the state's emphasis on the importance of motherhood was thus simultaneously snatched from her. At least mothers were still active; fathers found themselves outside the family as doctors became the authority figures in children's lives.

Propaganda consistently portrayed the forces of tradition as embodied in the female midwife. Traditional practices were thus feminized and contrasted with stronger, masculinized science. Although propaganda touted male doctors and men held posts in the upper echelons of the Department of Health, the actual battle for supremacy in matters of child rearing took place among women over an acknowledged woman's issue.[3] Women headed both the Russian and the Moscow branches of the Department for the Protection of Motherhood and Infancy—V. P. Lebedeva and O. P. Nogina, respectively. Large numbers of female volunteers carried out the majority of inspections. Women wielded the power to implement these ideas and challenged other women in an acknowledged women's realm. While hygienists railed against the midwife, they lacked the resources to replace her. The battle for supremacy in natal care was largely a symbolic one in which the chief offense of the midwife may have been not her care but her lack of recognition of the legitimacy of Soviet power and institutionalized scientific authority.

Believing that the size of a nation could set it on a path toward dominance, practically all industrialized countries instituted programs to increase population growth in the early twentieth century. Stimulated by the spread of bacteriology, the professionalization of medicine, and the rise of the social sciences, Britain, the United States, Italy, and other nations experimented with different programs to create healthier, larger, more stable populations. Increased nationalist competition and the greater sophistication of modern warfare made these moves important for state prestige and viability as well as internal stability. As states claimed the bounties of motherhood, the definition changed and mothers increasingly came under scrutiny. Germany, Britain, and the United States all attempted to lessen infant death rates and better educate mothers. These programs greatly accelerated after World War I. Despite extreme hardship Britain adopted natalist programs during the war, thereby recognizing the importance of population management. In Britain, Germany, the United States, and elsewhere concern for the health of the general population as well as infants led to eugenics programs to combat births from those seen as defective and to encourage the birth of pure racial stock.[4]

Nineteenth-century maternal health provisions also coincided with the move to protect mothers and children in the workplace. In the first half of the nineteenth century women and children were prevented from working in mining and other professions considered dangerous by Europeans. By the late 1800s, countries experimented with granting maternity leave and awarding subsidies to mothers in the hope of increasing the birthrate and boosting infant health. These efforts continued into the twentieth century. The 1920s saw the Viennese and Italians experimenting with aid to mothers. The British, French, and Americans also developed family welfare policies during this period.[5]

Concern for the care of mothers and children developed contemporaneously in Russia. The beginnings of natalist policy in Russia can be traced to Peter the

Great, who saw the need for more workers and taxpayers and therefore the necessity of caring for orphans and foundlings.[6] His programs concentrated on illegitimate or abandoned children and their care. Over the course of the eighteenth century, Russian ideas about the population and its meaning for the state shifted, and ways to control its growth, health, and productivity also changed. Catherinian foundling homes educated and molded children while they attended to their health needs. Catherine's much-touted concern for women's education contained more than a nod toward the crucial role of mothers in children's moral education and physical upbringing.[7] By the early nineteenth century, the military colonies of Arakcheev, under Alexander I, instituted programs to foster population growth. Organizers attempted to educate mothers in modern Western hygienic practices for their children. In doing so they hoped to ensure a healthy child who would grow up to become a strong member of the military. In the countryside almost half of all children reportedly died before reaching the age of five. These numbers led to increased interest in child welfare as a humanitarian concern, but it was also a matter of national pride. Russian infant deaths were higher than in any other European country.[8] Perhaps even more troubling for the state was the higher rate of infant deaths among Russians than among other ethnic groups.

While private interest in public health escalated during the nineteenth century, tsarist officials continued to shy away from action. In the early 1900s doctors and private individuals organized the first type of welfare for women in Russia, and by the 1910s the state had brought these programs under its umbrella.[9] Even with state involvement, the number of institutions remained small and the number of women reached was minimal. This lack of interest did not reflect a lack of problems with early childhood development. In 1914 the army was forced to reject nearly a third of draftees because of rickets, tuberculosis, or general unfitness.[10]

Revolution would eventually lead to the creation of large-scale programs for natal health. The interest in natal health may seem incongruous in a state that sanctioned abortion, but authorities did not legalize abortion because they considered it a right of women. Rather, they were more concerned about botched abortions. Indeed, social and medical authorities argued that abortion harmed women and that childbirth was a woman's civic obligation. New Soviet leaders desired a stronger, larger population to replenish the workforce and improve the birthrate. Legalized abortion and pro-birth policies would coexist for a time.[11]

Because of their importance as future workers and soldiers, children constituted a resource too important to be entrusted to parents. Indeed, even before the revolution, Lenin's wife, Nadezhda Krupskaia, had argued that women were unfit to be mothers because they were uneducated and unprepared for motherhood.[12] It was imperative for the state to intervene since, according to authorities, parents no longer represented the children's best interests. A housewife who was verbally attacked during an agitational trial in the 1920s railed against the new system and its invasiveness in words that likely echoed many women's opinions: "It was enough that they spoiled my husband. He forgot his faith, but I will not give them my children to spoil. . . . They are my kids. . . . I will do as I like." A young, female Komsomol member, representing the new order, rebuked her: "That is nonsense, Stepanovna. Your children are not your own. Children belong to the society of workers."[13]

To protect these youngest members of the society of workers, the government passed legislation to guard the health of mothers and children. Lenin ordered the establishment of the Department for the Protection of Motherhood and Infancy in 1918.[14] In 1925 O. P. Nogina, the head of Moscow's Department for the Protection of Motherhood and Infancy, summed up the importance of children's health and the heavily prophylactic nature of this work: "The health of every single person lies in his infancy and even before. Only a healthy mother can give birth to a healthy baby. The sanitation of the population begins with the protection of a pregnant woman and her infant."[15] Other departmental publications emphasized the strategic importance of neonatal and maternal health. In a postrevolutionary collection edited by B. S. Ginzburg, which was sent out to all the district departments, Ginzburg compared the new, European-wide fears of population depletion in the twentieth century with the Malthusian-inspired fears of overpopulation in the nineteenth century. The book included multiple tables and graphs of birth and death rates throughout Europe to underscore Russia's dangerously low population growth compared to other European countries.[16] In response to the needs of its population and of its subdepartment, the Moscow Department of Health devoted 16 percent of its budget to the protection of mothers.[17]

The Department for the Protection of Motherhood and Infancy supervised orphanages, nurseries, homes for mothers and children, maternity homes (for normal births, problem births, and for homeless mothers), abortion clinics, and consultations for nursing children and pregnant women.[18] While many new institutions were featured in this ambitious list, because of budgetary constraints the bulk of work took place in cities and came from the consultation and propaganda.[19] Since the state could not provide professional care for every child, hygienists found propaganda a cheap alternative that permitted them to train mothers to perform essential tasks until the state could find the resources to take over.[20] Natalist literature and visual propaganda grew steadily throughout the 1920s. In 1921 over 30,000 copies of various publications were printed by the department, and by 1931 150 titles appeared in 5 million copies.[21] Many of these pieces would be distributed by workers in the consultation system; sanitary enlightenment theorists contended that it was the best place for propaganda.[22]

Hygienists attempted to reach women in innovative ways, including lectures, talks, agitational trials, and even short movies and radio broadcasts. Department members organized schools of motherhood and infancy within the consultation, maternity home, and at factories employing large numbers of female workers. Worker clubs tried to spread the message through lectures and question-and-answer nights. Audiovisual presentations were encouraged, with the first film for the department appearing in 1919 and slides being sold to accompany lectures.[23] The museum offered a unique forum for instruction. In 1919 A. V. Mol'kov, director of the Narkomzdrav Museum of Social Hygiene, organized a Moscow health exhibition, with areas devoted to "Hygiene of Mother and Child." In 1923 the State Institute for the Protection of Motherhood and Infancy opened its own exhibition.[24] The Institute for the Study and Teaching of Infant Welfare opened a child care museum where the mother could see a model home complete with posters, wax displays, and ideal rooms. The museum organizers reproduced some of its posters on postcards—a convenient way to let women carry home the lessons of the exhibits (figures 5.1, 5.2). To reach women in their own neighborhoods, smaller traveling exhibits consisting of posters and wax displays of food, toys, and other objects toured consultations and maternity homes. The public was not left to its own devices in these presentations. To ensure proper interpretation of the exhibits, handbooks described exactly how to lead groups, including sample dialogue and even stage directions.[25]

The department claimed to be involved in an exhausting array of activities. A list of departmental actions for 1924 noted that it presented lectures, placed articles in publications, organized excursions, and printed 720,000 copies of books on maternal and natal health.[26] Another report pledged to use "lectures, meetings, exhibitions, conferences, handouts, posters, brochures, etc.," in support of the cause.[27] According to a brief account of natalist activities covering July through September 1924, the department presented 4 lectures together with the film *Children—Life's Flowers,* placed 22 articles in women-targeted journals, and led 119 excursions totaling over 8,000 visitors through the child care museum.[28]

The scope of activities, while large considering the limited resources of the department, could not begin to include the entire population. For those who did not see posters, exhibits, or plays, the department spread its message through its institutions. Consultation workers "instructed [pregnant women] in all

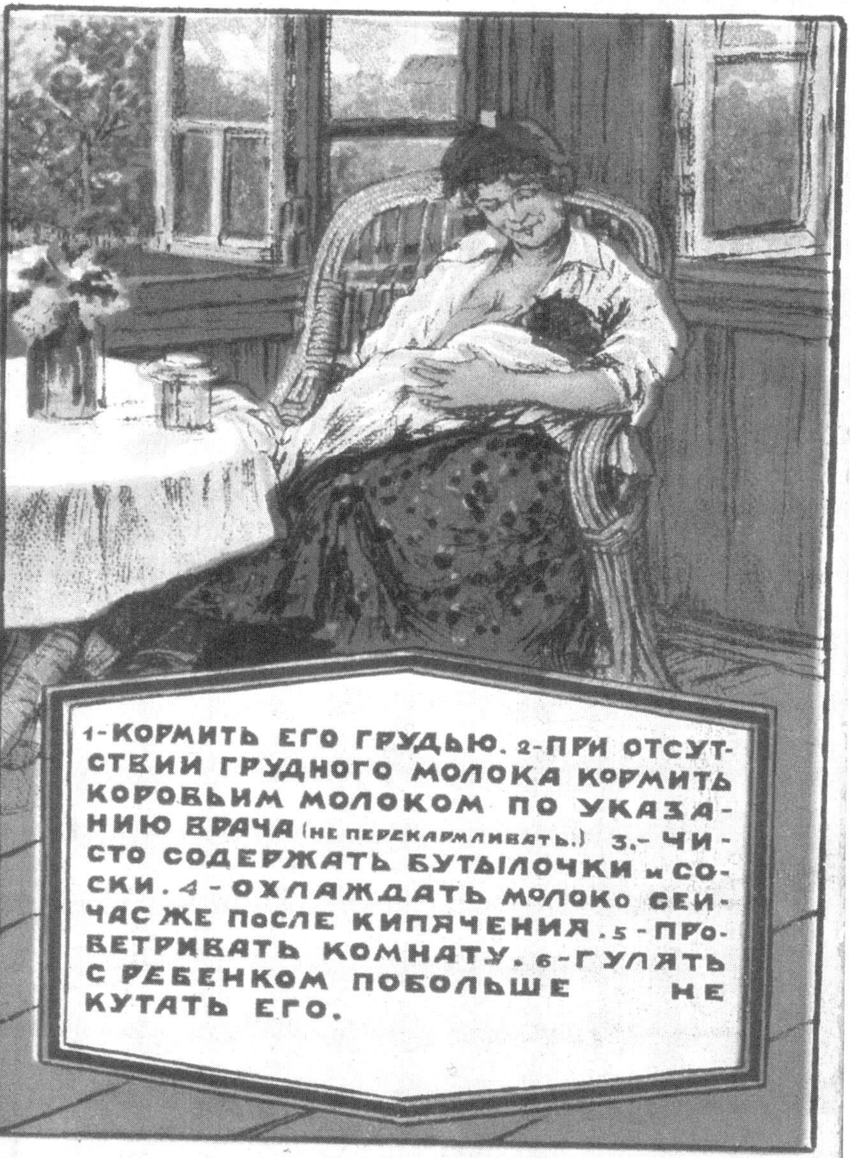

FIGURE 5.1. "Breast Feed." V. V. Spaskii. Pub. 50,000. Courtesy of the Russian State Library.

matters of hygienic living and child care" and provided detailed directives for prenatal care in terms of diet, exercise, and so on.[29] The Home for Homeless Mothers went even further, combining maternal instruction with vocational training, thereby enabling women to care for their infants while earning enough for a healthy life. The homes drained the budget for women's health care as NEP policies led to more unemployed women and budget constraints for such health programs. A support body was developed in 1922 to help the department's programs with fund-raising activities and other makeshift solutions to help keep these programs afloat.[30]

At the Home for Mothers and Infants, expectant mothers received more intense and prolonged instruction. In theory, they could stay anywhere from one month (before birth) or two months (after birth) to a full ten months. Organizers stated the twin goals of providing a hygienic environment for mother and child and teaching the mother proper care of the child.[31] A Moscow article stated: "A mother living two months in the Home for Mothers and Infants sees through action that she can and must live without old women's tales, that fear of the evil eye, fear of colds, spirits, and the swaddling of the baby cripples his life." While residing at the home, pregnant women learned how to "rationally spend the time until birth." After the mothers gave birth, "instruction on feeding and care continued."[32]

The message remained consistent: scientific care must replace traditional practice. Soviet authorities, acting as science's midwife, touted cleanliness and order as the epitome of correct care. Authors constantly stressed that mothers should keep all items coming into contact with the child clean. Experts recommended that toys be free of sharp edges. Mothers were advised to wash clothing, bedding, and linens frequently and change them often. They were also instructed to store food products carefully and boil water.[33] Some authors emphasized cleanliness as the primary measure for ensuring infant health: "A cleanly kept room, a frequently washed floor, washing hands, daily bathing of the child for the first six months, the frequent changing of underclothes—these are the costs for a healthy child."[34]

No matter how tidy and clean the apartment was kept, the home provided only part of a healthful upbringing. Doctors prescribed large amounts of fresh air and sunshine for expectant mothers and newborns. According to one expert, the baby born in summer should be taken outside immediately and for the entire day. For children born in winter doctors recommended short outdoor exposure for the first month and then four to six hours a day after that.[35] If outdoor exposure could not be provided, the transom should be opened to air the apartment during sleeping hours and periodically during the day.

Hygienists extended their advice to all aspects of child care. Health care advocates uniformly promoted the superiority of breast-feeding over formula or even cow's milk, a stance that Russian health officials had been pushing since the eighteenth century.[36] Ginzburg blamed half of all infant deaths on improper feeding of children.[37] Experts decried the old chew teat (*soska*)—the practice of giving a child previously chewed food that had been strained through a piece of fabric—as too filthy to be tolerated.[38] In nineteenth-century Russia doctors saw digestive disorders caused by the early switch to solid food as primarily responsible for infant deaths, even as peasants claimed that breast-feeding did not provide enough food for infants.[39] A health department postcard warned that "so many nursing children die in Russia" because of early feeding with cereal and the "chew teat."[40] Another postcard outlined the many rules for those who chose bottle over breast (figure 5.1). According to B. S. Sigal's *How to Raise a Healthy Infant* (1927), "the 'chew teat' killed more people than shells and bullets during the war."[41] A. N. Antonov's book *Sanitary Enlightenment Patronage of Nursing Infants* (1925) listed breast-feeding as the most important lesson the nurse could pass on to the mother.[42] A commemorative postcard from the health museum credited breast-feeding of 92 percent of babies with saving the nation from massive infant deaths.[43] While the benefits of breast-feeding were many, doctors emphasized its utility as a protection against rickets. One late 1920s postcard credited poor feeding habits and poor living with "almost always" leading to "the English Disease (Rickets)" (figure 5.2).[44]

Percentages and outcomes—the language of production—infiltrated natalist propaganda, as did the measurements and charts of Taylorism. Pelvic measurements, accident charts, and labor restrictions focused upon the relationship between women's production and reproduction.[45] Just as all aspects of Soviet life were being scrutinized and Taylorized, so, too, was suckling. Mothers were to nurse not based upon the demands of their own bodies or the cries of their children but according to the rigid schedule laid out by doctors. Doctors maintained that feedings had to be based on scientific analysis. Mothers were to nurse their children every three hours.[46] Some handbooks even prescribed the duration for nursing (twenty minutes) and the proper posture for breast-feeding—left foot on a bench, baby on knee, one arm along spine, with four fingers below breast and one above—implying that women did not even do this small activity correctly.[47] A late 1920s photo series issued by the Department for the Protection of Motherhood and Infancy illustrated proper and improper feeding. On the left was the correct proffering of the breast, with the incorrect feeding posture on the right (figure 5.3). An illustration of the Taylorization of breast-feeding graced the cover of a 1927 issue of the journal *To a New Life!* It

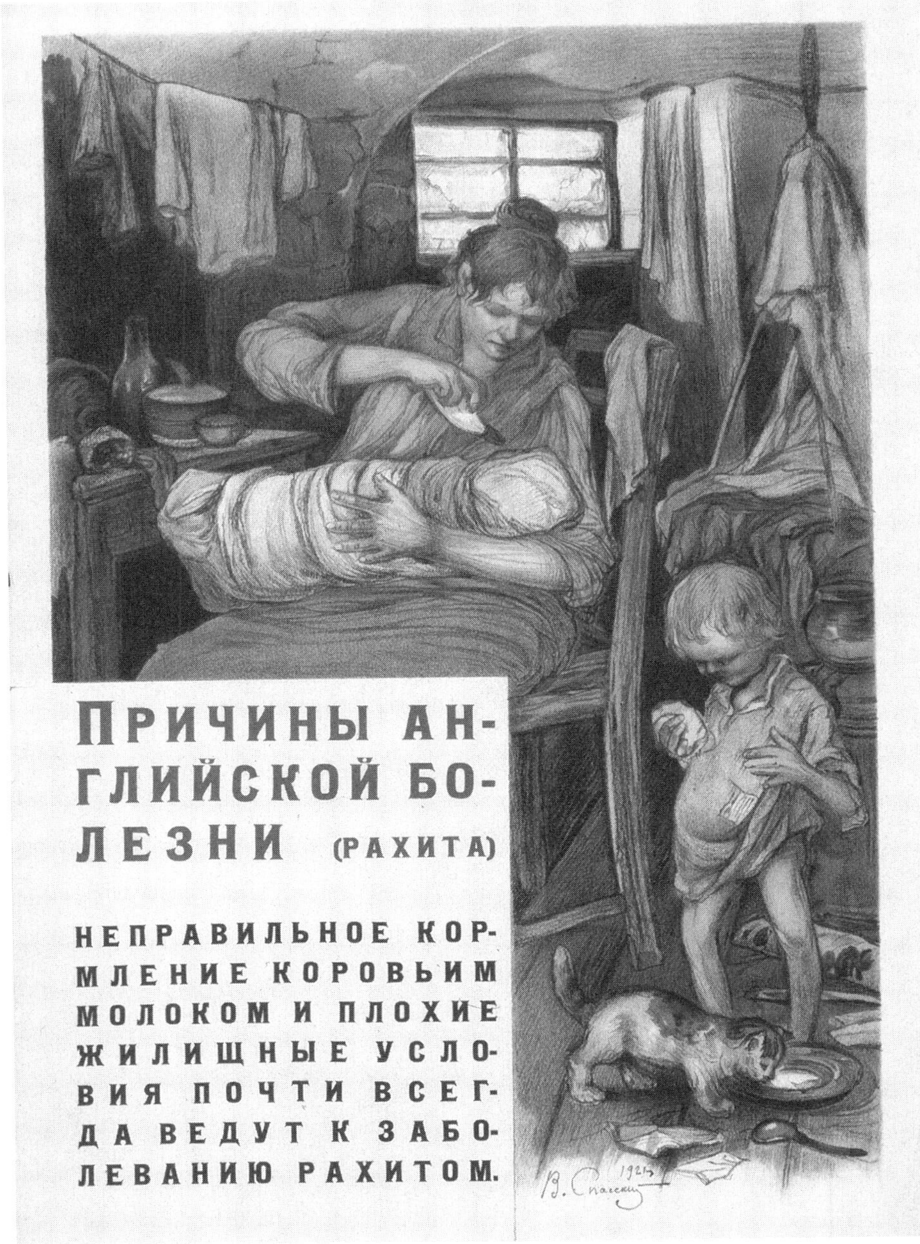

FIGURE 5.2. "The Causes of the English Disease (Rickets)." Moscow: OMM, 1926–29. Pub. 4,000. Courtesy of the Russian State Library.

featured four mothers, all from the Home for Homeless Mothers, nursing their infants. Maintaining the same position—even down to the tilt of the head and the prescribed proffering of the breast—each mother held her baby at the same angle and nursed in unison. Their heads were bent downward at such an angle that only a portion of their faces and hair were visible. Only the children had faces and hence personalities.[48] Official derision of women's input at this early stage of infant care was evident. They did not do even the simplest tasks correctly, and once they had been instructed in the correct technique, they became faceless conduits. Women were merely cogs in a feeding machine.

The feeding schedule had been arrived at scientifically and could therefore not fail. Experts discouraged individual initiatives or following the advice of others even if a mother swore that the schedule was not working. Any problems that resulted were solely the fault of the mother. Accused of negligence in a mock trial, one mother cried out to the judge: "But those books, father [*batiushka*], are not for our kind. Keep him clean, feed him by the clock, and take him outside. . . . I tried to do it that way, but then Kol'ka cried all the more."[49] After probing questions, the judge ruled that the woman had incorrectly followed the doctor's recommendations and ordered her to master the regimen, confident that it would overcome all problems.

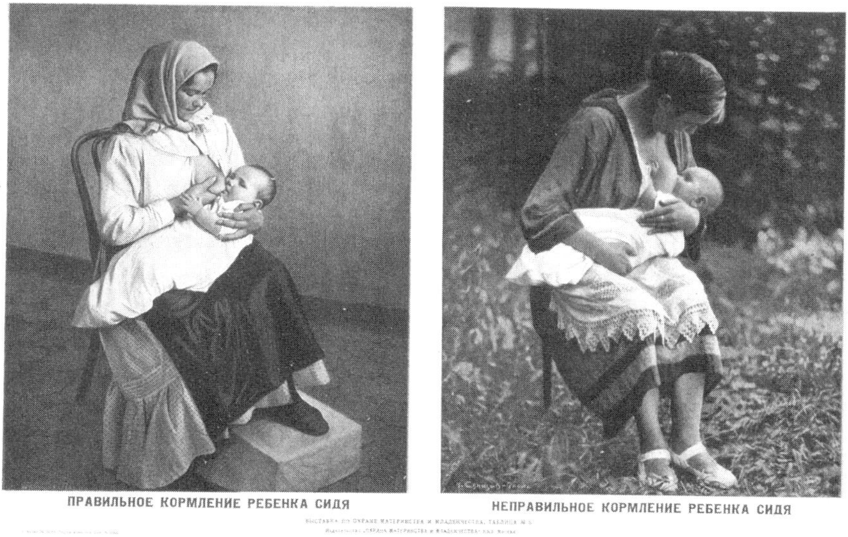

FIGURE 5.3. "The Correct Way to Feed a Three-Month-Old Child." Moscow: OMM, 1926–29. Pub. 4,000. Courtesy of the Russian State Library.

Just as a mother's complaint was disregarded, so children's cries were not permitted to interfere with the schedule. The wordy late 1920s poster "Why Do Infants Cry?" insisted they did so because of improper care (figure 5.4). In an article entitled "Why Babies Cry" the author explained that "infants never cry evilly, without cause," and that they only cry due to poor care, such as "clutter, insect stings, uncomfortable positions, extremely warm bundling (causing sweat, weakness, and unnerving the child), chills, a tight diaper, which binds the child. . . . All of these—and even more large and small offenses of care—are already well-known reasons for a baby's cry." If the mother remedied all these "offenses of care" and the baby still cried, she was to take it to the doctor, who would probably determine that it had gas. If the child continued crying, the fault lay with the parents. "There are children who exhibit an especially restless nature, and they are called nervous children. Children most often get this quality from their parents."[50] Even for this condition the regimen was the cure. As one article noted, a stronger application of the regimen certainly would cure this irrational and unwarranted crying.

According to propaganda, children subjected to a correctly executed regimen invariably conformed completely to behavioral standards. In a story about a specialized House of Leisure for mothers, a young child displayed the positive effects of the scientific system of child care: "Twenty-five nursing children are all sleep, but suddenly through the netting the black eyes of a youngster are visible. He doesn't sleep, but the House of Leisure has already taught him to lie quietly during predetermined times."[51] Soviet doctors and their invincible regimen had cured crying and taught obedience. In another conversation reported by Haines, the enthusiastic American nurse, a mother of twins gushed as she exited the consultation that her neighbor had been correct when she said that "'consultation babies did not cry and were not sick' and now all was well."[52] The propaganda assured reluctant mothers that Soviet science had ended crying.

With so much effort expended in the spread of information on rearing children, it should come as no surprise that authorities insisted that infant mortality arose not from poor conditions—and certainly not as a result of fate—but through women's laziness and ignorance. In one show trial set in 1925, a mother accused of inadequate care defended herself by saying: "Every mother herself knows how to care for her child. My mother, without consultants or doctors, raised me healthfully." She insisted that the child had died because of "God's will."[53] The court found this defense, including the accumulated wisdom of generations, inadequate since a nurse had visited the mother and told her how to change her life. Failing to recognize the superiority of Soviet techniques after an official had shown the way could not be excused. In summation, the defense

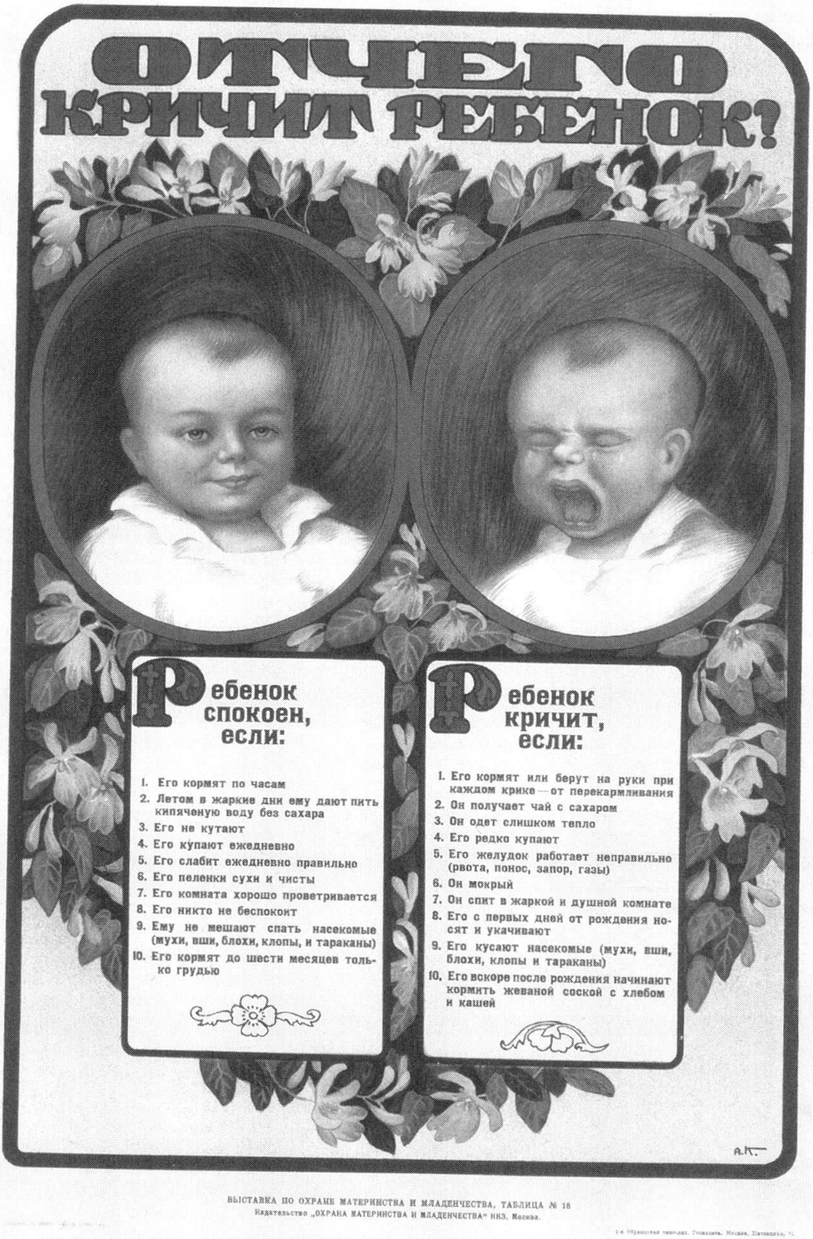

FIGURE 5.4. "Why Do Infants Cry?" Moscow: OMM, 1926–29. Pub. 4,000. Courtesy of the Russian State Library.

admitted that after eight years of revolutionary power even they could not accept such ignorance of Soviet techniques as a justification. The court was lenient, however, and instead of jail time it ordered the mother to enroll in courses to learn the necessary rules.[54]

Mock trials and other propaganda transformed motherhood from a natural preserve of women to a skill taught by health professionals. Doctors prescribed the proper way for mothers to maintain a healthy environment for themselves and their children, how they should conduct their daily lives, and even how, when, and what to eat. One particularly patronizing photo series actually demonstrated how to hold a child properly (figure 5.5). Health professionals vilified and ridiculed the networks women had traditionally relied upon for advice and counsel. Authorities rejected a woman's own experience as inadequate in the face of new medical information. One journal article even noted that mothers could be a source of infection for their children.[55]

Although authorites insisted that women were incapable of caring for their children or even posed a danger to them, they never suggested that men take over. Instead, women were instructed to care for their children under the supervision of men.[56] At the same time that the radical feminist theorist Alexandra Kollontai urged the liberation of women from child care so they could become

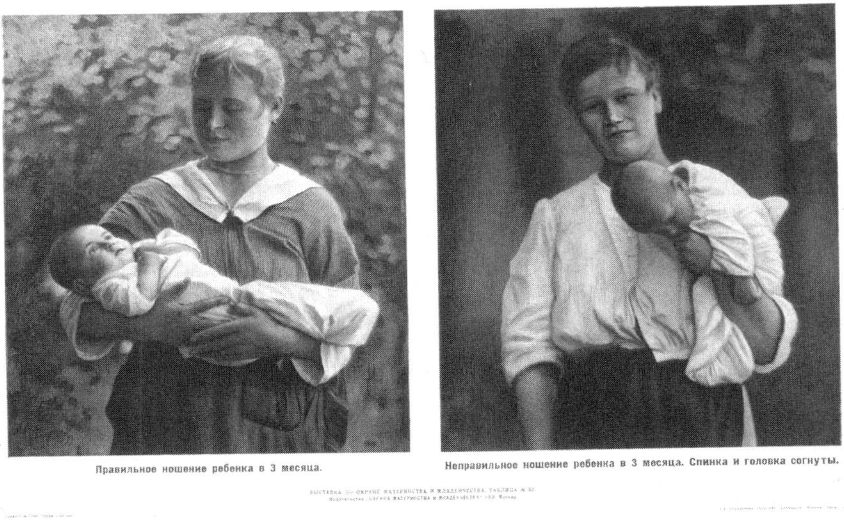

Правильное ношение ребенка в 3 месяца.
Неправильное ношение ребенка в 3 месяца. Спинка и головка согнуты.

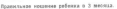

FIGURE 5.5. "The Correct Way to Hold a Three-Month-Old Child." Moscow: OMM, 1926–29. Pub. 4,000. Courtesy of the Russian State Library.

fully functioning members of society, doctors wished to seize child care because they deemed women incompetent. According to the American nurse Haines, specialists attempted to take children and place them in homes, to be brought up by trained nurses, "which was expected to show better results than the clumsy efforts of the untrained mother." The experiment ended quickly because "it was found that infants did not respond well to this regimen. . . . The department has now definitely adopted the policy of encouraging all mothers to keep their infant children at home."[57] No other records of this program appeared, and perhaps nurse Haines confused a reference to the heroine of Gladkov's novel *Cement* with reality. The heroine sent her child to an orphanage so she could pursue revolutionary work. The child's death fueled debates during the NEP era. Though there was no official program, many revolutionary women did hand their children over to relatives or Soviet care in order to pursue political work.[58]

Activists for women's emancipation and the expansion of medical authority could agree that women needed more options for child care. Institutional care did more than free up women to pursue political activity. For authorities it offered a way to supervise mothers and let medical personnel take over the care of the child. One observer of the Home for Mothers and Infants praised its ability to place children into the competent, skilled hands of the trained nurse.[59] Ultimate authority still rested with the doctor, but the nurse-practitioner fulfilled the duties of daily care.

Once the child and mother left the Home for Mothers and Infants, they were immediately placed under the purview of the nursery and its system of home visitation. Though not apparent at first, the nursery was vital to the observation, control, and treatment plans of medical authorities. The nursery gave physicians access to older children. Doctors urged mothers to place their children in day care centers. In addition, nurseries served as a cornerstone of Bolshevik plans for liberating women and enabling them to participate in the workforce and in political groups. Even temporary care was beyond the department's scope. In 1927 there was space for only 5,145 Moscow children in 102 nurseries.[60] Even these numbers were most likely inflated.

Mothers were often reluctant to accept nursery care for their children. Older women reportedly objected to paying for the care of other mothers' children when they had gone without support. One woman wondered about the nursery's safety since the doctor was summoned so often. Village women worried that their children might be held hostage for ransom or that the nurseries would be used to turn their children against traditional religious and cultural practices. Official faith in the institutions, of course, was strong. A 1926 report of the Moscow Department of Health noted that the city's seventy-five nurseries had been very involved in prophylactic work, plus the fact that these nurseries served as "schools of child care for the mothers."[61] According to authorities, mothers had to send their children to the kindergarten, the school, and the Pioneers or abandon them to education on the streets.[62]

Authorities attempted to instill in the public the proper ways to rear children, a sense of responsibility to the state as parents, and faith in the teachings of medicine. An entire system of checkpoints emerged to monitor children's health, including nurseries, prophylactic institutions, and physical culture groups. All depended on strict doctor supervision. In this quest, the physician's role often eclipsed that of an authority figure and became that of a father figure.[63] The father—already supplanted as an authority on child rearing by the consultation system's complete lack of attention to his caregiving skills—was further disempowered in family relations by depictions in the press that attributed fatherly pride to the child's doctor rather than to his or her father. Under this new, scientific father figure, the mother—and, in certain situations, even the nurse—would serve as a conduit for the knowledge of the doctor.

In a description of a 1927 baby contest, a practice copied from the West, the reporter claimed that the contest would test both the care given the child by the mother and the strength of the consultation as a program. The contest would examine everything, including "physical development, growth, teeth, weight, and, most important, the lifestyle and housing conditions in which the child grew and developed."[64] Even though the child's environment and development were a concern, the birth father was not even mentioned. In another contest description, the doctor, who represented the soul of the consultation, worried about the rating of the children under his care.[65] The article presented the two parental figures as the nurturing mother and the knowledgeable doctor, totally neglecting the birth father as a member of the parenting team even though he was present. The doctor father figure exhibited all the nervousness and pride in achievement usually attributed to the father. The doctor as father acted as the head of the family by receiving credit for his charges, and the mother fulfilled his plans for society's children. A description of the winners of the baby contest brought this idea home: "The conducting of the concourse is the best example of how, solely with the help and assistance of the consultation, many mothers knowledgeably bring up a child and prepare him for the 'contest of life' that still lies before him."[66] The mother merely functions as a helper to the doctor—his representative in the private home.[67]

Birth fathers suffered in comparison with these doctor father figures. Either they were evil creatures with "bad habits"—drunkards who beat their wives (the politically active woman ultimately left such men)—or, if well-intentioned, they were powerless to effect change when faced with recalcitrant wives and grandmothers. In *The Trial of a Housewife* the wife gossiped, maligned others, sought comfort from the church, and held back her children from public life—while the husband stood by helplessly. In the trial of an unlicensed abortionist, the husband, a clinic worker, actually lost his wife when she sought the midwife and ignored his attempts to make her accept the new medicine. The traditional healer proved to be too formidable for these politically active men. The only individual virile enough to challenge the authority of the old midwife was the doctor. While she did not back off immediately and perhaps would scrap with him during the agitational trials, she ultimately conceded defeat in the face of his greater logic and skill.[68]

In presenting new practices, propagandists decried the old, especially the mother's dependence upon the traditional healer or village midwife, the incarnation of the regressive, unscientific tsarist past. All blame fell onto her shoulders. As one author declared, "The biggest reason for infant deaths is not the poverty of the population—it is the midwife."[69] According to Soviet writers, the midwife compounded her offense by "torturing" the women throughout the birthing process. Authors also vilified midwives for their postnatal care and reputation as back alley abortionists. Doctor Ginzburg contended that 95 percent of all Russian women gave birth under the traditional healer's care and that this accounted for thirty thousand deaths a year.[70]

In a dual condemnation of gender and generation, visual propaganda invariably portrayed the midwife as a withered old woman with a skull-like visage. Usually hunched over and frail, she worked in filthy conditions. Posters depicted traditional healers delivering babies in rooms filled with hanging laundry, animals, and the occasional farm implement, thus connecting them with agricultural life and implied premodern habits. The patient was depicted in a pose that spoke of suffering and exhaustion, with hair falling in her open, screaming mouth or across her lips slack in unconsciousness. By contrast, a doctor-assisted delivery was portrayed as serene. The obstetrician, dressed in white, stood in a bare room obviously not used for anything but birthing. The postpartum woman assumed a tranquil, contented pose. The message of the propaganda was clear: a doctor-assisted birth produced a healthy baby and a happy mother.[71]

According to authorities, the midwife preyed upon politically unsophisticated or timid women and tried to steer them away from the new health facilities and programs. A mock trial charged the midwife Lopukhina with causing a woman's death as a result of a botched abortion. Lopukhina's first offense was presenting her services as being "for secret pregnancies" or for women who were ashamed to be pregnant (a supposed impossibility in the new state).[72] Lopukhina's charge mirrored those leveled at other traditional healers accused by authorities of magnifying the ignorance of the population by playing on the general mistrust of new medical authorities, exploiting the popular fear of the hospital as a place of death, and claiming that male doctors could not understand "women's business."[73] Furthermore, the midwife's ignorance endangered mother and child. The judge disregarded Lopukhina's thirty years of experience in delivering children and providing abortions. Experience was not adequate. Like the anti-midwife campaigns in Western nations, only institutionalized learning was acceptable. The midwives did not possess the ability to use the instruments considered essential by doctors. Instead of a thorough knowledge of medicines, traditional healers relied on what hygienists derided as herbs, prayers, holy water, bootlegged liquor, and, in extreme cases, a large log.[74]

Authors emphasized traditional healers' shortcomings in subsequent care for women and their children. One woman in an agitational trial lost two of her children to scarlet fever because of her faith in folk medicine.[75] In another mock trial the mother lost her child after visiting the old woman Buranova.[76] Health officials blamed midwives for infant deaths and blindness because they did not properly attend to venereal diseases such as syphilis and gonorrhea. In addition, agitational trials condemned traditional methods for calming children—including the use of opium tonics and alcohol.[77] The posters "Never Give a Child a Chew Teat" and "Do Not Go to the Midwife" emphasized the dirt and disorder of the crone and associated them with squealing children. In the individual frames desiccated old women in squalid conditions puttered around, apparently indifferent to the cries of the children. "Do Not Go to the Midwife" contrasted the traditional methods with the new consultation, showing a midwife's rooms and the Soviet response. In the second frame the mother appeared in the spartan and clean consultation with other happy women and a contented child.[78]

Not only was the midwife cruel and incompetent but—most damning in the eyes of many—she was also dirty. Writers eagerly detailed the filth of the midwife. As one reformer insisted, "The midwives do not know about the maintenance of cleanliness and really do not believe in it much. . . . Under their long fingernails they always have a lot of dirt."[79] Traditional healers did not keep their tools in cabinets or sterilize them and used methods that doctors found grotesque. One author claimed the traditional healer would cut the head off a live chicken while sitting between the mother's legs in order to frighten the baby out of the womb.[80] A series of posters from the Moscow Department of Health featured the filth and danger of the traditional healer. The poster "Vasilli

Went to the Midwife and Not the Hospital" depicted a hunchbacked, feeble crone and displayed her methods for "healing" venereal disease (figure 5.6). Images of filth, religion, age, and poverty accompany captions ridiculing her techniques by emphasizing their religious tone. She tells Vasilli, "Take this morning and evening and cross yourself while facing east." Other practitioners—the "Chinese" and the priest—are presented in the poster in lesser positions. The female practitioner remained top and center as both a threat and a target.

Department officials spread this message, overseeing its enforcement through home visits of the consultation. Visiting nurses were to investigate their patients and instruct mothers regularly. The visiting nurse entered the home not to treat an illness but to inspect a newborn or monitor a pregnancy. The government thus took upon itself the right to enter the homes of private citizens even if no illness prompted their visit. In addition to eroding privacy, the new doctors reconfigured the relations of the home. They deemed women responsible caregivers and undermined the authority of the father. As they investigated homes, doctors, nurses, and volunteers spread the message of Soviet natal health with varying success.[81]

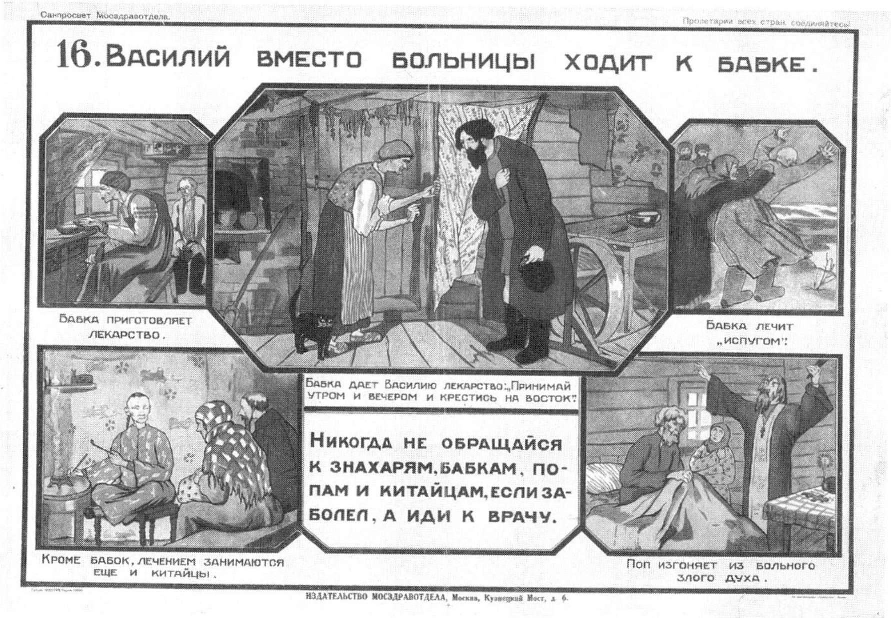

FIGURE 5.6. "Vasilli Went to the Midwife and Not the Hospital." Moscow: Sanprosvet MOZ, 1921–25. Pub. 10,000. Courtesy of the Russian State Library.

In 1921 Commissar of Health Semashko pointed out: "The affair of protection of mothers and infants has entered a new phase among us. Now it is no longer enough to agitate and propagandize that we must protect the mother and child. [The time] has arrived to explain how to do that and to give active, practical, concrete advice."[82] Semashko emphasized the importance of the dispensary in this work: "It did not wait for the mother to come to it with her needs but persistently reached out to the masses and awakened their minds and wills."[83] Contemporary accounts noted the power of the home inspection in the West, in particular the work of English nurse inspectors, credited with the significant decline in the death rate of infants.[84] The image of the powerful nurse also graced Soviet magazines and pamphlets. According to hygienists, the home visit afforded great opportunities to observe the origins of illness and to agitate for the prevention of further problems. In addition, the nurse educated women in cleanliness, house cleaning, and encouraged them to care for their own health by abstaining from work and sex during advanced pregnancy. Ideally the visiting nurse entered the patient's life to "uplift her."[85]

In connection with nurseries, in 1922 Moscow doctors conducted 18,611 home visitations and nurses 27,499. In 1927 doctors visited 42,300 homes and nurses 76,309.[86] Although health officials wanted doctors and nurses to carry out the home visits, a shortage of qualified professionals forced many of the investigations to be conducted by members of the party, *zhenotdel* activists, or other volunteers. While male doctors occupied positions of authority in Narkomzdrav, women influenced the organization and running of the department. Women also made up 70 percent of the Moscow Soviet's section for health care. Women's involvement was strong, probably stemming from the traditional association of women with the home and children as well as a devaluation of these tasks by society, which made them perfect for women's oversight. For instance, Komsomol activists considered anything linked to the home or health as beneath serious concern and unworthy of real effort.[87]

This devaluation of work involving mothers did not mean it was easy. Nurse inspectors gave the same conflicting reports when inspecting families as they did when inspecting homes. Caught in the middle, nurse inspectors reprimanded mothers for the poor care of their children while at the same time pointing to examples of problems that complicated tasks. Admiration for the often herculean efforts of mothers to provide for families, children, and homes crept into some reports. For example, one nurse inspector detailed the offenses of one woman yet simultaneously concluded: "On the other hand, it is easy to see from the house budget that [the mother] buys milk for the baby even when there is not enough money to buy bread for the adults."[88] Despite such compassionate moments, being of the same gender did not automatically create a strong bond between inspector and mother. According to one set of complaints, many of those sent in to teach were unable to work with children of a young age, did not have a strong knowledge of how to feed or clothe children, and "generally committed a sizable number of rude mistakes in their work."[89] It is doubtful that such incompetence met an audience primed for compliance. In the characterizations of nurses in the propaganda, however, no such weakness appeared.

In theory it should have proven difficult for women to avoid the influence of the consultation and nurse inspector. If a woman did not seek out the consultation within two or three weeks of giving birth, the nurse was sent to fetch her. One text recommended visitation within no less than three days of giving birth.[90] Sometimes neighbors turned in those who were reluctant to visit the consultation. In one brief article the author recounted the story of a female worker who came early to the consultation to notify them of the birth of a child to another woman in her building. The mother had given birth to the child two weeks earlier and had still not come to the consultation. The worker was worried because the mother was getting "absurd" advice from some "old lady relative." As a "cultured" worker she "urgently" insisted that a nurse be sent to the mother.[91]

Once they identified the new mothers and gained entrance to their homes, the nurse inspectors agitated vociferously for hygienic measures. According to one description, "The nurse, going to the home of a child of the nursery, acquaints herself with the family structure. . . . She uses every good opportunity in order to persuade those around the child of the necessity of upholding proper sanitary hygienic measures to show the mother how to wash the child or prepare kasha or kissel, to help the mother clean the room, and so on. The nurse appears to be a friend of the family and the parents relate to her with complete confidence."[92] The nurse thus infiltrated the normal running of the home by demonstrating how to cook or clean properly. Plus, the nurse had to have extraordinary bedside manners to elicit "complete confidence" from her subjects. Though the author probably overstated the "friendliness" of the relationship between the nurse inspector and target family, the home visit facilitated the development of a very intimate, if coerced, relationship between the agents of the state and individuals.

The home visitation provided instruction not just through lectures and demonstrations but also by the example of the nurse herself: "The nurse of the consultation must be not just a good nurse but also a cultured person. She must be a good advocate for the conducting of life and the necessity of the scientific care of children." Through her example she fought the residual powers of the "midwives and old aunts" because "she must be able to counter their arguments and strengthen her own. She must be able to answer questions on law, housing, cooperation, and Soviet construction. . . . It is a bad nurse who cannot answer these questions."[93] A 1922 survey in Petrograd maintained that mothers changed their care in the following ways after visits from the nurse: mothers who fed their children improperly declined by 62 percent; those who diapered their child poorly declined by 12 percent; those who bathed their children incorrectly declined by 12 percent; those who did not care for sense organs correctly declined by 60 percent; and those who gave improper suckling dummies declined by 6 percent.[94] The small percentages attested to the great difficulty of effecting any lasting change in child care habits.

While the nurse wielded great power during inspections, she consulted with the doctor regularly and followed his directives. Although she expressed her own opinions in her reports, the literature repeatedly noted her inferior status. According to Antonov, the nurse served as "the eyes of the doctor and occasionally his hands." His description assigned the nurse the role of a passive observer who was active only as a vehicle to serve the doctor's will. The nurse was important as an extension of the doctor's authority. Equally important was the quick submission by the mother to the doctor's scrutiny. According to Antonov's text, the nurse was to urge new mothers to visit the consultation immediately in order to see the doctor. If the mother did not appear within a week, the nurse should visit her again and deliver the same message.[95] Ideally the nurse inspector functioned as an emissary of the state, a source not just of medical knowledge but also of political messages. Not wholly political and not completely domesticated, she occupied a unique position. This allowed her to break down the barrier between public and private, enter the home, point to the future, and serve as an ideal of feminine political involvement. She was an authority figure, albeit restricted to power within traditional female arenas and only under a doctor's supervision.

The strictures of the health regimen for children would have added considerably to women's household chores. If social services such as nurseries, communal kitchens, and laundries had been implemented on an adequate scale, the burden on women would have been less. These services were scarce, however, and there remained a great many tasks for women to perform. Undoubtedly many women regarded the new rules as a waste of time, luxuries they could ill afford. Popular fiction indicated there was some resistance. In one short story a "cultured" factory worker suggested to an old woman caring for some children that the crying baby probably wanted to be fed. The old woman responded that she could go get the mother from work and bring her to feed the child and then "he would stop crying—but these are not gentry children." And when the cultured woman recommended that milk and water be boiled, the old woman complained there was no time for such things.[96]

Authorities inadvertently recognized the problem, for they consistently cured troubled homes or families by ridding the home of children and sending them out of the house to the nursery, the Pioneers, the factory kitchen, or elsewhere.[97] The problems started at birth. The Home for Mothers and Infants aimed to soften the impact of this new burden on women by immediately giving them help in caring for the child right after delivery. One author praised the home because it allowed women to recover "physically and morally [*moral'no*]" from the difficulties of childbirth and rearing."[98] This perceived burden on women did not change as the child aged. Hygienists viewed child rearing as so detrimental to a woman's health that they developed a special House of Leisure in 1926 to allow women to take their yearly vacation away from their children. They argued that the normal course of leisure did not restore the working mother because "she does not spend her holiday in relaxation but instead stays connected to her child and her regular habits of daily life. She also shoulders not a small load of housework."[99] Although mothers and children traveled to the House of Leisure together, once there they split up into different areas. Children aged six months to three years stayed in a separate facility with a special dacha for nursing infants. The mothers of nursing children would see their children solely to nurse them. Older children remained completely out of reach.

Though set up to "shield" mothers from the influence of their children, the organizers must have encountered some difficulty in persuading women to spend time in these facilities. Most accounts of the program take great pains to present it as a tremendous resource for mothers, while also admitting that many mothers came to realize this only after an initial reluctance. Indeed, separation seemed to be quite an issue for most of the women involved. One article sarcastically joked: "The belief that no one except mothers or grandmothers can care for an infant caused several to sacrifice their relaxation and return, refusing to stay in the House of Leisure for even one day."[100] The author added that these women were "non-nursery" mothers to explain away their rejection, implying that they had an unnaturally strong attachment to their children and that they were nonworking mothers who were therefore less politically astute.

While attempting to point out the benefits, even the most flattering accounts noted the strong resistance of women to these vacations. Reports concentrated on the *eventual* joy they brought the mothers. One article described the first day as the worst, but by the second most mothers had calmed down and by the second week they felt better. Of course, in these propaganda pieces the women ultimately applauded the House of Leisure. In an "overheard" dinner conversation one woman remarked "in a timid voice: 'It's good that the children are taken to a separate dacha. Good that you see the children rarely or otherwise the kids would only be upset and act up and the mothers would cry bitter tears.'"[101]

Sanatorium stays, intended to combat an illness and not just provide a rest, similarly fortified women, according to propaganda. In a laudatory article one mother who had just completed a stay at a sanatorium voiced sentiments implying that returning home was injurious to her health: "I've become accustomed to it here. . . . I will not willingly go home. At home I cannot live so calmly and cleanly. There it is children, housework, and overcrowding. As soon as I leave . . . I will again be taken ill."[102] Statistics supported her assertion. According to data collected on women who had been in the night sanatorium, only 40 percent of cases achieved long-term recovery. In the other 60 percent the benefits were "short-lived." The researcher concluded that "no more than three weeks after release from the night sanatorium they worsen again under the combined influence of professional work, domestic work, and the unfavorable standard of living."[103] Interestingly, these articles in support of sanatoriums actually underscored the hopelessness of their efforts in the face of horrendous living conditions, perhaps setting them up for charges of being useless, wasteful expenditures.

Theorists voiced distaste for children and domestic life that revealed a certain amount of ambivalence toward parenthood. This contradiction sprang from conflicting feelings toward fertility. Although the state needed more children, the fecund, female body unnerved philosophers and health advocates. They depicted pregnant or menstruating women as diseased, frail, or contaminating. Following the birth, the relationship between mother and child caused concern that went beyond health care. Theorists deemed the love of a mother for her child irrational and antisocial. The close and closed bond removed children from state control and placed them totally in the private sphere. This distaste for the "egoism" of motherhood was quite evident in the works of hygienists.[104] They constantly urged women to enter into more social relationships in which the needs of their own children would be passed over in favor of those of society at large. Political involvement would solve social problems, allow the state to gain greater access to children, and foster communal feelings over selfish, individual love.

The maternity home served as a means of getting out the call for women's social activism. It was not merely a place to give birth hygienically but a place where patients could be transformed. Activists noted: "The mother herself undergoes the educational effect of the cultural, socially conscious atmosphere of the institution, which presents the typical selection of cultural enlightenment offerings like the club and lectures, discussions for the improvement of sanitation, as well as the social literacy of the mothers. . . . The mother learns not just the correct way to care for a child but also acquires social experience and an understanding of her deficiencies."[105] Certainly vulnerable, frightened, new mothers provided a ready audience for criticism of their "deficiencies." Other arenas also served as bases for these messages of societal duty and citizenship. In one short story about a factory worker who returned home to enlighten her village, the politically conscious female used the nursery as her headquarters and taught the children's mothers their social responsibilities through literacy lessons.[106]

Though the peasant women feared a "confiscation" of their children or something dire in the American model, the resources of Narkomzdrav and, to a lesser extent, the Department for the Protection of Motherhood and Infancy assured them that this would not occur. What nurse Haines witnessed was probably not so much a reality of daily life for every Soviet mother as a Potemkin clinic set up to impress foreign visitors. Those involved, however, claimed they had made great strides: "On the vast front of achievements on the tenth anniversary of the October Revolution, successes in the protection of mothers and infants occupy an important place."[107] Nevertheless, maternal and child welfare institutions declined by nearly half in the early years of NEP. Despite economic recovery, services remained inadequate.[108] For example, between 1919 and 1923 the number of children served by nurseries rose by 63 percent, while the number of working women rose by 121 percent. In 1925, under the aegis of the Moscow Department of Health, there were 102 nurseries with spaces for 5,145 children; only 2 homes for mothers and children that cured 570 children and 522 mothers; and 20 birth homes that served 50,311 mothers.[109]

Birth homes probably came closest to caring for the entire population. In 1923 statistics for Moscow reported 50,474 births, which slightly outstripped the resources available two years later.[110] The consultations were much more active, with thirty-one consultations for children with 599,852 visitors and twenty-seven consultations for mothers with 181,434 visitors. Despite these low numbers, Moscow institutions generally accounted for roughly a fifth of the total number of institutions in each category in the Russian federation.[111] Even the most dedicated activists recognized that it would take a long time for services to meet the needs of women in urban areas and even longer to reach rural women.[112]

While services remained inadequate, Soviet health care activists declared the campaign against the midwife a success. Organizers claimed that by 1927 Moscow maternity homes housed 90 percent of births in the city. The number of women going to the consultation also increased. According to supporters, it was the "rare" woman who did not visit the consultation for pregnant women.[113] They also rated the work of the home visitation as highly effective. According to statistics from one district in Moscow, 75 percent of the nurse's suggestions were carried out by those visited.[114] Due to a lack of personnel and popular preference, even optimists admitted that the campaign in the countryside was not nearly as successful.[115]

Despite the low numbers, hygienists claimed that the programs succeeded in their primary objective of lowering the infant death rate. According to official statistics, in 1913 28 percent of children died before the end of their first year. By 1926 the infant death rate reportedly dropped to just 13 percent.[116] If so, protective labor legislation also contributed to the decline in infant mortality, as did an improved food situation. Increased and better urban sanitation obviously improved the living standards for thousands of Muscovites. The programs of the Department for the Protection of Motherhood and Infancy, while certainly important, constituted just one part of the sanitary improvements in the city.

Propagandists urged women to provide cleaner environments for their children and entrust them to Soviet care. To spread this message and help raise a plummeting birth rate, Narkomzdrav set up institutions for the aid and instruction of mothers and children. The importance of strong infants to the Soviet state stimulated the involvement of health care authorities in private life.[117] The consultation and the attendant visiting nurse spread the message of natal health throughout the city and parts of the countryside. Not completely satisfied, organizers claimed a qualified success. In her ten-year assessment, Nogina, head of the Moscow Department for the Protection of Motherhood and Infancy, stated: "Though we cannot say that we have completely changed the lives of mother-workers, the lives of nursing children have undoubtedly changed."[118]

Spotless homes, well-scrubbed children, and rigid schedules represented the ideal. Activists urged mothers to implement these changes at home even as they were being told to abandon their four walls to mother all of society. Although reformers emphasized child rearing as a social responsibility, they also encouraged volunteerism, claiming that by denying the egoism of the private family, women would emerge from darkness and be more fully integrated in society.

As an added benefit, through volunteerism women would become politically aware Soviet citizens. Instead of the double burden of laboring and mothering that Lenin had associated with capitalism in 1899, activists created a triple burden for the ideal Soviet woman, who now had to be a laborer, mother to her child, and mother to all of society.[119] In 1923 Lebedeva, head of the Russian Department for the Protection of Motherhood and Infancy, admitted that while it would take time, she predicted that ten years hence women would happily become mothers once they were freed of their obligations relating to child care.[120] Ironically, hygienists argued that women would happily become mothers only when they were free of their children.

6 The Body

Hygiene, Modernity, and Mentality

The clock ruled life—or at least that was what the 1927 poster "8 Hours for Leisure—8 Hours for Sleep—8 Hours for Work" implied (plate 4). While pictures of daily activities obscured the fact of it, the overarching reality and template against which these activities were measured was the clock. A giant twenty-four-hour timepiece, it formed the background to, and synchronized the rhythms of, daily life. The man's factory workstation connected him to a machine belt, suggesting that at work he joined a timepiece, his rhythms dictated by the turning of the drive and the pace of the factory. For life beyond the range of the factory whistle, clocklike circles of action framed images of leisure, sleep, and club, thus subjecting these actions to the clock's rule as well.

While the poster's final slogan declared "Physical Culture Proceeds 24 Hours a Day," only two of the fourteen scenes depicted athletic activities. Instead, the viewer beheld an entire day rationally laid out: cleanliness recommendations—a morning wash in the basin, washing hands before meals, brushing teeth, and showering at the factory or *bania;* nutrition advice—a light breakfast and dinner with a factory cafeteria luncheon; and leisure time suggestions—reading in isolation, skating, calisthenics, and reading aloud at the club. The pie sections of the clock were color-coded to show their level of usage: blue for sleep, dark red for work, and lighter red for leisure. This device implied that all activities during one's waking hours should be "red-centered" and devoted to communist concerns.

Beyond the clock's realm, to the left and right, were slogans denouncing those activities that remained alien to a Soviet life, namely, heavy drinking and smoking. Not forming part of the vision, they were not illustrated. The poster's artist also omitted other aspects of daily life. Even though the poster was intended for both urban and rural areas, the healthy life was not on the farm but in the factory. To the exclusion of many, the healthy individual was male, Russian, and literate. While showers and eating took place in communal areas, the worker slept and lived in a seemingly private room with a single bed—highly unlikely in the overcrowded city. The sole female figure appeared in the factory cafeteria. No women were featured in the club scene or on the factory floor, not to mention in the worker's insular home.

This poster, including its omissions and overarching vision of health as a twenty-four-hour pursuit, represented the main themes of propaganda concerning individual behavior. Orderliness, abstemiousness, and physical conditioning were prescribed as promoting well-being for the individual and the entire body Soviet. This poster as well as other propaganda argued that the perfected individual, as both a citizen and a worker, could streamline government, increase production, and speed the transition to communism. Regularized, mechanistic behavior served as the ideal in a society focused on production as a result of its governing ideology and the necessity of postwar recovery. Militaristic calls to action and drill-like physical activity functioned as the model for proper behavior, with political implications for those who did not produce. Indulgence in alcohol, sex, or tobacco did not fit the definition of proper comportment, and those who so strayed had to be "cleansed" through physical activity and by eschewing licentious behavior. Activists' assumptions of their audience—basically male, urban, and industrial—colored their vision. Others did not escape instruction but instead were inscribed with inferiority. Women, softened by their pulsing, productive center, could not triumph over their biologically determined, scientifically affirmed inadequacy. Peasants, ignorant and infantilized, could not learn outside what was the province of workers. When urban males became the ideal, women and peasants fell to an inferior status that did not permit them to attain their full productive potential and active political citizenship.

This message, however, was not received by a compliant population. Material problems guaranteed that there would be difficulties for all—even among those willing to follow the hygienists' restrictions—and that resistance, contention, and rejection would greet the other recommendations. Some saw echoes of revolution in filthy clothes and argued for different definitions of dirt. Still more saw no reason to wear simple yet clean clothing when fashionable clothing could serve as a marker of identity. Rules governing behavior were similarly contested. Abstention from drinking, smoking, and sex were not merely inconvenient. Many thought that such behavior marked true revolutionaries. Hygienists did not cast propaganda onto cleared, fertile ground. The Soviet body was a battlefield.

In a society obsessed with progress and industrialization, the machine, the ultimate symbol of the modern age, became a metaphor for the perfection of humanity. The pervasive concern for industrial growth and a strong working class ensured that simple mechanistic metaphors would be understood by the general populace. Hygienists readily applied the language of the factory to commentaries on the body and adapted the rhythm of the industrial clock to health prescriptions, just as it had been used by industrialists the world over.[1] With his 1918 collection *Poetry of the Worker's Blow*, Aleksei Gastev became the prophet of the clock in Russia. Although initially critical of Taylorism, which he considered the triumph of capitalism's application of science to production, Lenin himself thought the technique could be adopted by the Soviets; he even put a Gastev poster up in his office.[2] With high-level backing and a ready audience, Gastev inspired over eight hundred cells and eight laboratories for the Scientific Organization of Labor (Nauchnaia organizatsiia truda [NOT]) by the end of 1924.[3] Gastev's courses, based on European biomechanics, were studied by over half a million Russians. Although his ideas came under official fire for too closely tying man to machine, his concept of the mechanized body remained popular throughout the 1920s. Other theorists and groups also conceived of the body as a machine, such as the Time League, which focused on wasted time rather than mechanized man. The Time League was disbanded in 1926, while NOT remained active until 1929.[4]

Inspired by the rhythmic lines of Gastev's poems, NOT cells sought to improve production by regulating the body at work. Drawing upon socialist ideas of the nature of labor, Gastev depicted work as integral to human development. He noted, however, that if done improperly, work strained the body. By modifying movement, training the body, and rationalizing work, Gastev hoped to make labor more efficient, thereby getting the most out of each worker. As he observed, "We live the best parts of our lives at work. We must learn how to work so that work will be easy and a constant school of life."[5] Gastev theorized that in this "school of life" mimicking the movement of machines would transform men into more efficient and productive human/machine hybrids, attaining rationalized thought as they became rationalized in movement.[6] In one of his mechanistically paced poems, Gastev hammered away at this theme:

The machine-automat works precisely,
QUICKLY AND EXACTLY
—as is its habit, so does it proceed—
and the factory depends upon the regulations.
With a human it is just the same
the regulation of the body
the regulation of nerves
the definition of movement
the definition of labor skills.
In the beginning movement (work) proceeds with difficulty.
But just begin to work out
REG-U-LA-TION,
movements proceed surefootedly, exactly, quickly.
Regulation gives step-by-step
TRAINING.
This training may exactly calculate and
EASE
Training can develop
QUICK TRANSITIONS
from one directive to another.[7]

Gastev emphasized the repetition of actions as a way to condition reflexes, nerves, and the mind to perfected movements and also rapid change. Adaptation would take time but would eventually develop into habit. The poem concluded by explaining the political benefits of rationalized movement. A conditioned body moved easily from one point to the next, from one system to the next. Ultimately labor training would impel revolution.

Machines and their inherent control became a powerful vision for a people obsessed with disorder. Health writers incorporated the metaphor of the body as machine into recommendations for leisure, nutrition, and rest. In *Labor and Health of Worker Youth* (1925), Doctor Sigal devoted an entire chapter to the theme "How the Living Machine Works."[8] A 1922 program circulated as part of an adult enlightenment curriculum recommended that during the first fifteen hours of class, students be instructed in the concept of "the human machine carrying out work . . . and the skeleton and muscles of a man as a mechanism."[9] Gastev further extended the machine metaphor to fueling the body. In his 1923 collection *Youth Come Forward!,* Gastev warned: "The body must be cared for like a working machine," that it had to be carefully monitored by the clock and in terms of fuel.[10] Gastev outlined a fifteen-day work, rest, and food schedule:

III. 15 Spring Days in 1921
A. Organism's Activity:

	per day	*total*
Mental labor	9 hrs. 32 min.	143 hrs.
Physical labor	1 hr. 28 min.	22 hrs.
Hiking	1 hr. 30 min.	22½ hrs.
Sleep	5 hrs.	75½ hrs.
Unaccounted	– hr. – min.	– hr.
Domestic labor	6 hrs. 30 min.	97½ hrs.
	24 hrs.15 min.	360 hrs.

B. Quantity of Food:

Black bread	8½ lbs.
Onion	4 lbs.
Potatoes	4 lbs.
Nuts	2 lbs.
Dried apples in water	1 lb.
Water	18 lbs.[11]

Not a minute was wasted; not a second left unconsumed by sleep, labor, or physical activity. Gastev expanded the hours of the day and did not allow for any unaccounted time. Hence one may conclude that such a possibility as unexploited time was not within his idealized vision.

In his exhausting schedule, which was devoid of leisure time, Gastev made no allowance for gastronomic excess or, seemingly, enjoyment. Regulation of time, body, and food intake were combined in Gastev's advocacy of a simple, meat-free diet. The mechanistic turn merged with an already present interest in food both within and outside Russia. Consumption rarely concerns just the maintenance of the physical body. As John F. Kasson points out regarding the Victorian diet, "The ways people feed their physical bodies express larger concerns about the needs and perils of the *social* body."[12] In Russia food and politics intertwined in visions of politically active eating. Chernyshevskii had his ideal revolutionary Rakhmetov eat simple fare—such as ham, black bread, and nearly raw beefsteak, which he gnawed methodically—while eschewing luxuries like fruit, veal, poultry, and sugar.[13] The emphasis on chewing—an obsession of nutritionists worldwide—may have come from a concern for cultivating controlled, genteel behavior even as it was cloaked in admonitions about care of the digestive tract. Rather than wolfing down his food, the new man controlled his intake in quantity, quality, and speed by cultivating the solitary virtue of mastication.

The prophylactic benefit of dietary management was an issue that crossed international borders at the end of the nineteenth century. The importance of nutrition in combating diseases like tuberculosis was first recognized at this time and increased as statistics from distressed countries during World War I made the links between disease and diet self-evident. In addition, European theorists linked diet to productivity and investigated how much food intake would yield the maximum amount of work output. German theorists in the 1880s conducted careful studies of the calories needed to complete tasks. In the early twentieth century research on vitamins in Britain and the United States led to even greater interest in dietary health.[14] Dietary regulation arose from this interest in diet and the acknowledgment of food-borne pathogens as a cause of many diseases.

Even before these scientific forays into food quality, the mouth was a charged site—a portal to bodily pollution and possible contamination. Utopians, already worried about the purity of the environment, now concerned themselves with bodily purity and the protection of those areas subject to penetration—the mouth, the eyes, and other orifices. As early as the 1500s utopians had declared dietary regulation a key not just to temporary good health but to the prolongation of life and the creation of an ordered world. In the nineteenth century doctors began to express concern over diet in an attempt to define a proper lifestyle for the middle class. Prophets of whole foods, vegetarian diets, and other permutations of healthy eating emerged throughout Europe and the United States.[15] For the Bolsheviks consumption of food, like any type of consumption, had greater meaning since they suffered from what Eric Naiman terms "revolutionary anorexia." For example, in *For Love of Worker Bees* Kollontai detailed her heroine's diet of birdlike portions of simple foods and contrasted her slight, wiry frame with the fleshy NEP women.[16] The characters passed on more delectable dishes in a symbolic rejection of all pleasures associated with capitalism. Not merely an issue for novelists, dietary control also obsessed reformers during the 1920s, with nutrition-related pamphlets and posters readily cautioning against improper dietary fueling of the machine man. For proper digestion, Soviet reformers recommended serving food at medium temperature, eating slowly and in small bites, and thoroughly chewing before swallowing. In addition to avoiding spirits, pregnant women were advised to avoid meaty, salty, or spicy foods.[17]

Hygienists expressed concern not only about what was eaten but also how much. Writers recommended limiting the intake of water. According to Commissar of Health Semashko, "The most common method through which infection enters the body seems to be our mouths and our digestive organs.

Most often this infection comes through water."[18] Zheleznyi advised drinking only four to five glasses of water a day.[19] This emphasis on curtailing water intake stood in sharp contrast to American advice to youth at the time, which recommended a minimum of four glasses of water a day. Given the prevalence of water-borne diseases in Russia, it seemed a sensible suggestion.[20] Semashko recommended the boiling of water to eliminate infectious agents.[21]

For the ill, beginning in 1924 cafeterias specifically geared to dietary regulations served the needs of the community, either at hospitals or other health institutions. They all required that patients be admitted by a doctor, adhere strictly to the regimen, and submit to supervision. As with other prophylactic institutions, these cafeterias offered indoctrination along with treatment. Within five years the staff of such cafeterias in Moscow had given five thousand lectures on food-related themes and seen more than forty thousand patients.[22] According to a questionnaire given to workers on the first anniversary of these cafeterias, the majority of the respondents said they had learned "'how to eat in order to be healthy, to wash hands before eating, to not rush eating, to chew food well, and to pay attention to the work of the intestines."[23] Clean hands and regulated consumption figured prominently in these laudatory results. The success of the cafeterias, according to these statements, lay as much in *how* the patrons ate as in *what* they ate.

Food preparation met with similar in-depth discussions since it had special meaning for nutritional health, women's liberation, communal life, and management of resources. The communal dining hall was a fixture of the utopian vision. Chernyshevskii wrote of huge communal dining halls in his utopia, as did Bellamy.[24] Communal dining liberated women from kitchen duty, freeing them for political participation while fostering a communal spirit. During civil war and famine, the Soviets experimented with communal dining halls. To committed communists communal dining, which optimized the preparation of scarce goods, seemed the ideal method of feeding the population. The cafeteria could also help in the civilizing mission by supplying clean tablecloths, placing fresh-cut flowers on tables, and providing musical accompaniment while dining.

It would take far more than posies and a piano to make diners ignore the highly unpalatable offerings of the communal cafeteria. In 1923 People's Nutrition (Narodnoe pitanie [Narpit]) was established to oversee the feeding of the general population. From the very beginning it battled funding problems and unsanitary conditions.[25] The Soviet press printed lurid details of the filth, poor ventilation, and health problems. One well-publicized outbreak of scurvy was associated with a Kremlin cafeteria. By 1926 Narpit fed only about 11 percent of workers and 5.5 percent of the Moscow population as a whole because of inadequate funding, a bad reputation, and limited working kitchens; those that did work produced inferior food at higher prices than home-cooked meals. Worries about food preparation, quality, and care led to the assignment of health inspectors to restaurants and grocery stores.[26]

Home dining was hardly more pleasant or hygienic. The persistence of shortages meant high prices and a limited selection. The average worker existed on a starch-heavy diet of bread, soup, kasha, and potatoes. Even this spare diet cost more than it had before the revolution, and the time needed to forage for these meager provisions was substantial.[27] Hygienists' exhortations to eat moderately meant little to the average worker, who was forced to subsist on a miserable diet. Dietary advice engaged those who had greater access to resources and who perhaps felt the need—because of this relative luxury—to show off their revolutionary fervor in their eating habits.[28] Possibly, activists recommended eating modestly to make people feel better about the diet they were forced to accept. Overall, attempts to revolutionize food consumption had only a limited effect. According to the 1923 all-union health survey of worker youth, the majority ate at home and only around 10 percent ate in cafeterias or artels.[29]

In addition to describing the fueling of the "machine man," reformers often employed militaristic rhetoric. The military, like the machine, served as a popular image of efficiency and strength, but it had the additional benefit of denoting struggle and heroism. For a population recently emerged from war, as well as one warned of the inevitability of a coming war, military metaphors certainly toned portentiously. Moreover, military imagery recalled the camaraderie and bravery that was important to those who had made sacrifices in the civil war and proved attractive to young men and boys who had not participated in the revolution.[30]

A fiery call to arms that asked Pioneers to remember their fathers' tales of valorous sacrifice prefaced the 1925 pamphlet *How Does One Live to Be Healthy?*, in which Zheleznyi cautioned that it was time to take stock in this period of rest before the inevitable storm. He continued, "And we would be poor combatants if we were unable to use this reprieve to prepare for a new attack. We must necessarily rejuvenate and save our physical strength—it is our gunpowder. . . . And tomorrow, for the new attack, we must be able to send into the battle iron groups of young and old Leninists—healthy, courageous, and strong in battle—for the enemy is strong. No one knows when that 'tomorrow' will be. Perhaps after a year, maybe after five, but we know one thing, namely, that Pioneers must come to the relief of the Komsomol and the party, and those reinforcements must be healthy."[31] Zheleznyi's thundering prose elevated health to an issue of defense and citizenship. The text also drove home the point that

NEP represented a temporary respite. The real battle of building communism and struggling against capitalism still lay ahead.

The poster entitled "All Athletes to the Front Lines of the Lenin Workers!" (1921–25) used similar military metaphors, together with images of industrial might, to connect the strength of the individual body with that of the country (plate 5). The slogan evoked martial imagery by ordering workers to assemble at the "front lines," with the purposeful group of athletes marching together resembling a military parade. Male and female athletes hiked, biked, and ran toward the forge, where men in red athletic outfits stood at anvils tempering this raw, human metal for the industrial cause, symbolized by smokestacks at right. These gigantic blacksmiths dwarfed the masses. Dressed in unusual work attire, these red-infused personages functioned as a portal to a new life by showing how bodily maintenance paved the way to industrial productivity and eventual state triumph. Physical fitness characterized the makers of the new, industrial state and prepared them to take their positions. The red color of the metalworkers denoted the political consequences for the individual during this transitional period. The white clothing of the marchers symbolized a state of physical purity as they prepared for their political transformation.

Military metaphors were applied at the cellular level, with the body the arena where battles between sickness and health were waged. In a poem published in the magazine *To a New Life!* in 1925, the healthy body itself became a line of defense requiring fortification:

Know and remember all—
These are not just simple phrases.
Every healthy person
Is an unassailable fortress
Against tuberculosis.[32]

Although disease and microbes attacked the body, people could buttress themselves against this onslaught by maintaining good health. Semashko employed the "fortress" metaphor in his book *Social Illnesses* (1926). Cautioning readers not to partake of things that weakened the body, he declared: "If you sleep around [*polunochnichaesh'*], dragging about to different places, then it is self-evident that you destroy your fortress."[33]

Whether it was a call to arms or the clock, recommendations for change followed. To improve health, authors of propaganda pamphlets recommended regimentation and cleanliness, with special attention paid to clothes and teeth. If readers followed these suggestions, they predicted a future without disease, where technology and prosperity benefited everyone. This belief in the powers of a proper regimen echoed conceptions of conduct and health by religious and secular philosophers. Medieval monastic orders in Russia and Europe expounded at length on the regulation of the body as part of their codes of conduct. European Enlightenment philosophers resuscitated the Hippocratic philosophy, which preached that life could be prolonged and preserved through healthy diet and exercise. In the nineteenth century utopian communities sprouted up everywhere. They advocated an ordered lifestyle as a way to transcend present woes and move on to a better life either in this world or the next.[34] Soviet ideology continued to emphasize the links between behavior and health.

Keeping to stringent schedules emerged as the essence of a healthy life.[35] Zheleznyi told Pioneers, "The first step is to put your day in order—when and how much to sleep, to work, to eat . . . therefore the first step is keeping track of time."[36] The pamphlet *Workers Take Hold of Your Health* argued that the way one lived during scheduled times was equally important: "A normal way of life demands work in a healthy situation, correct leisure, adequate sleep (no less than seven hours every twenty-four hours), and exercising all parts of the body." Within this schedule moderation was key: "Labor, correct leisure, adequate food intake, normal sex life for adults, and sports for all ages—these are the foundations of a healthy life."[37] All activities had qualifiers to show their corrrect utilization. The term "correct" or the ubiquitous "normal" denoted not just the duration of these events but their proper completion. In their sample schedules hygienists made sure every moment was usefully employed. The rule of the clock regulated lives down to the second, implying that unscheduled time was wasted—and even unhealthy—time.

The regimen involved not just scheduling of when to sleep and wake but how to perform these activities and others throughout the day. Following bathing, sleep was to be accompanied by fresh air in a clean, single bed free of bedbugs.[38] Some advice literature went even further, instructing readers to lie down at the same time every night and avoid anything that might cause too much excitement before bed, such as reading, eating, working, or fighting. They must wear nightclothes (the writers did not specify whether this was in preference to nudity or street clothes), sleep on linens changed every two weeks, and use a firm mattress aired weekly.[39] Schedules were quite detailed. Pioneers were to train themselves to wake at the same time every morning (7:30 a.m.) and to rise quickly.[40] The following activities could fill their healthful day:

7:30–9:00	After getting up, do calisthenics; make bed; wash/dress accurately; tighten belt. Breakfast. Walk quickly to school.

9:00–1:00	While in school: campaign for cleanliness; sit up straight; care for eyesight; organize games during breaks.
1:00–2:00	Home: Wash hands and eat without rushing.
2:00–3:00	Rest. A walk.
3:00–5:00	Reading (or lessons); light handiwork.
5:00–6:30	Housework: Agitate for sun and clean air and against dust and insects.
6:30–7:00	Dinner. Walk to group.
7:00–9:30	Group.
9:30–10:00	Walk home from group. Prepare for bed by washing hands and legs and brushing teeth.
10:30	Sleep.[41]

Catriona Kelly argues that these recommendations for children were not just intended to teach them about regimens but also to infuse their lives with a sense of time and its passing.[42]

Schedules stressed daily cleansing and credited a good wash with benefits beyond the removal of dirt. After rising, washing with room-temperature water and briskly drying oneself with a rough towel assured "very good spirits," according to *The Path to Health* (1926).[43] Contemporary Europeans recommended a cold-water splash to increase circulation, improve skin tone, and calm nerves. They insisted that hot baths contributed to poor constitutions and laziness.[44] Soviet writer V. Sukharev similarly noted the ability of a cold-water wash to "strengthen health [and] . . . calm the nervous system."[45] The emphasis on cold water fit in with calls for austerity and necessity, given the problems of finding not just water but warm water in the capital. The cold-water wash was integral to the Soviet battle for *zakalennost'*, or steeliness, and this brisk morning adventure helped to improve physical and mental health, especially in men.[46] Aside from these effects on the mind, bathing combated skin diseases and parasitic infections.[47] People were advised to wash their hands before eating and do so several times a day.[48] During the morning wash, the subject needed to scrub the "face, neck, hands, and even the torso to the waist" with soap.[49] Campaigns where the population was urged to use the *bania* for free were shown to increase attendance and fight social diseasess.[50] Organizers saw the *bania* as a frontline defense to promote civilized living. Hygienists urged readers to "Get into the Cultured Habit—Change Underwear and Go to the *Bania* Weekly" (figure 6.1). The *bania* was "a necessity—to cleanse the body of sweat and grease secreted by the skin and also from casually acquired lice, which, if caught quickly, did not have sufficient time to multiply."[51]

Maintaining healthy eyes, ears, and nose were a distinct concern since they were viewed as delicate. "If you ruin your eyes, you cannot buy new ones," advised Mol'kov.[52] Another pamphlet recommended reading with adequate lighting and at a proper distance, always wearing glasses (if prescribed), and using only a sanitized cloth to cleanse the eyes. The writer warned that one should read from no closer than thirty centimeters, with the light source on the left or straight ahead.[53] These detailed recommendations for eye care accompanied instructions for ear and nose care, including never putting matches or sharp objects in either orifice.[54]

Questions of dental hygiene occupied an inordinate amount of space compared with that for eye and ear care because of presumed links to stomach ailments, fertility, and general nutrition. Almost every pamphlet recommended brushing twice daily, with a visit to the dentist every six months to round out the regimen.[55] An ode to dentistry published in the magazine *To a New Life!* instructed readers to brush twice daily for three minutes at a time, while *Take Hold of Your Health!* advised in which direction to brush upper and lower teeth.[56] Mol'kov emphasized brushing's connection to good nutrition and good eating habits, since without strong teeth workers could not chew food completely.[57] Hygienists also warned that rotting teeth led to stomach ailments and could harm the fetus of pregnant women.[58]

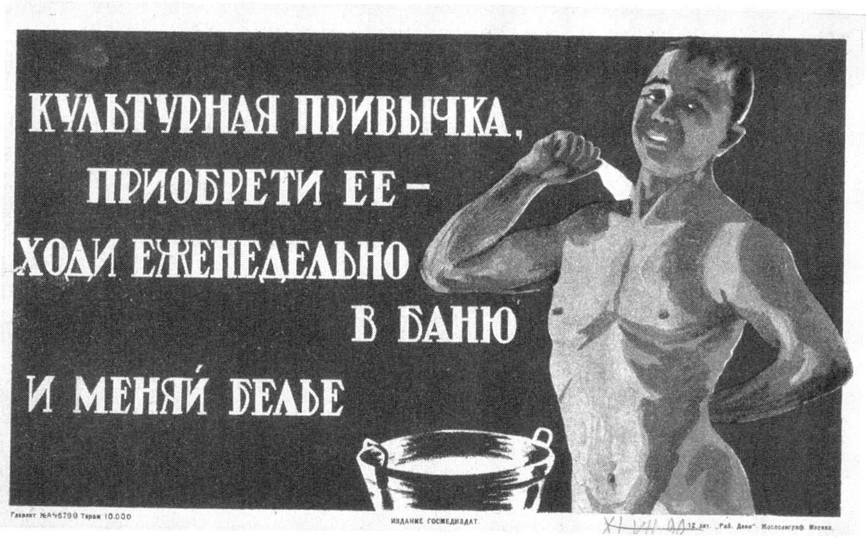

FIGURE 6.1. "Get into the Cultured Habit—Change Underwear and Go to the *Bania* Weekly." Moscow: Gosmedizdat, 1926–29. Pub. 10,000. Courtesy of the Russian State Library.

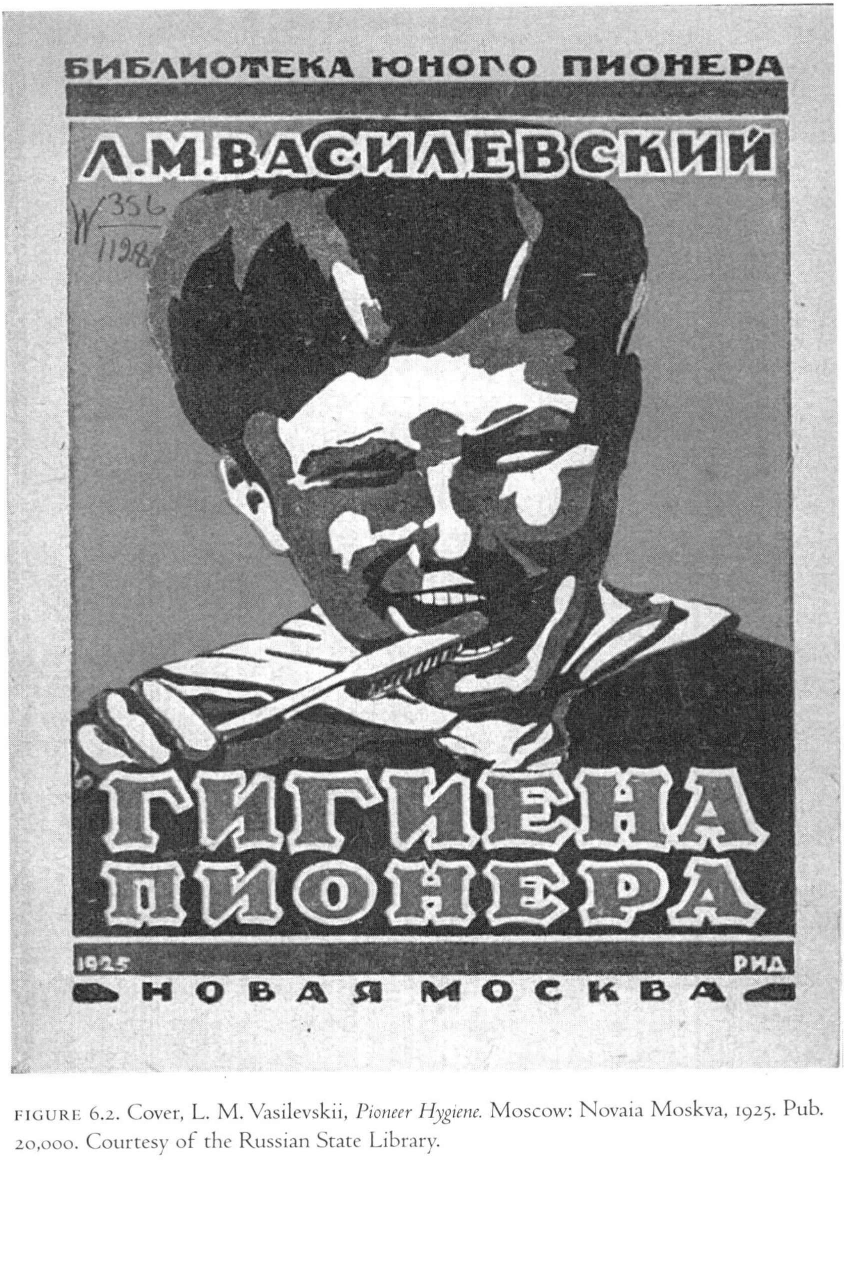
БИБЛИОТЕКА ЮНОГО ПИОНЕРА
Л.М.ВАСИЛЕВСКИЙ
ГИГИЕНА
ПИОНЕРА
1925
РИД
НОВАЯ МОСКВА

FIGURE 6.2. Cover, L. M. Vasilevskii, *Pioneer Hygiene.* Moscow: Novaia Moskva, 1925. Pub. 20,000. Courtesy of the Russian State Library.

Brushing one's teeth also reflected a cultural attainment. The cover of *Pioneer Hygiene* (1925) summed up the book's message with a smiling Pioneer wielding an enormous toothbrush, thus privileging this habit above all other hygiene issues (figure 6.2). One hygiene poster equated brushing with personality traits of precision and vigor: "Be Accurate. Don't Be Lazy. Clean Your Teeth—Daily" (figure 6.3). Workers themselves recognized brushing as a sign of advancement. At a meeting in 1927, one worker declared, "The cultural level of the working masses has risen markedly and therefore the needs of the working class for medical help have also risen. Who among the workers would have cared earlier for their teeth? Now, when a tooth just starts to darken, we are already at the dentist's because we understand the connection that exists between tooth pain and gastric illnesses."[59] For this worker interest in dental health signified enlightenment and the progress of science. The rising cultural level of workers was reflected in frequent visits to the dentist.

In propaganda posters and pamphlets hygienists portrayed the male body as normative. In fact, the cover of Vasilevskii's *Hygiene of Women's Labor* (1925) featured a man doing work as part of the series's seal.[60] Pamphlets set out different strictures for men and women on the subject of cleanliness, implying that women suffered from unique problems. Hygienists betrayed a distinct discomfort with women's bodies and their sexual function by delineating sex-specific

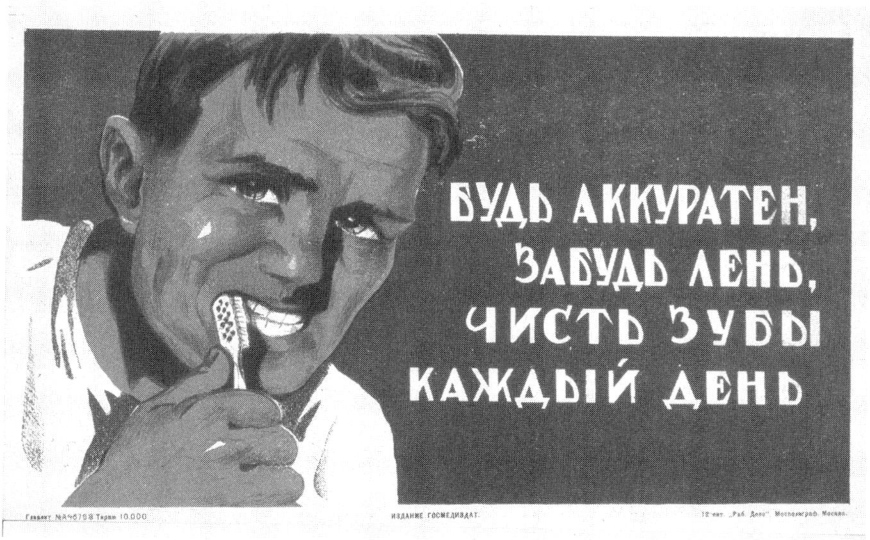
БУДЬ АККУРАТЕН,
ЗАБУДЬ ЛЕНЬ,
ЧИСТЬ ЗУБЫ
КАЖДЫЙ ДЕНЬ
ИЗДАНИЕ ГОСМЕДИЗДАТ.

FIGURE 6.3. "Be Accurate. Don't Be Lazy. Clean Your Teeth—Daily." Moscow: Gosmedizdat, 1926–29. Pub. 10,000. Courtesy of the Russian State Library.

cleansing needs since menstruation made women dirtier and more vulnerable to infection. N. Iu. Lur'e opened the 1927 pamphlet *The Hygiene of Girls, Young Women, and Women* with instructions on how to maintain the procreative health of young girls, addressing the danger of the female body to the newborn child, and noting the risks of women's sexually transmitted diseases to newborns. Lur'e detailed the special strictures that menstruating women must follow to maintain cleanliness and reproductive health. She decried the traditional treatment of menstruation, where, she contended, the changing of underwear was not considered necessary. Furthermore, Lur'e described the secretion of blood by a woman as a means of infection for those who came into contact with her. A threat to others, menstruation weakened the woman's own ability to resist infection. Sexual contact could lead to infection since during menses "the very womb becomes like an open wound" through which "every manner of microbe" may infect the woman.[61] In the pamphlet *Women's Sexual Health* (1927) Dembskaia wrote that during menstruation "the blood, flowing from the womb, serves as a kind of bridge" for microbial infection.[62] In the West doctors similarly cautioned women about their weakened state during menstruation.[63]

While writers of Soviet health pamphlets warned women of these dangers, they also advised them that emanations from the womb discomfited others. Menstrual blood, if not properly contained, could "flow down on the hips, quite often emitting a nasty [*skvernyi*] smell." All this caused "an unpleasant feeling in the woman menstruating and in those around her."[64] Vasilevskii, concerned about this "unpleasant odor," insisted that "one of the most important hygienic concerns in a girl's life" was proper care of her body.[65] Hygienists legitimated popular repugnance concerning women's procreative functions by giving medical credence to long-standing assumptions regarding women's cleanliness; these cautions reflected miasmatic fear of odors as well as traditional religious prohibitions against menstruating women.[66] Because of the heightened danger of menstruation to the woman and to those around her, the standard cleansing was insufficient. Instead of the cold-water wash recommended for men and nonmenstruating women, Dembskaia prescribed a hot-water wash.[67] This may have reflected a perceived weakness since cold water invigorated and strengthened, but here warm water was recommended. For pregnant women the strictures were even more detailed, indicating that it was not simply the emission of bodily fluids that endangered women. Perhaps this anxiety reflected concern over the hidden, and therefore suspect and dangerous nature of women's sexual organs. The aroused male organ was evident, but female arousal—and vaginal activity—was not always obvious. In any case, cleanliness strictures for pregnant women reflected concern over sex organs in operation. Antonov recommended that pregnant women go to the *bania* twice weekly and clean themselves with boiled water and soap daily.[68]

Women's health manuals addressed more than just the cleanliness and mechanics of the body. They also advised on beauty and fashion as aspects of health. V. E. Dembskaia's *Individual Hygiene for Women: Caring for Health and Beauty* (1927) opened with a chapter on beauty. She deemed makeup unnecessary, "from either a hygienic or aesthetic point of view," but she stressed the need for women to accentuate their natural beauty.[69] For healthy skin, women must wash with warm water and soap and expose their skin to clean air and sunlight. The author of *The Young Woman and the Komsomol* (1927) opposed makeup and artificial beauty enhancements, noting that the joys of powder and perfume were short-lived.[70] Other articles observed that rouge and lipstick, which were necessary in capitalist countries, where women had to hide their pasty complexions, lost their necessity in a country ruled by and for workers.[71] In addition to health considerations, writers attacked makeup as a waste of time, emphasizing an ideal of beauty not tied to work, strength, or any Marxist attributes. Instead of makeup, health manuals equated beauty with cleanliness.[72]

All these special strictures for the washing of face, neck, hands, and torso meant little if a woman or man wore dirty clothing. The pamphlet *Hygiene and Health of the Worker and His Family* (1925) argued: "The soiling of the skin and clothing may serve as a source of different illnesses, so it is necessary to keep this from happening by maintaining careful care of skin and clothing."[73] In 1926 in his *Science of a Healthy Society (Social Hygiene)* Semashko wrote: "Dirty clothing pollutes and infects our body. Infection of all kinds is transferred by dirty clothing and underwear. That is why among dirty people skin diseases are so widespread."[74] Clean clothing prevented infection and became a matter of social duty. The pamphlet *How Does One Live to Be Healthy?* argued that clothing was the body's "mobile dwelling" (*podvizhnoe zhilishche*). It insisted that underwear had to be changed at least once a week and that outerwear should never be worn without a protective layer of linens.[75] Outer clothing could be reworn if cleaned with a brush, but underclothes had to be changed.[76] Dirty clothing did more than endanger the wearer; it made others uncomfortable. Semashko concluded, "It can be unpleasant for all those around if somebody sits down at the theater or movie in dirty, stinking, greasy clothing." He further noted that cleanliness was "a sign of culture [*kul'turnost'*] and respect for oneself and others."[77]

It seemed that clothes did make the man, and better clothes made for a better man. Soviet designers theorized that clothing could alter personality and action. For example, one book advised pioneers: "Comfortable clothes facilitate work, while dirty, torn clothes put the imprint of untidiness on study and work. That is why the military demands from its Red Army men that they are always dressed smartly and accurately."[78] Semashko commented upon the same idea in his *Art of Dressing* (1927), where he applauded the use of color, arguing that "the more cheerful and joyous life will be, the more cheerful and joyous clothing will be."[79] Hygienic clothing permitted free movement and circulation.[80] Vasilevskii counseled Pioneers to wear clothing that was open at the neck, exposed hands, and covered legs to the knee, and to go barefoot during the summer.[81] For women the choice of garment was tied to health as well as political fitness. Reformers cautioned women to avoid fashionable dress, such as unstable high heels, constricting waistlines, and long skirts that gathered up dust. Instead they recommended loose jumpers (*sarafani*) and low shoes.[82] Thus, reformers attacked both earlier and contemporary fashions. They also disparaged jewelry as bourgeois and primitive.[83] According to Vasilevskii, "In terms of beauty and in terms of health, the best adornment for a girl is her natural freshness and the attraction of her youth."[84] Here again reformers based their recommendations upon internal traditions and reflected worldwide trends in health. Chernyshevskii's revolutionaries preferred simple clothing. Vera Pavlovna even counseled loose-fitting, Greek-style clothing.[85]

Whereas propagandists hailed positive behavior, they warned that negative habits would lead to a host of problems. Reformers singled out smoking, drinking, and sexual activity as particularly degrading to the body and campaigned vigorously against all three. Smoking was not part of a proper regimen. According to antismoking advocates, smoking destroyed the body in a number of ways. In its pure form the nicotine from cigarettes could kill. Over an extended period it stunted growth and destroyed teeth, lungs, stomach, vision, and nerves. According to the 1924 pamphlet *Hygiene for Propagandists,* smoking harmed the propagandists' most important tool, namely, the voice.[86] The cover of the pamphlet *The Truth about Smoking* suggested that cigarettes enslaved the heart and vanquished the will (figure 6.4). In more dire situations, smoking could lead to heart problems, blindness, hearing and memory loss.[87] Smokers also became infected with tuberculosis.[88] A poster with the Maiakovskii-penned slogan "Quit Smoking. It's Paper-Wrapped Poison" (figure 6.5) summed it all up. The look of the youth in the poster conveyed disgust. At the same time, the disembodied cigarette focused attention on the object rather than the addicted person.[89]

According to *A Dangerous Habit (Tobacco Smoking)* (1929), smoking impacted women more severely than it did men and could have drastic effects on her progeny. Another article implied that a smoking, expectant mother could hurt her child or end up miscarrying.[90] While women directly harmed children

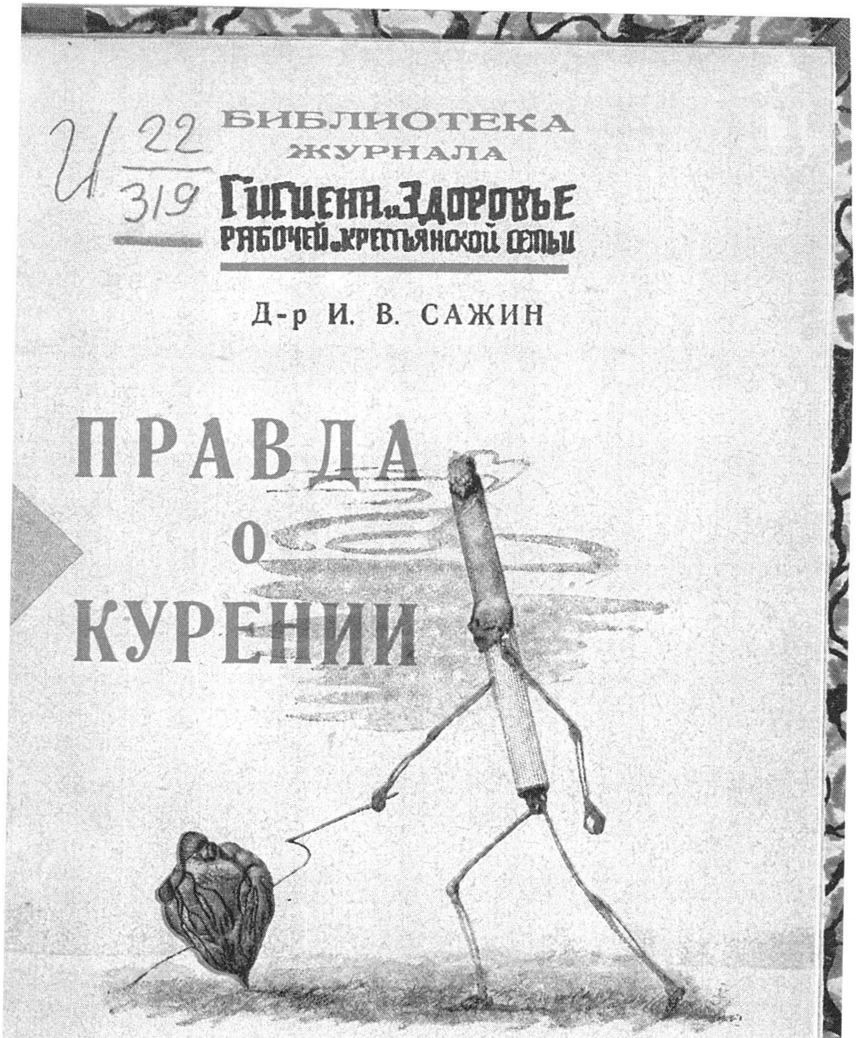
БИБЛИОТЕКА
ЖУРНАЛА
ГИГИЕНА и ЗДОРОВЬЕ
РАБОЧЕЙ и КРЕСТЬЯНСКОЙ СЕМЬИ
Д-р И. В. САЖИН
ПРАВДА
о
КУРЕНИИ

FIGURE 6.4. Cover, I. V. Sazhin, *The Truth about Smoking.* Leningrad: Leningradskaia Pravda, n.d. Pub. 10,000. Courtesy of the Russian State Library.

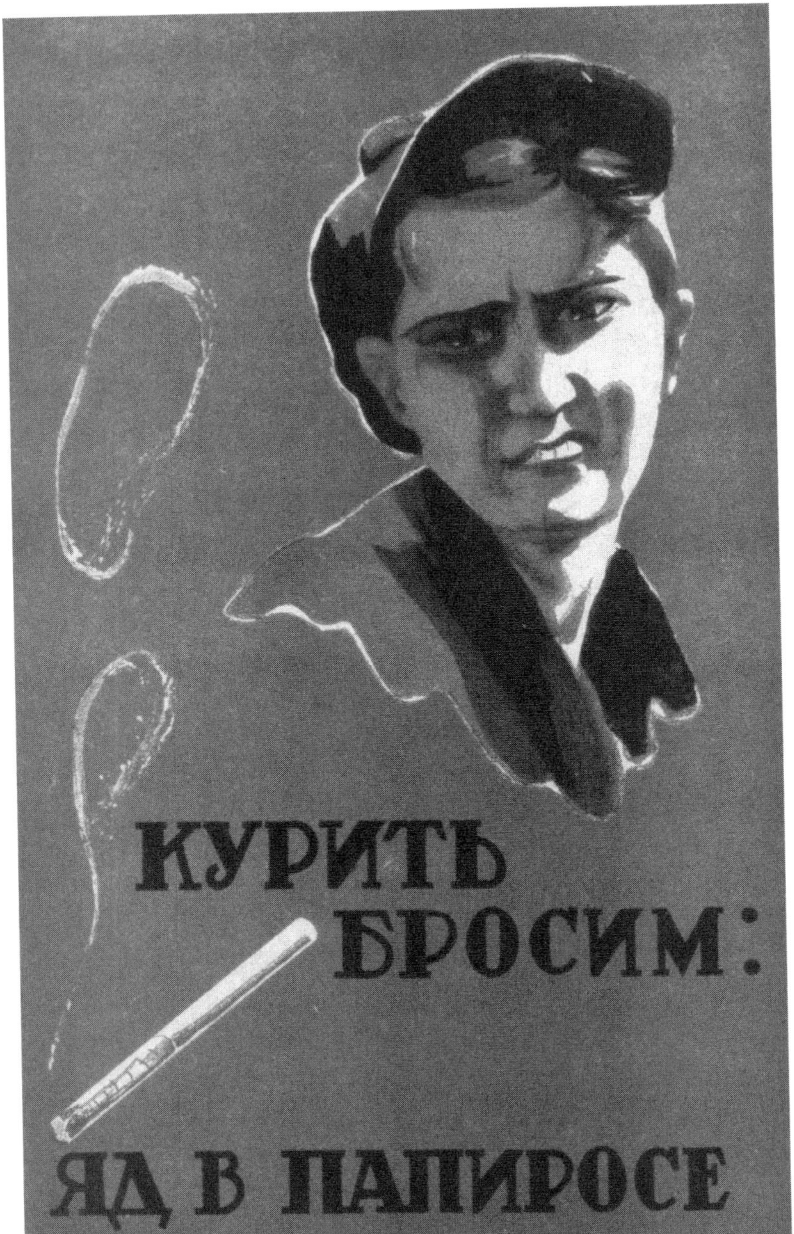

FIGURE 6.5. "Quit Smoking. It's Paper-Wrapped Poison." Moscow: Gosmedizdat, 1926–29. Pub. 10,000. Courtesy of the Russian State Library.

through their actions, fathers took the blame for glamorizing smoking and acting as models of bad behavior. In the 1927 mock trial of a smoking Pioneer, the judge pointed out that although the Pioneer had ignored his pledge and expert advice, the blame must be shared with another. The judge reprimanded the father for setting a bad example.[91]

As with other "bad habits," reformers portrayed the harm to the individual as secondary to the harm done to society. Of particular concern were the female tobacco workers victimized by the production of tobacco products. In studies cited in *The Truth about Smoking*, the handling of tobacco products caused severe complications in pregnant women, harming both present and future generations. According to anecdotal evidence, women had healthy children before and after they worked in the cigarette factory but miscarried while there. The study noted that workers in tobacco industries suffered higher death rates than other workers.[92] The production of cigarettes killed workers and their offspring. Smoking supported an industry that crippled this generation and the next.

Soviet hygienists' harangues echoed worldwide disgust with the demon weed. Cigarette smoking rose in the late nineteenth century as a result of lower costs due to mechanized production, with the product becoming even cheaper in the twentieth century. Seen as au courant, energizing, and masculine by some, cigarette smoking increased. With the rise in the consumption of cigarettes, attacks against tobacco increased. In the 1920s German doctors vilified tobacco as a financial drain, a detriment to female reproductive health, and a sap to male virility. American prohibitionists attacked smoking alongside alcohol.[93] In the 1930s the Germans pointed to cigarettes as causing ulcers, gastritis, heart disease, and sexual dysfunction. Health problems aggravated societal problems. According to German hygienists, cigarette eventually led to a loss of military prowess and the compromising of a citizen's allegiance, the weakening of the will, and abuse of cocaine or morphine.[94]

NEP-era pamphlets similarly expanded cigarette smoking from a private indulgence to a public problem. Reformers argued that smoking wasted resources and contributed to societal fragmentation. Smoking caused fires and wasted farmland. One text correlated tobacco use with the criminality.[95] Hygienists argued that smokers at work endangered their coworkers, they were given special treatment in the form of separate smoking lounges, and they were permitted smoking breaks from work.[96] *Take Hold of Your Health!* listed the threats: "The smoker harms not only himself but also those around him, forcing them to breath air saturated with smoke. The smoker presents a rather harmful example to youth and juveniles since smoking generally begins with imitation." The pamphlet concluded with a call to the tobacco industry to assume some responsibility: "The smoker supports the tobacco industry, one of the most harmful to the health of workers."[97] In 1926 N. Bukharin stated in the Komsomol's *Alphabet* that smoking was an old habit dating back to the old regime. It had served as a sign of rebellion, but now it did nothing: "It spoils the air; ruins the smoker; disturbs our living together, and fouls one's mood [*dobro*]." He concluded that it was not stylish in any way.[98]

Other justifications for smoking fell on deaf ears. Sazhin noted that smoking under the capitalists made sense, whereas the current hard times provided no such excuse. Women, he concluded, had a much harder life yet smoked considerably less than men.[99] Semashko argued that Lenin was offended by smoking and forbade it in meeting halls. During lengthy meetings Lenin permitted smoking only around the fireplace, where the smoke could go up the flue. He reportedly referred to smokers as the "smoking cockroaches."[100] Picking up the message, some groups expressed antismoking messages. In one Moscow factory workers began an antismoking circle in 1925 in cooperation with the dispensary. A score of workers testified that they had given up smoking for six months.[101] Letters to the magazine *To a New Life!* protested smoky conditions at work and in clubs, which they insisted needed to be changed.[102]

Reformers paired alcohol with smoking as twin "bad habits" that destroyed body, mind, and society. Russia's temperance movement emerged in the late nineteenth century even as the state's monopoly on alcohol ensured continued production. Still, in the midst of war state interest led to prohibition in December 1914. Internationally activists had long battled alcohol. In Canada reformers linked alcohol to tuberculosis. Later the Nazis campaigned against alcohol, linking it to poor fetal health and cancer. They also perceived it as an economic drain that encouraged vice and weakened the will. While the Bolsheviks destroyed liquor supplies in 1917 and further attempted to prevent its manufacture and sale, their efforts merely led to widespread bootlegging. By 1925 restrictions on alcohol production had essentially been lifted, and there was evidence that traditional binge drinking had returned. Perhaps most striking, between 1923 and 1928 the number of alcohol-related deaths in Moscow multiplied by almost fifteen times.[103]

Semashko pointed out that alcohol "ravages all human organs."[104] In another pamphlet he commented that alcohol "ruins the protective forces of the organism. For instance, it destroys the heart, which regulates everything; destroys the liver, which also influences a person's general constitution and health; destroys the kidneys; destroys the blood vessels, and leads to arteriosclerosis." He made abstaining from alcohol the first rule of personal hygiene.[105] Specialized dispensaries catered to the alcoholic, but ultimately psychologists would beat out social hygienists in the treatment of the chronic alcoholic.[106]

Although alcohol maimed the individual, for health advocates this problem paled in comparison to that visited upon society.[107] Alcoholics made bad examples for children, and children of alcoholics suffered, according to hygienists, from idiotism, psychosis, and susceptibility to criminal behavior.[108] The author of one pamphlet posed the rhetorical question "Do drunken parents have the right to bear children and to produce sickly, unneeded people?," and responded "No, they do not. . . . If a husband or wife is a drunkard, they should not have children. Their children will not only be sickly but drunkards just like their parents."[109] As the prolific Doctor Sigal noted, whereas the United States sterilized drunkards, this was not an acceptable solution in the Soviet state. In the new workers' paradise they had to be educated.[110] Although reformers preached education, punitive measures were prevalent. In party organizations drinking could lead to dismissal for "discrediting the party," and the Pioneer code listed both drinking and smoking as unacceptable. In a few districts the Committees for the Sanitation of Labor and Life obtained police records of people charged with public drunkenness and hounded them until they had agreed to get to a dispensary. Activists claimed this led to the recovery of approximately four thousand people.[111]

Other pamphlets pointed to economic problems. The alcoholic squandered his money, which could be used to purchase products to fortify rather than destroy the body. Posters showed the quantity of goods that could be purchased for a similar amount of money.[112] Pamphlets noted not only how alcoholics wasted their money on drink but also how they imperiled their productivity since drunkards made poor workers: "His hands shake. His eyes are poor. He is completely incapable of detailed work."[113] Factory committees regularly discussed alcohol and poor behavior in the workplace.[114] The scientific literature highlighted the rampant absenteeism and frequent accidents of the drunkard. Doctor Sigal noted that "there are more accidents on Monday than any other day of the week." He admitted that this effect on productivity could be due to other elements: "True, one component of this is that after a long rest the organism has not yet readjusted to the work process, and attention is therefore weakened. But a far greater factor is alcohol."[115] Missed Mondays had been a problem in industry for some time. Prior to the revolution Moscow metalworks paid wages on Saturdays to limit this problem.[116]

The poster "Drive out the Drunkard from the Thicket of Workers" brilliantly conceived alcohol's effect on the factory and the economy (figure 6.6). A sickly, jaundiced, hovering figure sloppily pours himself a glass of liquor. By

В МАЛЕНЬКОМ СТАКАНЕ
В ЭТОМ ВОТ
МОЖЕТ УТОНУТЬ
ОГРОМНЫЙ ЗАВОД
ИЗ РАБОЧЕЙ ГУЩИ
ВЫГОНИМ ПЬЮЩИХ!

FIGURE 6.6. "Drive out the Drunkard from the Thicket of Workers." Moscow: Voprosy Truda, 1929. Pub. 15,000. Courtesy of the Russian State Library.

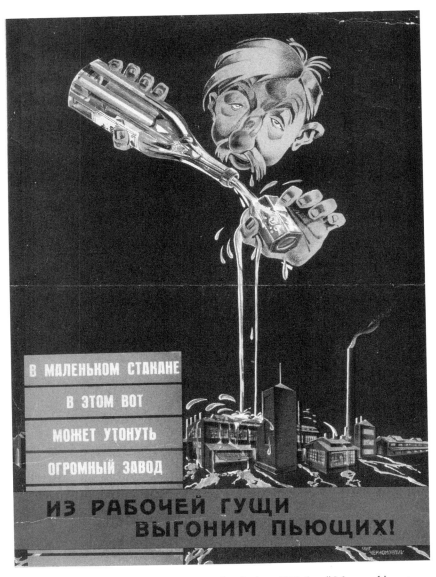

making the worker larger than life-size, the artist relayed the fact that one individual could be very powerful. The contents overflowed the glass, dousing the factory below. The poster appended the phrase: "In a small glass there is enough to drown a huge factory." In the yellow-colored skin of the drunkard, the poster linked his sickliness with other societal burdens, inasmuch as the color evoked both the yellow-ticketed, prerevolutionary prostitute and the yellow of the Russian madhouse.

The late 1920s poster "Down with Religious Holidays," in addition to making a similar connection between alcohol and its effect on society in terms of decreased productivity, added the specter of religion (figure 6.7). In the central image two workers—one of whom has a crucifix hanging from his neck—stumbled in front of a large work calendar with nearly all the dates blocked out by the words "skip" or "illness," which connected alcohol with decreased productivity. Once again the figures were drawn larger than life-size, suggesting the far-reaching impact of one person's actions. The poster showed a drunken man molesting a woman on the streets of the city in one panel and storming away from his sobbing family in another. Most distressing, the drunkard was crushed by a streetcar in the upper-right-hand panel, a "victim of the religious revelry" that actually seized hold of the transportation arteries of the busy city. The streetcar stood still while crowds milled about, the rush of urban life brought to a halt by the irrational, antisocial behavior of a single man.[117]

The 1922 poster entitled "The Workers of the USSR Do Not Have the Right to Poison Their Strength, Body, and Mind, Which Are Needed for the Collective Work of the Socialist Construction of the Proletarian State" presented a bleak picture of the effects of alcohol (plate 6). Criminals and haggard prostitutes framed the alcoholic life depicted on the left, which contrasted with the sober existence on the right. In the pivotal center position a worker who is drawn larger than life-size must choose between stupor and sobriety, dark and light, bad and good, destitution and prosperity. The worker's immense size argues for the massive effect of the individual's poor choice. Beatings and poverty accompanied the alcoholic at home instead of the ordered, well-appointed room of the sober worker. With sobriety came the rewards of more children, greater economic prosperity, and even technological advances, as evidenced by the curtains, tablecloth, table settings, sewing machine, and gramophone. At work the alcoholic mutilated himself and destroyed the entire establishment, in contrast to the productivity symbolized by the smokestacks on the right. The faceless, impersonal symbols of productive industry underscored the larger social benefits of individual sobriety. On the next level, the poorly lit, violent city of the alcoholic loomed dark and violent in contrast to the electrically lit,

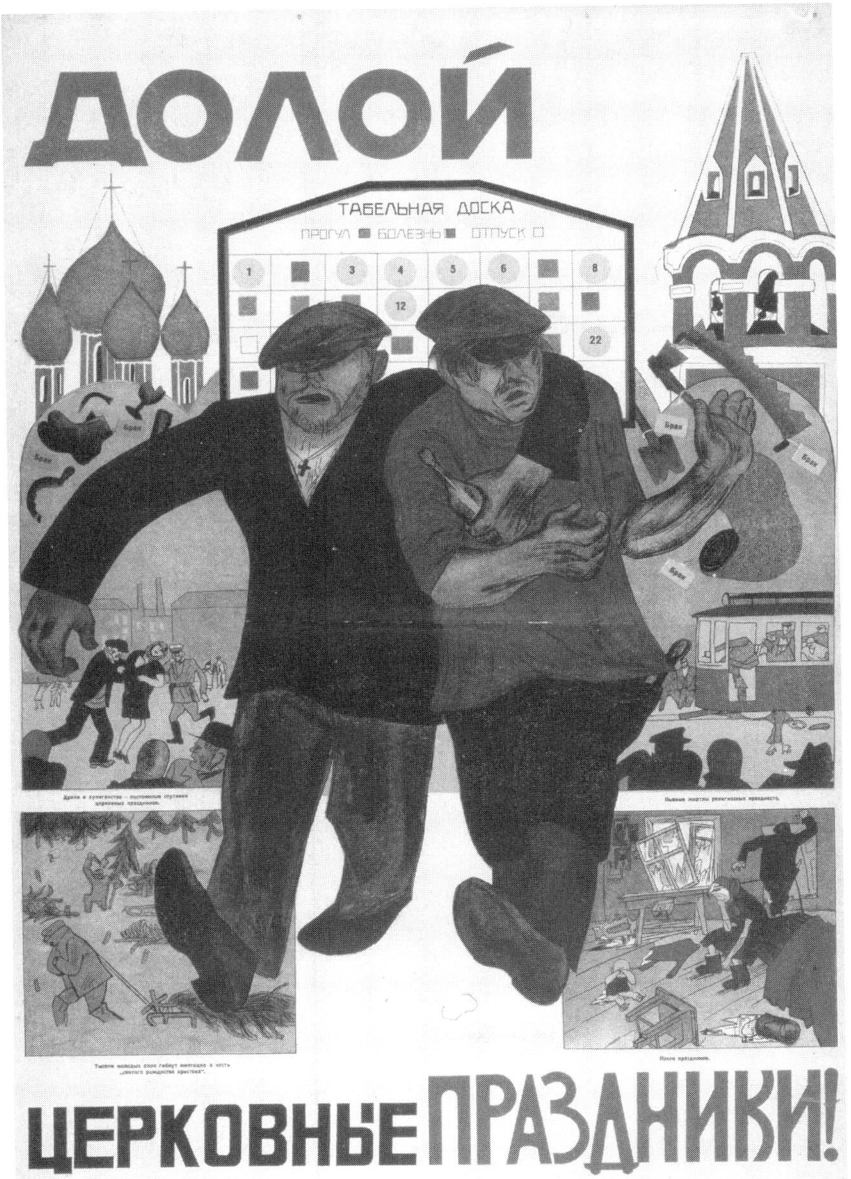

FIGURE 6.7. "Down with Religious Holidays." Moscow: Glavlit, 1926–29. Pub. 20,000. Courtesy of the Russian State Library.

cultured city of theaters, movie houses, and clubs on the right. In the end, the drunkard enjoyed the company of prostitutes and sickness, choosing suicide over the healthful route of sex-segregated, sober activity. Without sobriety, personal and social life collapsed. In its slogan and visuals the poster emphasized the duties of citizens and the dangers to society of poor individual choices.

In the late 1920s the message regarding alcohol consumption remained consistent, with a greater emphasis on education through demonstrations, films, and plays.[118] Drink endangered workers and society. Even more serious, reformers saw it as a gateway to narcotics, juvenile delinquency, prostitution, and venereal disease. In a 1927 mock trial a fatherless, teen-aged poet started with alcohol but graduated to the more addictive cocaine, and from there to antisocial behavior and hooligan activity.[119] Furthermore, drink ruined the hopes of the next generation. As the trial pointed out, "Every husband and wife, of course, wishes to have a child, but it is not always possible—for instance, if they are syphilitic, which, more often than not, occurs because a drunk person does not have the willpower to abstain from sexual intercourse, falls in with prostitutes, transmits the infection to his wife, and that infection is then passed along to the children."[120] While both spouses are addressed at first, by the end it was clear that men were the target. Drink so degraded the husband's will that he visited a horrible disease on his wife and children.

Women under the influence could serve as the locus for infection for the entire family. In the agitational play *Trial of a Syphilitic* (1923), the worker Platonov raped and infected a friend's wife while she was intoxicated. Returning to her husband, the woman infected him.[121] Complete blame in the trial did not fall on the abusive friend because the wife compromised herself through drink. Reformers further implicated drink in fostering prostitution and the spread of venereal diseases.[122] The agitational trial of a prostitute and a madam claimed that alcohol had so impaired the judgment of a country boy who had left his wife at home that he slept with a drunken prostitute and caught syphilis from her.[123] In short, from the Soviet perspective, descent into alcoholism initiated the following chain of events: abandonment, absenteeism, illicit sex, disease, and death.

In propaganda, sex and alcohol led to venereal disease. Because they were deemed "secret diseases" by the population, sexually transmitted diseases were an even more dangerous social evil than most, this according to Doctor Sigal.[124] Discomfort with sexuality did not stem solely from concerns about venereal disease. According to experts, social problems and other ailments that were not always venereal in nature resulted from sexual contact. In the 1920s theorists regarded sexual activity with great concern since they saw within it the seeds for the corruption of utopia and society generally.[125] Even Kollontai, unfairly demonized as an advocate of "free love," did not support sexual contact outside of strong, loving relationships or that interfered with the work necessary for constructing the revolution. Ideally, the revolutionary sublimated his or her sexual urges to work. In a continuation of the mechanistic metaphor of the body as machine, sexual discipline was necessary to conserve the "energy" of the body.[126]

All manner of sexual release occasioned anxiety, but certain types of behavior were viewed as especially dangerous. Homosexual activity, treated with some ambivalence by the state, concerned hygienists, who felt it was destroying society.[127] Hygienists discouraged men from engaging in sexual activity outside marriage, which inevitably led to syphilis.[128] Throughout the propaganda, the message was that sexual arousal and pleasure had no place in the revolutionary lifestyle. Sexual release—associated with the bourgeois, the feminine, and the individualistic—did not connect to the communal, ascetic ideas of revolution. Even as pamphlets emphasized the dangers of transmission, the individual sex act of masturbation was also perceived as a danger. Reformers opposed masturbation because of its social distancing (the solitary sin) and presented it as a dangerous alternative to abstinence because it weakened the body.[129]

Reformers urged parents to discourage children's sexual awakening by withholding tea, coffee, and alcohol; monitoring their sleep; and making sure they slept on hard, individual beds, with their hands placed chastely above the covers. Parents were responsible for waking them early, washing them using cold water, encouraging them to engage in proper physical activity (which kept blood from pooling in the sex organs), and doing work in the fresh air. Children were to be shielded from lascivious entertainment. Activists considered children to be in a transitional state and therefore more malleable as well as more vulnerable to maladies of all types, including poor behavior. Soviet pundits regarded the sexual activity of youth as especially perilous; considering their disinclination to follow abstinence programs, this was not surprising. According to contemporary surveys, youth believed abstinence led to psychological problems and felt that sexual release—especially for males—was necessary for continued health. Hygienists were not swayed and continued to comment upon youth living *A Life Out of Control* (1929), as one book title insisted melodramatically.[130] Though adults were stronger, the risk of infection remained and health advocates counseled abstention for them as well.

Not even marriage protected one against sexual disease. One article noted that 75 percent of sick women began their sexual life with their husbands and that 71 percent of dispensary patients were infected by their spouses.[131] In fiction, male characters grew impatient and did not complete the full course of treatment offered by the dispensary, returning home to infect their families. In the 1925 mock trial *Statute 155 of the Law Code of the RSFSR*, the wife became infected through such means.[132] The propaganda guaranteed full recovery if patients underwent a full treatment. If sex was contemplated, health care advocates recommended soap and water, condoms, or slathering the sex organs with calamine lotion and then washing with soap to ward off infection.[133]

For women sex never existed without complications, nor was it discussed as pleasurable. As Frances Lee Bernstein shows, in contrast to sexual advice in other countries, Soviet doctors took little interest in male sexual pleasure and even less attention was devoted to female arousal or frigidity.[134] The propaganda claimed that for women sex performed without the intent of procreation or outside the confines of marriage always resulted in venereal disease or unwanted pregnancy. According to Sigal, "the healthiest and most stable men and women are those who are able to sublimate" their desires until maturation or "the solidification of the organism."[135] Other pamphlets warned women that without sex they would waste away, age prematurely, lose their attractiveness, and sicken: "How great an effect sexual life has can be seen in how quickly, even by age thirty or thirty-five, a woman who has not known the joys of sex [*polovykh radostei*] withers away."[136] Other European sex experts spread similarly contradictory messages for women. French hygienists predicted a loss of beauty and other physical problems, as well as mental instability, for women who abstained, though sex outside of marriage was always risky.[137] Italian physicians claimed that reproduction was essential to a woman's nature.[138]

The Soviet pamphlet *Mother and Infant* (1925) upheld this concept of essential motherhood and the transformative power exercised by carrying the fetus: "Motherhood and the birth of an infant—in particular the first—occupy a large place in the lives of women. . . . From that moment when a woman begins to feel the movement of a new life [within her] she is, in a sense, reborn. The woman and the wife are transformed into the mother."[139] The mother worker and the mother activist were subsumed, with the woman becoming incapable of resisting the power of the fetus within her.

Just as motherhood was considered natural, so infertility was viewed as an abnormality. A marriage that was not immediately fruitful required medical intervention by proper authorities. The emphatically titled 1926 pamphlet *Girls as Future Mothers* presented conception as a necessary conclusion to normal, marital sexual relations: "A woman beginning to live a sexual life usually must become pregnant by the first or second month. If pregnancy does not occur, then she needs to go to the doctor in order to discover the reasons for infertility."[140] Soviet reformers told women that sex was necessary for continued health and beauty. While celibacy or sex without progeny endangered women, propaganda portrayed motherhood as a basic element of womanhood as well as a duty. One doctor advised: "Motherhood is a woman's most important societal obligation. To give birth to and raise a healthy child is a woman's duty to the proletarian state." He further stated that female health should be carefully monitored because of the importance of mothers. Special attention needed to be paid to those diseases that threatened a woman's reproductive abilities. He explained that while legal, abortion should not be undertaken without serious thought: "Abortion never occurs without punishment. Abortion presents danger and brings damage to women's bodies even when performed by a doctor in a hospital environment."[141]

For women or men who were smokers, alcoholics, addicts, prostitutes, or infected with venereal disease, salvation lay in the institutions of Narkomzdrav. The vendispensary and narcodispensary were medical institutions devoted to those suffering from venereal disease, narcotics abuse, and alcohol addition.[142] In the 1927 poem "To a New Life" the female protagonist declined from responsible work to alcoholism and streetwalking until a dispensary doctor told her:

"In the prophylactory they're able!"
Though the living there is hard
All the same life there is better
Than on the boulevard.

Working there you'll see
That in life there is hope
And there you will soon forget
All the wine and other dope. . . .

The fight for life in history
Moves on in the U-S-S-R!
To the prophylactory
Partner to the dispensary.[143]

The dispensary system promised recovery to the heroine by placing her within the labor system of the prophylactory, which provided the medical supervision and regimen of the dispensary, combined with a living space and job training. Established in 1924, the prophylactory attempted to address the social conditions that gave rise to prostitution by providing political and cultural enlightenment to women, as well as the economic means to fight the lure of the streets. In the facility women were subject to rigid schedules, close observation, and strict labor discipline in addition to literacy education and cultural activities.[144]

Women learned a trade and redeemed themselves through physical labor. In the 1927 film *Prostitutka* the prophylactory served as a crucial lifesaver for one of the women, who had been forced by economic circumstances into a life on the streets.[145] The prophylactory proved very popular, with applicants outstripping available spaces. The vendispensary and narcodispensary were in similarly short supply. In 1924 there were only thirty-nine vendispensaries in the RSFSR as a whole.[146] Authorities presented this gap between need and provision as temporary and noted that this was a program unique in scope even if inadequate in number.

While labor could cleanse the body, redemption through physical exertion imbued the rhetoric of physical culture. Physical fitness figured heavily in the Soviet mission of *kul'turnost'*, with well-toned bodies forming the basis of hygienic advice. Sports had attained a high status internationally in the late nineteenth and early twentieth centuries as a means of national rejuvenation.[147] For the Soviets physical culture was more than just part of a healthful regimen. Physical activity imparted character, strengthened the will, and curbed dangerous sexual urges. It was also essential to the military preparedness of the young state. The first organization involved with physical training was charged with bringing men up to the level necessary for conscription.[148] The reasons for exercise, however, also included productivity as well as other issues. Instead of following unhealthful pursuits, workers needed to engage in physical activity. According to Semashko, even Lenin participated in physical exercise in the form of cycling. The commissar of health went so far as to declare that thanks to this activity Lenin survived the assassination attempt of 1918. According to Semashko, Lenin understood the broader meaning of physical culture.[149]

Reformers credited physical activity with economic and cultural benefits, while Semashko considered it a panacea. The proper use of physical culture, he said, "does not only lead to the improvement of the population—in particular the young reserves—but helps solve the basic questions that modern life poses."[150] In his recommendation for regimentation and exercise, Semashko was following the Hippocratic philosophy, which gained renewed popularity under the Enlightenment.[151] Other reformers claimed that activity would "make workers healthy and increase production of worker and peasant labor," thereby ensuring a "bettering of the economic situation of the country and a rise in the cultural level of the population."[152]

Hygienists used the term "physical culture" rather than sports, recalling prerevolutionary debates on the need for and nature of exercise. The development of sports in Russia was influenced by state, military, and foreign ideas. Peter the Great introduced exercise to Russia as a form of military training, and eighteenth-century military and civil colleges continued to use physical training to produce fit men whose skills could also serve the army, navy, or civil service.[153] Later authorities hoped it would curb worker and student discontent as well as provide assistance in military training.[154] During the late nineteenth century Russian physical exercise expanded greatly, with particular emphasis on building character; competitive sports were disparaged as producing antisocial attitudes. Women were encouraged to engage in physical activity as a means of liberation. Many of the ideas of the 1920s emerged from these prerevolutionary foundations, including a dislike of competition and a perception of physical activity as emancipatory, although competitive sports eventually overcame this less hierarchical concept.[155]

By the turn of the century, a healthy desire for physical exercise and fresh air penetrated almost all of society except for the peasantry, which got more than enough of both, and the workers, who could not afford to find either. Such sports figures as Sandow the Magnificent popularized bodybuilding in Russia and the world and typified a movement for control and building of the male body as a way to ensure the stamina of an entire society. Following the revolution, with the government facing serious health problems, physical culture became a cheap, quick way to improve health.[156] Although Semashko argued that the primary goal of physical culture was to increase labor productivity, he insisted that it must also enter into the entire day's activities.[157] The Higher Council of Physical Culture agreed and highlighted "physical culture in the broadest sense of the word . . . employing the correct personal hygiene, using the forces of nature—sun, air, [and] a correct regimen of labor and rest."[158]

Although sport was overwhelmingly identified with men in the nineteenth century, peasant women were ideally robust and often engaged in weightlifting and wrestling. By the end of the century, there was a push for female physical training. Encouraging sports for women continued after the revolution, with Lenin viewing it as a way to socialize women. While the Soviets democratized the pursuit of sports, the reasons for physical exercise remained gender-specific.[159] Exercise reduced sexual urges for men, while strengthening procreative abilities for women. In both cases physical culture increased potency. Men who denied themselves physical pleasure but exercised increased their stamina and strength, while also improving their leadership qualities. Exercise made women healthier mothers. According to one book, during pregnancy women required physical exercise more than men, thus testifying to its energizing qualities.[160]

The 1927 poster "Among Women Displacement of the Internal Sex Organs Is Frequently Observed" (figure 6.8) concentrated on physical culture, reproduction, and women. The central diagram, featuring a bisected woman, underscored the visible, knowable nature of woman's most inner mysteries before man and illustrated how the recommended exercises would prevent a prolapsed uterus.[161] The poster presented exercises directly connected to pregnancy as taking place inside the home, thus constricting the women's sphere. In addition, the poster cautioned that heavy exercise should not coincide with menses, when a woman's constitution was weakened. During menstruation women should only do light exercises and take short walks.[162] The poster noted that even nonmenstruating women could never attain the physical strength of men and advised healthy women never to participate in certain sports: "Soccer, Weight Lifting, Wrestling, Boxing, and Diving from Great Heights Is Forbidden!" The large figure of the sportswoman suggested that hockey was acceptable.

In a companion poster entitled "Sun, Air, and Water—The Best Rest from Labor," the artist presented men's relaxation as integral to their contribution to the state in terms of production, not reproduction (plate 7). Participation in sunbathing and water activities in the first two panels led to the muscular, chess-playing males of the third panel. In their homosocial world men participated in exercise to tone their bodies and improve their minds, albeit not for any procreative function. In a society resonating with martial metaphors, the homosocial environment may have prompted viewers to link physical fitness with military experience. In addition, the poses, glances, and lithe, naked male forms imparted a homoerotic tone. Although hygienists condemned homosexual activity as abnormal, it could be testimony to either the artists' longings or a general reverence for the male form.

The cover for the pamphlet *Physical Culture as a Part of Cultural-Enlightenment Work* (1924) illustrated the same message of men's empowerment through exercise (figure 6.9). The silhouette of a finely turned male figure presented in stasis, with book in hand and weightlifting equipment idle, connected physical vigor with intellectual acuity. The posture and bearing intimated strength and command. Replacing the dumbbell with a globe, the pose of the shadowy male figure recalled portraits of historical men of power. Physical culture prepared men for leadership and domination. The calculated display of musculature indicated that while cultural enlightenment was the purported goal, a body worth looking at was not an undesirable offshoot.

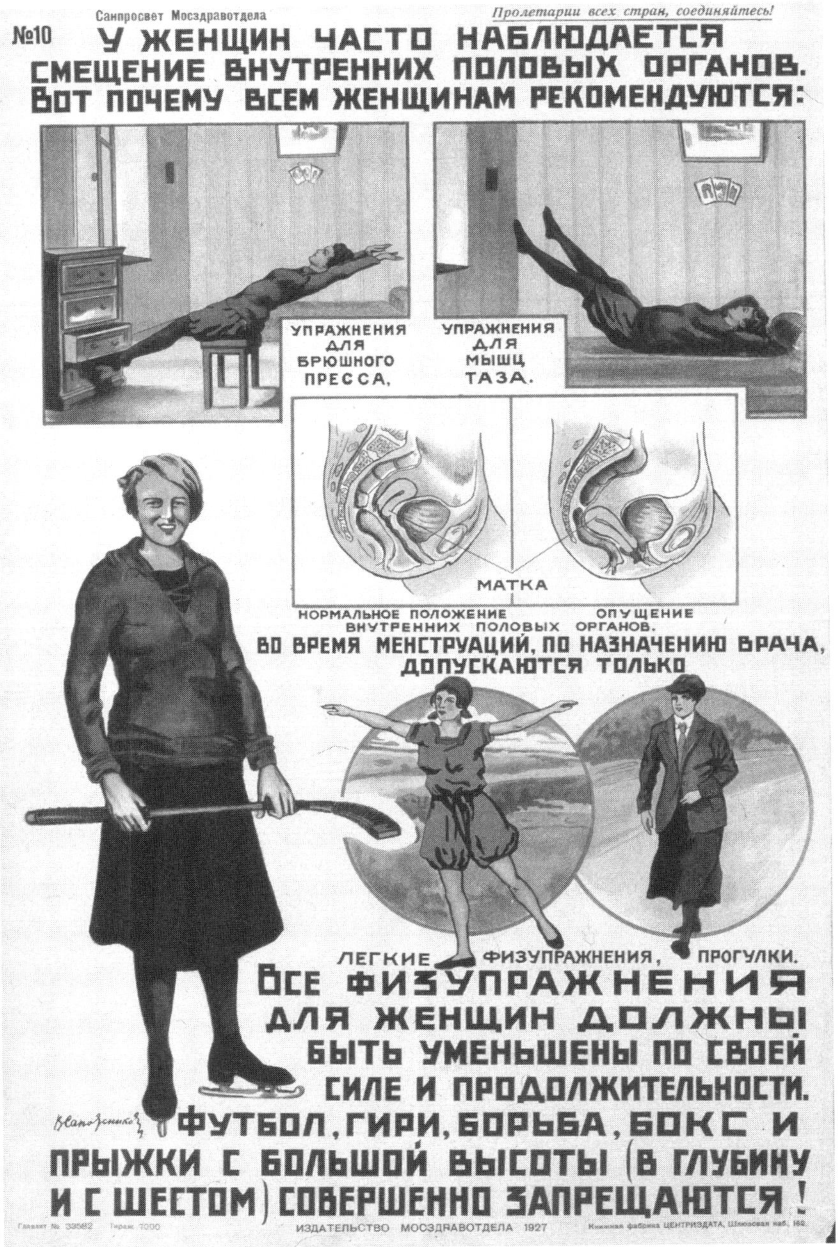

FIGURE 6.8. "Among Women Displacement of the Internal Sex Organs Is Frequently Observed." Moscow: MOZ, 1927. Pub. 7,000. (Note the bottom comment next to the female hockey player: "All Physical Exercises for Women Must Be Decreased in Their Strength and Length. Soccer, Weight Lifting, Wrestling, Boxing, and Diving from Great Heights Is Forbidden!") Courtesy of the Russian State Library.

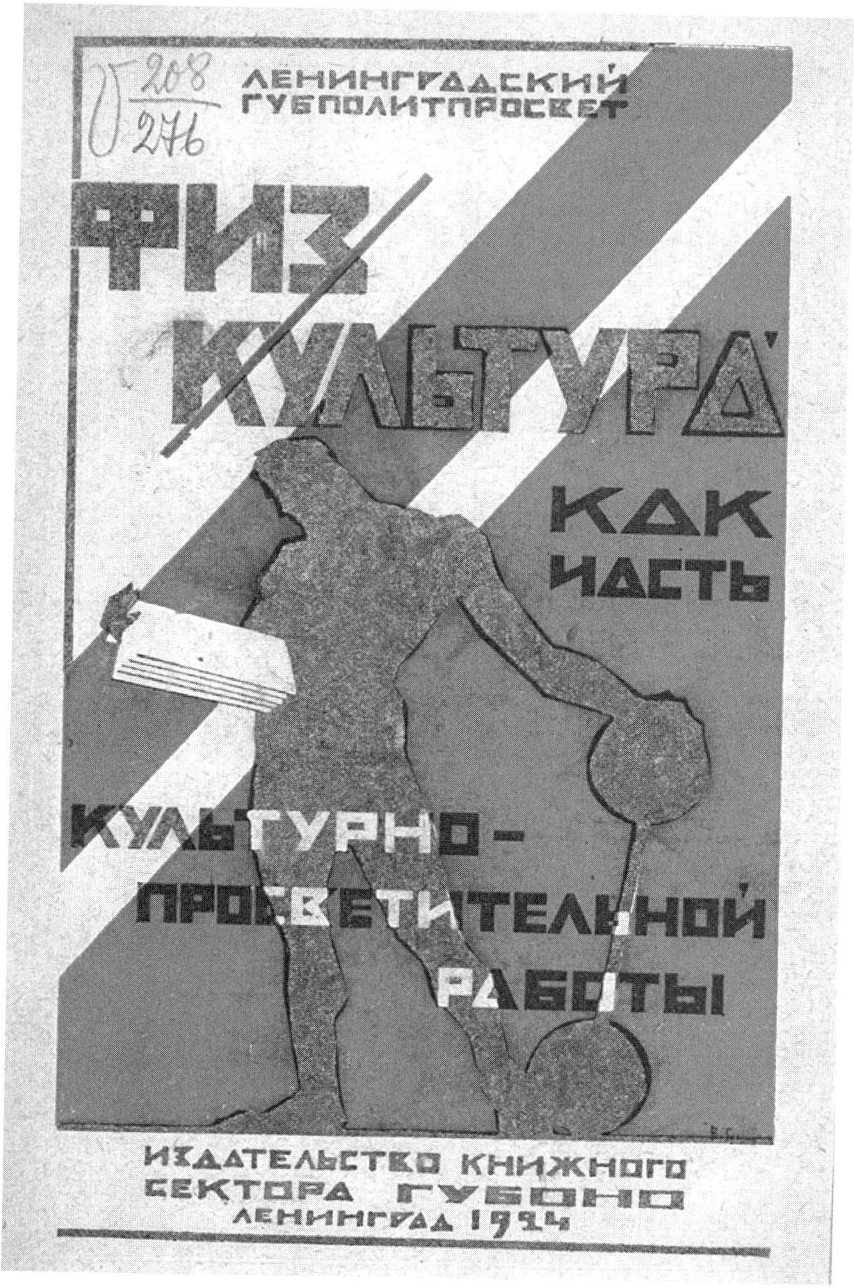

FIGURE 6.9. Cover, D. A. Kradman, *Physical Culture as a Part of Cultural-Enlightenment Work*. Leningrad: Knizhnyi Sektor Gubono, 1924. Courtesy of the Russian State Library.

Pleasure in viewing the male body may have inspired the proliferation of taut, sinewy male figures—often partially nude—in propaganda posters (figures 6.1, 6.3; plates 5, 7). Nudes, internal views of bodies, and the idealization of their energy and force had preoccupied the avant-garde before the war and continued to be of interest to artists and the state in the 1920s. Nudes depicted in hygienic posters undoubtedly reflected a general interest by artists in costume and the body. The nude torso also served as an outlet for social anxiety by allowing viewers to contemplate the trained, controlled male body, which remained vigorous despite the fears of neurasthenia and dissipation that accompanied modern life. The image of the well-formed figure became a source of shame, prompting viewers to gauge the state of their own bodies, yet it may also have been an object of desire.[163] In addition, each representation's dependence upon the white male asserted the primacy of Russian men over women and non-Russians.[164]

Posed pictures in other venues suggested that workers enjoyed contemplating and displaying their bodies. Particularly compelling are the number of photographs of workers in synchronized-gymnastics routines and carefully staged tableaus used to promote physical culture and the House of Leisure system. For example, an early 1920s photograph entitled "Second Group at the Lenin House of Leisure" (figure 6.10) taken at the facility at Serebriannyi bor was not simply a physical exercise or even a tower of flesh. Rather, it was an article of propaganda, a display of pride, and an ironic commentary on 1920s health reform all rolled into one.[165] The spindly arms, bulging joints, and hollowed-out chests reflected the dire economic circumstances of the 1920s, whereas the triumphant—even defiant—pose attested to the high goals and determination to conquer adversity. The pose itself, dependent upon cooperation and balance, underscored the corporate interest of individual health. Even the fetishization of the machine emerged in the coglike tower and the recording of the entire event thanks to the technological wonder of the photographic print.

Posed photographs emphasized the physical benefits of exercise, while posters displayed powerful men and fertile women. Physical culture did more than simply develop a strong constitution; hygienists belived it strengthened the will to resist other temptations. A 1923 survey upheld this belief, revealing that those factories with less sports activity experienced heightened illness, alcoholism, and hooliganism.[166] The state of the body could both help and hinder the workings of the mind. Semashko cautioned that alcohol weakened the will: "Look at the person of a 'drunkard.' His hands shake. He is puffy . . . his eyes and face are red. He is dressed shabbily and . . . has already lost the feeling of human modesty. Children laugh at him."[167] Vasilevskii advised Pioneers to use

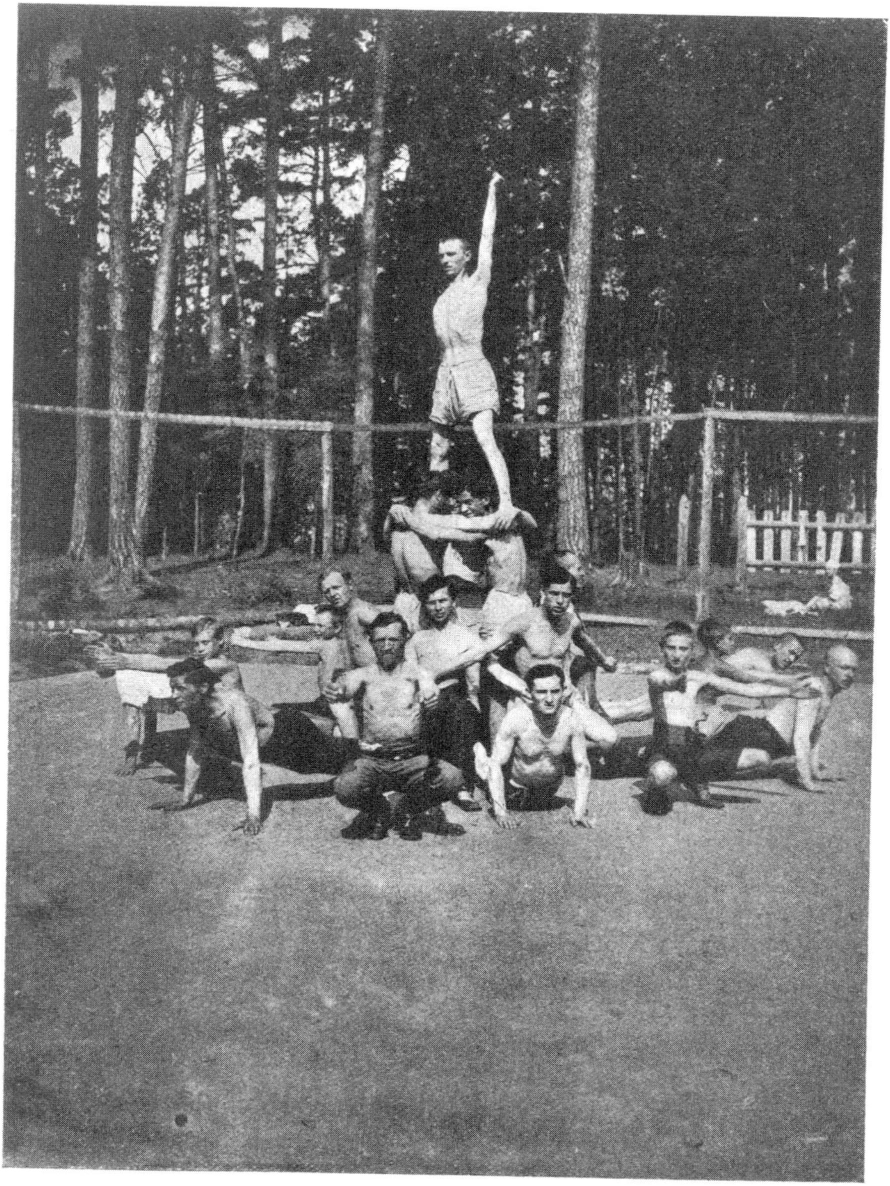

FIGURE 6.10. "Second Group at the Lenin House of Leisure." *Doma otdykha: Sbornik statei i materialov, 1920–1923 gg.* Moscow: Gosizdat, 1924. Courtesy of the Russian State Library.

this developed strength of will to regulate their bodies, suggesting they train themselves to defecate at the same time every day, "most advantageously in the morning, immediately after rising."[168] Semashko concluded that physical culture also thwarted sexual desire: "Physical culture destroys the physiological bases for sexual anomalies."[169] For Semashko physical culture allowed patients to sublimate improper urges and thereby avoid disease and moral dissolution.

Given the perceived relationship between body and mind, it is unsurprising that it was felt that succumbing to bodily urges would lead to mental debilities. For men onanism weakened the mind, although they could overcome the domination of their bodies over their minds by denying themselves sexual release.[170] For women, whom European and Russian philosophers had long depicted as being hindered by their anatomy, there was no remedy since the normal functioning of their bodies inevitably weakened them mentally. One female commentator who argued that the onset of menses overwhelmed young women recommended that steps be taken to offset the problems their bodies created for their minds: "During the period of sexual maturation of the female organism a complex work, a large rebuilding, occurs. During this time it is not advisable to increase stress with excessive work, whether physical or intellectual. No comparison should be made to boys of the same age. . . . Some of the forces of a girl are absorbed by internal reorganization within her. . . . It is better that during this period of sexual maturation the girl stay perhaps an extra year in class rather than undermine the womanly force."[171] The commentator made clear that women could not escape the draining effect their bodies had on them because of their glandular nature, making them "lazy, weak, timid, and lacking both stamina and concentration."[172]

Sex difference remained a cornerstone of Soviet and European health discussions in the 1920s. During the late nineteenth century French and British doctors similarly depicted menses as an extremely difficult time for young women. These concepts held sway into the 1920s as hygienists urged careful monitoring and rest for young girls in order to avoid damaging their procreative functions during this difficult time. This biological determinism seemed odd given the environmental and prophylactic emphasis of Soviet medicine. Theorists argued that because women's sex organs were larger (in proportion to their bodies) than those of males, young women were harmed more by puberty. Women were cursed, being constantly beset by biological urges and therefore unable to think or function reasonably.[173]

It seems than many citizens were unwilling to leave personal questions to be decided by the state. Theorist Pierre Bourdieu argues that identity is often articulated not just through political or cultural preferences but also through hygiene and bodily care.[174] While hygienists in the 1920s made the case for science, questions of care remained bound up with identity. For some this meant strictly adhering to hygienists' determinations. For others—especially many young male activists—the life recommended by reformers lacked the romance and mystique of the civil war hero, whom they credited with a certain lackadaisical attitude toward hygiene and admirable bravado in dealing with women.[175] More militant activists found such recommendations for sublimation and abstemiousness old-fashioned and criticized the Bolsheviks for becoming more bourgeois than the bourgeoisie, just as nineteenth-century militants and nihilists had decried orderly behavior as antirevolutionary.[176]

Instead of the cleaned-up image foisted upon them by hygienists, young people of the 1920s favored a rougher—and decidedly dirtier—public image. Authorities tried to combat this concept, but Semashko's comment ("There is nothing revolutionary in filth and rags") fell on deaf ears.[177] As one contemporary observer remarked, clothes "were assertions and proofs of proletarianism. In America we all try to dress like capitalists, and in Russia they all try to dress like workers."[178] This may also have reflected a peasant/working-class resistance to cleanliness as being the signifier of the outsider, whereas the presence of dirt was an inevitability in worker/peasant life and an instant badge signifying belonging.[179]

Politicized women adopted this attitude and promoted masculine styles to demonstrate their commitment to revolution. This trend particularly disturbed reformers, who accused women of pushing their male comrades into poor political choices. Reformers argued that men were forced to form liaisons with improper women because they were not attracted to overly masculinized, female comrades. They blamed politically conscious women for driving the men away rather than the men for choosing to engage in homosexual activity or visit a prostitute.[180] Despite such attacks, many female communists remained unswayed. Some activists avoided personal hygiene on principle.[181] Not all women wore their politics on their sleeves. Many women did not wish to sacrifice fashion to militancy. For these women a bit of powder or a flounce on a dress could serve as an escape from the harsh realities around them.

Material conditions made following clothing and cleanliness recommendations difficult if not impossible. Clothing, always in short supply, could be hard to find as well as expensive. It was easier to remain in rags than purchase a pair of shoes or a coat.[182] Simply finding enough water and soap for multiple, daily washings presented enormous difficulties. In 1923 only thirty-six *bania*, capable of serving 160 people a day and 130,000 a month, serviced all of Moscow.[183] The capital could not provide running water for most of its inhabitants, and the situation was even worse in outlying regions. Even in apartments that had running water, keeping up with all of the building's inhabitants proved difficult. In one instance workers reportedly used the single tub in the only bathroom of their building for washing laundry and bathed at the public baths.[184] Reformers occasionally acknowledged these difficulties. One 1923 article entitled "How to Be Clean without the *Bania*" described the ways in which one could do without soap or hot water for bodily washings by substituting soda or salt.[185] Even in the best of circumstances, the bathing that hygienists demanded involved a lot of labor and discomfort: hauling in cold water from outside; standing naked and shivering in the inadequately heated rooms; and probably bathing in front of children or other lodgers due to the crowded conditions in the home.[186] It is a small wonder that many did not see the reasoning for this.

Prohibitions against tobacco, drink, and sex met with similar resistance. Antismoking advocates continued to combat the public's perception of cigarettes as manly and revolutionary. Workers viewed alcohol consumption in the traditional sense as a masculine, invigorating pursuit; those who shunned alcohol were seen as effeminate and alien to the worker's milieu.[187] Despite such resistance, the pleas and enforcement tactics of the Bolsheviks made some inroads in drinking culture. According to some figures, in St. Petersburg alcohol consumption and missed Mondays decreased during the 1920s and alcohol consumption increasingly took place outside factories.[188]

Hygienists presented regimentation as a cure-all for personal and societal illnesses. The pamphlet *What You Must Know about Cancer*, published in the late 1920s, stated that "a simple, healthy life, simple foods, abstention from smoking and drinking keep a person young and protect him from cancer."[189] Responding to commentators who feared that years of civil war, revolution, famine, and epidemic diseases had drained the population of vital energies, in his 1922 article "The Fight against Fatigue" Maslov theorized that the Americans fought fatigue through studious attention to the clock—waking at the same time of day even on holidays—and thereby training away tiredness.[190] In 1926 Semashko postulated that the question of fatigue, "which now disturbs the party," could be settled by organizing time and regulating life.[191] Schedules, clock watching, regimentation, discipline—these were the medical miracles of the new Soviet society, the therapeutic remedies of the communist state.

Reformers had greater goals than maintaining clean skin or defeating disease. Hygienists pressed for a complete overhaul of life through the manipulation of habits and made sure that personal choices were also political ones.

Indeed, if maintenance of a proper regimen could enhance industrial productivity and military capability, it became a social and political duty to follow these strictures. As the 1922 poster "The Workers of the USSR . . ." (plate 6) bluntly stated, workers did not have the "right" to drink. In her modern contemplation of illness and its meaning, Susan Sontag argues that changing concepts of disease made illness appear not as a personal tragedy but as a personal failing.[192] The Soviets attempted to create a similar nosology. Since illness could be avoided through proper behavior, it became a transgression against Soviet ideals to suffer from disease. Regimens, schedules, and physical activity could not, however, overcome the widely accepted biological inferiority of women. The consistent focus on urban, mechanized males similarly cut peasants out of the picture of health. Nevertheless, both women and peasants were urged to follow similar prescriptions—if not to attain perfection then at least to better themselves.

Perhaps more intangibly, following correct habits led to the triumph of culture. One improved habit threw open the window to utopia. By cleansing one's body, maintaining a strict schedule, abstaining from polluting activities, and engaging in physical culture, citizens could triumph over biology and resist the temptations and pitfalls of modern, urban life as well as the enticements of the flesh. They could transcend the untidy political and social environment of the 1920s and advance directly to utopia.[193] The political, economic, and cultural battle for a new state—a body Soviet—could proceed in this most humble of venues with the most meager resources. One individual—making the correct choice to brush one's teeth, wash one's hands, or exercise on the weekend—became not just a healthier person but the embodiment of the future success of the Soviet experiment.

Conclusion

The February 1929 issue of the satirical magazine *Krokodil* included a cartoon parodying children's games for a very adult purpose (plate 8). The "Puzzle Picture for Party Children of a Young Age" challenged the reader's purity and their perspicacity with a depiction of two common types. On the right a smiling, capped figure whose coveralls, hands, face, and legs were smeared with grunge was unquestionably dirty, but visible dirt was not the question. Instead, the caption asked the viewer to assess the inner qualities of the figures rather than their outward appearance and to determine the following: "Which of the two is cleaner? And which of them should be cleaned up?"

The figure at left, placed in opposition to the worker, intimated his class background, political affiliation, and threat to Soviet construction through none too subtle, embedded markers. Sporting a natty suit and round glasses, plus a red portfolio, he represented the bureaucrat-intellectual-specialist rolled into one, creating a plum target for the campaigns of the cultural revolution initiated during the First Five-Year Plan, which was at full steam. Already politically suspect, further evidence from the picture pointed to this bureaucrat's other offenses. The portfolio, filled to bursting, and the fountain pen in his pocket indicated a purveyor of the dreaded bureaucratic red tape. The eyeglasses signaled the taint of an intellectual—perhaps even a Trotskyite—conspirator. Furthermore, a red kerchief in the pocket over the heart carried with it overtones of a political affiliation assumed for presentation to the outside world but not reaching to the core of the individual. This play on outward appearance versus inner desires hinted at the dangers of the fellow traveler or "veiled" enemy.

Although these meanings flowed easily from the image, references to physical health were more subtle. Even though he possessed a cleaner body, the bureaucrat's physical appearance was less virile than that of the worker. Whereas the worker's chiseled face and easy smile exuded health, the bureaucrat's simpering smirk, along with porcine cheeks, gave little indication of a healthy constitution. In addition the worker displayed firm, distinct musculature in his arms and the sliver of chest visible under his v-neck shirt hinted at a powerful male torso. The bureaucrat's physique suggested infirmity, his spectacles indicating poor eyesight and his frail hands insinuated effeminacy. The delicate, filter-tipped cigarette signified an infraction of hygienic teaching and brought the bureaucrat's virility into question. Rather than a hand-rolled worker's smoke, the bureaucrat chose a factory-rolled cigarette with a filter tip commonly associated with women's and bourgeois brands. In place of a cigarette, the worker held a pipe fitters' wrench—symbolic of work considered useful in the industrial march of the country—as opposed to the bureaucrat's drain on production through an addictive, decadent habit.

The transparency of the clothing revealed still more of each subject's interior life. Both were "visible" beneath their clothing, their physical bodies providing silent commentary on the strengths and weaknesses of their differing political orientations. Looking past their public display to their respective levels of fitness, the superficial appearance of cleanliness melted away, revealing the spindly, emasculated frame of the lollipop-headed bureaucrat versus the discernible narrow waist, full chest, and broad shoulders of the worker's body. What at first appeared to be a simple question of visible dirt became a lesson in political hygiene etched upon the individual body.

While a child's game served as inspiration, the language of cleansing and purging made the commentary anything but lighthearted. The tag line ominously suggested: "Send answers to the nearest control commission." This cartoon cunningly revealed how the Stalinist cleansing of society through the excision of undesirable class elements assumed the language of hygiene. Though anxiety over purity had been aggravated by the soft line of NEP, the elimination of the capitalist compromise and the launching of the Stalinist plan had not shielded the Soviet people from the pollution of the past or the world. Throughout the 1930s and following the war the danger of the past still oozed into the present, threatening the body politic.[1] Legacies of class and blood both served as the basis for impurity.[2] Worries over the politics of the population—in particular the difference between "visible" and "hidden" agendas —infected society and inspired phases of state-sponsored decontamination. As V. M. Molotov later pointed out: "We have no ready-made pure people, purged of all sins."[3]

Against the background of the battle over specialists, another conflict was brewing. From 1927–28 onward the per capita expenditure on health in Russia decreased.[4] In the summer of 1929 a battle erupted over the hygienic campaign.

Hygienists primarily favored need-based care, while the party demanded worker-centered benefits. The following winter the Central Committee reprimanded Narkomzdrav for not carrying out party directives to reorient the commissariat along class lines and subsequently restructured the health departments.[5] In January 1930 Semashko—comrade of Lenin, architect of Narkomzdrav, and champion of social hygiene—became a victim of his own rhetoric. He ceded his post to a professional party man with bureaucratic rather than medical experience. Obukh, head of the Moscow Department of Health, was replaced by a bureaucrat with no medical education, and many other hygienists of the 1920s were turned out.[6] Just a few months after the satirical cartoon appeared, Narkomzdrav itself was subjected to a "cleansing."

Before his dismissal, Semashko had witnessed great progress. In 1927, on the tenth anniversary of the revolution, he assessed the work of Narkomzdrav. Comparing the Europe of the present and the Russia of the past, he declared: "The death rate of the population has dramatically dropped. Epidemic illnesses, which were the historically pathetic difference between our country and the rest of Europe, sharply decreased." He pointed out that infant death rates fell from approximately a quarter of all births to about a fifth, while in Moscow and other urban areas they amounted to a little over a tenth of all births. Not only did Russia now compare more favorably with Europe, but Narkomzdrav had dramatically changed the situation from that which had existed in the prerevolutionary era: "All of [these indicators] in general and each separately have fallen far below the prewar levels." He concluded that the nation's course was true.[7]

Although pleased with his statistical display of victory, Semashko was forced to admit that not nearly enough had been done. He offered examples of what he felt marred Narkomzdrav's successes: inadequate care for the peasantry and an insufficient number of institutions. Semashko admitted that in the city need still outstripped services and outside the urban centers medical practice had made little, if any, progress. He could have offered still other statistics to raise further caveats had he included the numbers of institutions built on a per capita basis. Dispensaries, consultations, and other prophylactic institutions could serve only a fraction of the needy. Consultations could advise mothers but lacked the wherewithal to offer them milk or other types of support. Pharmaceuticals and vaccines remained in short supply and were not distributed efficiently. The House of Leisure, which exposed so many to the lessons of healthy living, lacked the facilities to treat every urbanite and came nowhere near to providing care for all Soviet citizens. The few doctors who ventured outside Moscow and Leningrad confronted equipment and supply shortages as well as a distrustful population. Even in the urban home, poor material circumstances and overcrowding conspired to limit improvements. The highly touted communal kitchens, laundries, and nurseries simply did not materialize. Despite the disdain of the propagandists for capitalist medicine, most ordinary Russians still remained far less healthy and well cared for than their European counterparts.[8]

While it might appear that Narkomzdrav and the dream of universal health care were sacrificed on the altar of steel, Stalin's course in health policy was not without precedent. After the epidemic threat of the civil war years abated, Lenin's enthusiasm for health initiatives slackened in the face of the pressing need for rebuilding. Lenin supported Semashko in the primary position of doctor to the body Soviet but offered him little financial support. Stalin's programs would continue to prioritize industrial funding over health financing. The dismissal of Semashko signaled ideological as well as economic changes in Soviet programs. It should come as no surprise that with Stalin's great turn there would be a similar turn in discussions of health. During NEP the reality had been one of differential care, but the ideal among social hygienists had always been to implement care for all.[9] No longer would such soft, classless idealism drive Narkomzdrav. New bureaucratic handlers advocated care for workers (and socialized peasants) first and foremost and deflected discussion of health issues away from investigating the social origins of disease. With its stress upon statistical research, social conditions, and the contextual nature of disease, social hygiene brought to light troubling facts about current industrial policy, and these insights often conflicted with official stances.[10] In 1934 Stalin declared the class war over.[11] Opposing voices were silenced.

With the removal of the most dedicated social hygienists, Soviet medicine turned from ideals of universal care to embrace a hierarchical system centered on worker health. Stalin's plan fulfilled certain elements of the revolution's promise to make the last become first and give concrete benefits to the workers.[12] It did so even as it shied away from the vision of universal, prophylactic care that had made Narkomzdrav so revolutionary. Even though the shift to industry diminished funding for health care, relegated medicine to a lower level of importance as a career choice, increased the feminization of care, and contributed to lower standards of training, the group of insured workers expanded with the industrialization drive, with more of the population now qualifying for and demanding health care.[13] The 1930s saw the consolidation of health benefits and its extension to the makers of revolution as its true beneficiaries. Not content with simply a gift from above, workers agitated for the greater fulfillment of promises by learning how to speak the language of the state. Medical benefits emerged in other ways as well. The curtailing of the length of medical training required and the lowering of standards for students permitted the entrance into the medical profession of a remarkable number of people from formerly oppressed and excluded groups, such as workers, women, and ethnic minorities.[14] Major difficulties, however, remained and some even intensified. As a consequence of the numbers of new, inadequately trained personnel, care at the lowest levels was often poor. Given that the bureaucrats at the top valued increased numbers served over quality of individual service, an assembly-line approach to health care predominated.[15]

In addition to the shake-up in personnel, the late 1920s would reveal greater obstacles to Narkomzdrav as the First Five-Year plan—which subordinated the needs of the citizenry to those of industry—forced dislocations for some, famine for many, and desperate flight for millions. From 1926 to 1939 over 20 million peasants emigrated from the countryside to the cities in order to fill the jobs of the expanding industries of the First Five-Year Plan, as well as to escape famine and collectivization. In Moscow the population burgeoned from a little over 1 million in 1920 to almost 3.7 million by 1933 and 4.1 million by 1939. In Leningrad the population rose by over 500,000 from 1926 to 1939.[16] Municipal authorities were unable to cope with housing and sanitation needs. The ebb and flow of the population led to overcrowding and shortages, which resulted in increased levels of infection and deaths.[17] Although more people received care, as a result of the disregard for the social origins of disease, more people needed care. The dismissed social hygienists were undoubtedly horrified that smallpox, typhus, and malaria reemerged in the late 1920s and early 1930s.[18]

Despite all these problems, health remained the most prevalent example of the success of the revolution as reflected in propaganda aimed at workers inside the Soviet Union and around the world. Foreigners granted a peek behind the red curtain were still likely to find a doctor on the other side. Even the most unlikely observers were impressed by what they saw. Despite the scarcity, the promise of Narkomzdrav's programs shone through. A generally unsympathetic English observer, Sir James Purves-Stewart, visited a Leningrad night sanatorium in the early 1930s. He found it—the former villa of a wealthy German sugar investor—"rank and neglected" and badly in need of repair. He nevertheless admitted that the organization of Soviet public health was "impressive" and "elaborate": "Some of [their programs] are dramatically opposed to the codes of social life in western countries. Others, however, constitute a challenge to capitalist governments, a challenge which they would do well to take up, and, if possible, to surpass."[19]

Hygiene remained an important cultural and political mission in Stalin's campaigns to spread revolution throughout the population, control the actions of its citizens, and manage them as a resource. The Stalinist leadership retained a commitment to social and cultural change and to that end pursued hygiene instruction. Advice literature continued to emphasize health, rationalization, and discipline in the quest for *kul'turnost'*.[20] Behavioral recommendations included an emphasis on cleaning as worries about dust also carried over into the later Soviet period.[21] Institutions for the spread of healthful ideas continued to multiply and retained their sanitary enlightenment programs.[22] The Red Army included strictures on personal cleanliness in its regulations and school textbooks promoted hygiene.[23] The mass festival culture of the 1930s encouraged participation by citizens who maintained hygienic behavior and eschewed drinking and other traditional holiday activities. Physical culture parades proved particularly popular and also led to the establishment of hierarchies of workers and industries based not so much on work output as on physical appearance.[24] Education through display was supplemented by further education on hygienic principles. The domestication of peasant immigrants began with instruction in the care of both the body and home.[25] Contests for the cleanest home joined baby competitions of the 1920s to promote hygiene.[26] The exhortations to workers to use their leisure productively endured, as did worker's clubs designed to provide a healthy alternative, and the club network expanded its offerings. While physical culture underwent changes favoring a more sporting style of gaming, the importance of physical activity was maintained. Houses of Leisure proved popular. Although their numbers and patrons increased throughout the period, exit studies showed that they had little lasting effect.[27] Throughout this expansion, volunteers carried on their battle. In the 1930s wife-activists assumed the role of the citizen inspector. These spouses of specialists and managers were urged to use their leisure time to edify the workers, order their lives, and beautify the city.[28]

As the institutions of health and hygienic culture multiplied, they expanded geographically as well. Hygiene activity on the periphery was used as a measure of the revolution's march and the reach of state control. In Central Asia health campaigns served as a way to bring cultural and political reform into people's lives. Naïve activists with overly optimistic plans, however, often behaved condescendingly or provided misinformation.[29] Not only did the institutions of health expand outward, but the political and symbolic meanings of cleanliness came to inform concepts of identity in the ethnic regions. Cleanliness became an important signifier of progress in self-critical tales of metamorphosis among minorities of the Soviet state. The overlap between material culture, hygiene, and political enlightenment emerged in literary accounts, where the transformation from native to Soviet often included a bath or haircut as outward symbols of inward conversion.[30] Pushing into Siberia, Central Asia, and the countryside, cultural workers promoted Soviet values to counteract what they considered the bizarre, unhygienic customs of the natives. Force was not always effective, however, in accomplishing such delicate ends as "civilizing" a people. The actual impact of these proselytizers of orderliness did not live up to the tales touting miracles of conversion. Cultural and medical activists in Central Asia met results as mixed as those of Moscow and Leningrad campaigners.[31] Shocked doctors reported that some patients even mocked their advice.[32]

Gendered distinctions regarding sex and the body became more pronounced in the 1930s as natalist campaigns, sparked by anxiety over the birth rate, took center stage.[33] In the campaign against the midwife, hygienists claimed great success. In Moscow huge numbers of expectant women took their business to the state rather than to traditional providers. Beyond the city center health facilities still did not meet local needs despite their increase in number.[34] Fears over birth rates continued to push policy. Abortion was outlawed except in cases of danger to the mother. While women were advised that they were not fully healthy without exercise of their reproductive capacities, medical authorities continued to describe a detrimental relationship between sexual release and mental acuity for men.[35] Birth, however, was merely one target of the programs aimed at mothers and children. Women, who were important to the work force and necessary for future progress, saw an increase in day care and greater support for their household needs, although facilities still failed to provide for the entire population.[36] Also, since shortages of goods paralleled the increased importance of domestic care, such women's tasks as cleaning, shopping, and raising children took more and more time.[37]

Certain campaigns disappeared altogether. The call for simplicity in home decor fell by the wayside, without reference to the earlier politically and hygienically themed arguments against curtains, rugs, and other collectors of dust.[38] Although campaigns against drinking and smoking slackened in intensity, statistics became a useful tool in the maintenance of the body Soviet. The statistical analysis of the population—used to justify the intrusion of the state into the private lives of its citizens for hygienic purposes—now targeted certain groups. People deemed contaminants, antirevolutionary, or anti-Soviet were targeted for treatment/terror or amputation/excision.[39]

Statisticians and officials may not have considered the purification of society a success, but with statistics as weapons they attacked the idea of Western superiority. They crowed that from 1910 to 1970 the number of physicians in Russia increased twenty-five fold. During the same period the number of doctors in the United States showed a little over a twofold increase. The per capita number of doctors in the USSR reached about twice that of the United

States.[40] With more doctors, improvements in sanitation, and a higher standard of living, it was not surprising that despite the low status of the medical profession and limitations on services, Soviet health continued to improve. During the prerevolutionary period the average age of death in European Russia was given as thirty-one for men and thirty-three for women. By the end of the 1920s the Soviets claimed to have raised this figure to forty-two and forty-seven, respectively, climbing to sixty-one and sixty-seven, respectively, in the postwar era.[41] By the 1960s the life expectancy of Soviet citizens paralleled that of citizens of Western countries.

Buoyed by the numbers and bolstered by the evidence of their seeming political, social, and medical superiority, some hygienists contemplated the possibility of near immortality in a communist state. If they could more than double the average life span in just fifty years, many believed there were virtually no limits to what could be accomplished. In the 1970s one gerontologist claimed that Soviet scientists possessed a different mind-set and economic background that made them better able to tackle questions of longevity, arguing: "Researchers in other countries have attempted—and are still attempting—to prove the imperfection of human nature, pointing out biological difficulties and defects." He saw this as faulty reasoning. Instead of man's biology, it was society that caused aging and infirmity: "The many centuries of mankind's history prove that the cruelest and most merciless enemy of human longevity is a society in which man is exploited by man."[42] Although international experts may not have agreed that the Soviets had almost triumphed over death, they did credit them with great success. Foreign public health advocates pointed to the capabilities of Soviet care and unprecedented state support. Other countries moved to increase state intervention and to provide greater welfare support to the population. The Soviets' early programs presaged a European-wide trend as state-sponsored care further accelerated in Europe following World War II.[43]

While Soviet researchers were confidently tracking heartbeats and calculating the "limits" of mortality, statistics on the health of the population reflected a disturbing change beginning in the 1970s. The Soviet Union became the first industrialized country to show a decrease in life expectancy and an increase in infant mortality.[44] Economic collapse in the 1980s took its toll on the health of an already ailing population, with dramatic declines in wages, sudden inflation, and economic hardship resulting in a decline in public health.[45] According to Murray Feshbach and Alfred Friendly, Jr., inadequate medical provisions and changes in lifestyle were exacerbated by environmental problems and official neglect, occasioning a precipitous decline in health after the fall of the Soviet Union.[46] The 1991 collapse ensured that the criteria of cleanliness used to divide and conquer the body politic would be redirected, but the Soviet health system remained in the sorry state it had been in at the time of the collapse and continued to decline. By the mid-1990s the average Soviet male could be expected to live into his middle fifties. The life expectancies of women extended into their middle sixties.[47]

Russia is now in the midst of a demographic crisis.[48] Increasing abuse of drugs, alcohol, and tobacco, coupled with a disregard for moderation, healthy diet, and exercise are all contributing to the failing state of health. Included in this laundry list of ills is an incomplete understanding of health issues by the population.[49] While an analysis of current health problems is certainly beyond the scope of the present study, many of the problems pointed to by demographers and analysts stem from what hygienists in the 1920s termed "lifestyle" illnesses. William C. Cockerham, a sociologist and specialist in behavioral risk factors, postulates that structural constraints—a dearth of information on health, a lack of control over diet and environment, and a society where heavy drinking and smoking are normative—may have so determined Soviet identities, and consequently self-direction, as to "leave people with little or no choice in exposing themselves to unhealthy conditions and practices."[50] According to recent surveys, many inhabitants of the former Soviet Union still feel their lives and their health are caught up in a system without rules and over which they have no control.[51]

Prophylaxis depended upon citizens taking control of their lives, making behavioral changes based on hygienic norms, and thereby lessening the frequency of disease. This requirement for popular action necessitated a faith that personal decisions could affect lasting change. In 1999 Cockerham concluded that the post-Soviet decline was the result of "poor health lifestyles," including drinking, high-fat diets, inactivity, and smoking, the exact choices that hygienists hoped the population would avoid.[52]

The message of decades of propaganda on hygiene and rational living had not achieved its intended outcome. The body Soviet was neither healthier, nor stronger, nor more physically fit than any other nation on the globe. Nor had surveillance, propaganda, and hygiene programs created the anticipated changes in lifestyle, the body, and the mind. The spirit of collectivism had not risen up to animate the purified bodies of the Soviet citizenry. Nor had the state triumphed. Even as metaphors of hygiene permeated Soviet and Russian society, health was—and remains—elusive.

NOTES

Abbreviations

AMO: Arkhiv Moskovskoi oblasti
GARF: Gosudarstvennyi arkhiv Rossiiskoi Federatsii
KOTiB: Komitet ozdorovlenie trud i byt
MOZ: Moskovskii otdel zdravookhranenia
Narkomzdrav: Narodnyi komissariat zdravookhraneniia
OMM: Okhrana materinstva i mladenchestva
TsGAODM: Tsentral'nyi gosudarstvennyi arkhiv obshchestvennykh dvizhenii Moskvy
TsGAMO: Tsentral'nyi gosudarstvennyi arkhiv Moskovskoi oblasti
TsMAM: Tsentral'nyi munitsipal'nyi arkhiv Moskvy
ZNB: *Za novyi byt*

Introduction

1. Lenin, "Report of the All-Russia Central Executive Committee and the Council of People's Commissars, December 5," in *Collected Works*, 30:228; also in N. A. Semashko, "Politika v dele zdravookhraneniia za desiat' let," in *Desiat' let oktiabria i sovetskaia meditsina*, ed. N. A. Semashko, 4. Lice were identified in 1909 as a vector for typhus, an epidemic in urban and rural areas by this time; see K. David Patterson, "Typhus and Its Control in Russia, 1870–1940," 361, 372.

2. After reading my project description, one Russian university official quipped: "We had hygiene?"

3. W. Horsley Gantt cited ten million dead for the period 1916 to 1923 in *Russian Medicine*, 144. Basing himself on E. I. Potova, *Bor'ba s infektsionnymi bolezniami v SSSR, 1917–1967*, 67–70, Gordon Hyde amasses statistics to point to cholera (368,390 deaths, 1918–21), typhus (5,763,470 deaths, 1918–21), typhoid (2,046,709 deaths, 1914–21), and dysentery (1,665,645 deaths, 1914–21); quoted in *The Soviet Health Service: A Historical and Comparative Study*, 48–49.

4. I. A. Slonimskaia, "V. I. Lenin ob okhrane zdorov'ia naroda," in *Ocherki istoriografii sovetskogo zdravookhraneniia*, ed. M. I. Barsukov, 13.

5. In early studies of Soviet health care, eager fellow travelers recounted in detail the benefits of socialism in contrast to the deprivations of capitalism; see: Gantt, *Russian Medicine;* Anna J. Haines, *Health Work in Soviet Russia;* and Sir Arthur Newsholme and John Adams Kingsbury, *Red Medicine: Socialized Health in Soviet Russia.* Others touched on health in a survey of all things Soviet; see, e.g., British Trade Union Delegation, *Russia Today: The Official Report of the British Trade Union Delegation* and Fannina W. Halle, *Woman in Soviet Russia.* Later surveys give health its due, but in these larger studies the revolutionary years and international context are not a focus. See Henry Sigerist, *Medicine and Health in the Soviet Union;* Mark G. Field, *Soviet Socialized Medicine;* and Michael Kaser, *Health Care in the Soviet Union and Eastern Europe.* Recently historians have returned to questions of professionalization and the creation of a civil society in discussions of medical care. Nancy Mandelker Frieden argues that health care professionals, essential to a civil society, were weak; see *Russian Physicians in an Era of Reform and Revolution, 1856–1905.* John F. Hutchinson focuses on the political struggle among medical professionals rather than on a binary of professionals vs. state; see *Politics and Public Health in Revolutionary Russia, 1890–1918.* Solomon and Hutchinson's edited volume *Health and Society in Revolutionary Russia* further complicates the understanding of professionalization and centralization. Mary Schaeffer Conroy addresses Soviet pharmacy in the 1920s primarily as a means of understanding the problems of Soviet pharmaceutical production, particularly in later periods; see *The Soviet Pharmaceutical Business during Its First Two Decades (1917–1937).* Michael Zdenek David investigates social construction and professionalization against the backdrop of tuberculosis care in "The White Plague in the Red Capital: Tuberculosis and Its Control in Moscow, 1900–1941." A recent set of works has brought to light the experience of health care outside the centers. Paula A. Michaels examines health care as a tool in Stalin's empire in *Curative Powers: Medicine and Empire in Stalin's Central Asia.* David L. Ransel intertwines questions of gender and ethnicity in his study of women's healthcare in the village through the Soviet period; see *Village Mothers: Three Generations of Change in Russia and Tataria.* Cassandra Cavanaugh investigates Central Asia in "Backwardness and Biology: Medicine and Power in Russian and Soviet Central Asia, 1868–1934."

6. Conceptualizing disease as a social problem—social hygiene—was the guiding principle of Narkomzdrav; prophylaxis was the cornerstone of social hygiene. See Susan Gross Solomon, "Social Hygiene and Soviet Public Health, 1921–1930," in *Health and Society in Revolutionary Russia,* ed. Solomon and Hutchinson, 175–99.

7. A number of works have investigated the intersection of lifestyle, politics, and creation in the 1920s. Richard Stites details the utopian philosophies of Revolution in *Revolutionary Dreams: Utopian Vision and Experimental Life in the Russian Revolution.* Lynn Mally reveals proletarian cultural experiments in *Culture of the Future: The Proletkult Movement in Revolutionary Russia.* Katerina Clark investigates the prerevolutionary origins of Stalinist culture in *Petersburg, Crucible of Cultural Revolution.* Eric Naiman shows that a disciplined, male body was crucial to utopia in *Sex in Public: The Incarnation of Early Soviet Ideology.* Anne E. Gorsuch examines how the quixotic dreams of youth clashed with the aspirations of the party elite in *Youth in Revolutionary Russia: Enthusiasts, Bohemians, and Delinquents.* Catriona Kelly engages the culture of the period in *Refining Russia: Advice Literature, Polite Culture, and Gender from Catherine to Yeltsin,* as well as in the edited volume *Constructing Russian Culture in the Age of*

Revolution, 1881–1940, ed. Catriona Kelly and David Shepherd. In both works Kelly mentions hygiene, in its critical aspect of ordering and rationalizing, as part of the cultural mission of the 1920s. Diane P. Koenker documents the intersection of socialist rhetoric and daily life among printers in *Republic of Labor: Russian Printers and Soviet Socialism, 1918–1930*. Most recently scholars have looked to questions of sexuality and control as part of the experience of health in the 1920s. See Dan Healey, *Homosexual Desire in Revolutionary Russia: The Regulation of Sexual and Gender Dissent*; and Frances Lee Bernstein, *The Dictatorship of Sex: Lifestyle Advice for the Soviet Masses.*

8. As Orlando Figes and Boris Kolonitskii argue in *Interpreting the Russian Revolution: The Language and Symbols of 1917*, certain symbols, like the red flag, became "polyvalent"; different groups "could project their own revolutionary ideals" onto these symbols (3). I argue that the fight for health was similarly drawing together different groups toward a seemingly common goal. In *The Dictatorship of Sex*, Gorsuch, working with didactic literature and programs for youth, uses the term "moralists" to cover the large group of people with overlapping programs—from social scientists, to youth-group organizers, to the youths themselves—who were interested in furthering the Soviet agenda. Many of these moralists held hygienic conceptions within their prescriptions (3–4). Like Gorsuch, I argue that although many individuals did not always work together, they were nevertheless united in a common goal—in this case a balanced, rationalized, ordered, hygienic lifestyle backed by scientific justifications. Jean-Pierre Goubert, in *The Conquest of Water: The Advent of Health in the Industrial Age*, similarly argues (146–68) that in the European context government officials, educators, doctors, state representatives, and the ruling class were united in their condemnation of dirt and exhortation to cleanliness and order.

9. Alphonse d'Houtaud and Mark G. Field, *Cultural Images of Health: A Neglected Dimension*, 9–12.

10. See Leon Trotsky's expansive attacks on "uncultured behavior"—"Attention to Trifles!" (1923), "The Struggle for Cultured Speech" (1923), and "Culture and Socialism" (1923)—in *Problems of Everyday Life: And Other Writings on Culture and Science*, 52–56, 73–76, 227–49.

11. Hyde, *Soviet Health Service*, details these early efforts of workers' commissions against typhus (50–52).

12. In *Refining Russia* Kelly argues for the centrality of hygiene in the *kul'turnost'* campaigns (265).

13. For publication statistics, see T. F. Makarova, "Meditsinskaia pechat'," in *Okhrana narodnogo zdorov'ia v SSSR*, ed. M. D. Kovrigin, 481–82. Wherever possible I have supplied publication figures for pamphlets. See: A. A. Ashikhmin, *Tuberkulez i zhilishche;* A. L. Mendel'son, *Vospitanie voli;* I. M. Barushkin, *Pochemy vreden tabak?* (pub. 15,000); Il'ia Rubanovskii, *Za knigu ili v pivnuiu?* (pub. 10,000); N. A. Semashko, *Iskusstvo odevat'sia* (pub. 15,000).

14. In the case of an alcoholic thrown out of the building for "incurable" alcoholism, the court rather than the inspectors made the decision; see TsGAMO f. 2129, op. 1, d. 97, l. 17.

15. Kenneth M. Pinnow notes this collapsing of private and public in "Violence against the Collective Self and the Problem of Social Integration in Early Bolshevik Russia" (653).

16. Peter Holquist argues that Soviet techniques were those of modern states and it was their ideology that distinguished their application. See his "'Information Is the Alpha and Omega of Our Work': Bolshevik Surveillance in Its Pan-European Context," 427–48; *Making War, Forging Revolution: Russia's Continuum of Crisis, 1914–1921,* 6–8, 206–40; "Violent Russia, Deadly Marxism? Russia in the Epoch of Violence, 1905–21," 643. For an analysis of Soviet control in the 1930s as a convergence of prerevolutionary, international, and revolutionary thought, see David L. Hoffmann, *Stalinist Values: The Cultural Norms of Soviet Modernity, 1917–1941.* Stephen Kotkin argues for the revolutionary essence of Stalinist control in *Magnetic Mountain: Stalinism as a Civilization.* Amir Weiner details the "purification" impulse of the state and its continuation well into the post–World War II era in *Making Sense of War: The Second World War and the Fate of the Bolshevik Revolution,* 17, 22. Francine Hirsch argues for the strong influence of ideology on Bolshevik policy in *Empire of Nations: Ethnographic Knowledge and the Making of the Soviet Union.*

17. Dorothy Porter, *Health, Civilization and the State: A History of Public Health from Ancient to Modern Times;* Roy Porter, *The Greatest Benefit to Mankind: A Medical History of Humanity;* George Rosen, *A History of Public Health.*

18. Michel Foucault's work on the rise of the social sciences in Europe greatly influences the analysis of Soviet hygiene in the present work. While historians have criticized Foucault for his dependence upon the "modern" era and "liberalism" as the origin of all things, scholars of the Soviet Union still find elements of his theories helpful. Here Foucault's use of Jeremy Bentham's panopticon as an example of surveillance of the individual and the creation of the invasive, medicalized "gaze" is particularly effective. See Foucault, *Discipline and Punish: The Birth of the Prison,* 195–228; see also *The Birth of the Clinic: An Archaeology of Medical Perception,* ix–xix. For Foucault in a Soviet context, see Kotkin, *Magnetic Mountain,* 157–237.

19. On subjectivity, see Jochen Hellbeck, "Working, Struggling, Becoming: Stalin-Era Autobiographical Texts," 340–359; and Eric Naiman, "Discourse Made Flesh: Healing and Terror in the Construction of Soviet Subjectivity," in *Language and Revolution: Making Modern Political Identities,* ed. Igal Halfin, 287–316.

20. In their study of Russian and Soviet culture, Kelly and Shepherd succinctly remark that "it proved a great deal easier to manufacture 'blueprints for identity' than to 'engineer human souls' in the envisaged manner." See "Introduction: Literature, History, Culture," in *Constructing Russian Culture,* ed. Kelly and Shepherd, 5. Igal Halfin details the anxieties over purity and "the Bolshevik hermeneutic of the self" in his *Intimate Enemies: Demonizing the Bolshevik Opposition, 1918–1928.*

21. Dale B. Martin, *The Corinthian Body,* xiv.

22. The political interpretation of dirt presented here relies a great deal upon Dame Mary Douglas's *Purity and Danger: An Analysis of Concepts of Pollution and Taboo.*

23. Even in the 1800s Moscow was recognized as a hub of disease and was the first to be attended to by authorities. Beginning in the 1890s, the Moscow duma worked to improve the city since the ruling class could not ignore the problems at their doorsteps; see Robert W. Thurston, *Liberal City, Conservative State: Moscow and Russia's Urban Crisis, 1906–1914,* 138, 181.

24. Lenin, "Speech Delivered at a Meeting of the Moscow Soviet of Workers' and

Red Army Deputies," in *Collected Works,* 30:410–16; N. A. Vinogradov, E. D. Ashurkov, and S. V. Kurashov, "Osnovnye tempy razvitiia sovetskogo zdravookhraneniia," in *Okhrana narodnogo zdorov'ia v SSSR,* ed. Kovrigin, 45.

25. Foucault describes these attempts to manage sexuality and connect procreation to the needs of the state as the "'responsibilization' of couples with regard to the social body as a whole"; *The History of Sexuality: An Introduction,* 105.

26. Christopher M. Davis, "Economics of Soviet Public Health, 1928–1932: Development Strategy, Resource Constraints, and Health Plans," in *Health and Society in Revolutionary Russia,* ed. Solomon and Hutchinson, 146–72.

Chapter 1. Revolution: Destruction, Cleansing, and Creation

1. Klara Zetkin, *Reminiscences of Lenin,* 45–46.

2. Douglas, *Purity and Danger,* 2.

3. See Phyllis Palmer, "Dirt and Divisions among Women," in her *Domesticity and Dirt: Housewives and Domestic Servants in the United States, 1920–1945,* 137–51.

4. In *Stalin's Outcasts: Aliens, Citizens, and the Soviet State, 1926–1936,* Golfo Alexopoulos uses the arguments of Clifford Geertz to bring out the underlying binaries of capitalist and communist used to diagnose alien "class" elements in the 1920s and 1930s. In *Petersburg, Crucible of Cultural Revolution* Katerina Clark distinguishes her own binary of the 1920s, arguing: "Much of intellectual life was driven by a version of a thirst for the sacred with a concomitant revulsion against the profane" (2). This duality between dirt and cleanliness is used in both of the above cases and in other contexts in discussions of what is acceptable and unacceptable.

5. Leon Trotsky, *My Life: An Attempt at an Autobiography,* 328. Although he directed this remark at the Mensheviks, the metaphor of defilement could also be applied to any political recalcitrant.

6. A. Zheleznyi repeated the Zetkin-Lenin conversation in *Kak zhit', chtoby zdorovym byt'?,* 27. (pub. 9,000).

7. For more, see Richard Stites's *Revolutionary Dreams,* which shows how enthusiastic youth and even their wizened elders indulged in such reveries.

8. See Roberta T. Manning, *The Crisis of the Old Order in Russia: Government and Gentry;* for more on the fragmentation of Russia in the late nineteenth and early twentieth centuries, see also Victoria E. Bonnell, *Roots of Rebellion: Workers' Politics and Organizations in St. Petersburg and Moscow, 1900–1914;* Edith W. Clowes, Samuel D. Kassow, and James L. West, eds., *Between Tsar and People: Educated Society and the Quest for Public Identity in Late Imperial Russia.*

9. There are too many excellent books concerning the Russian Revolution to list here. The following works provide a good starting point for more detailed accounts—Sheila Fitzpatrick's *The Russian Revolution* addresses the revolution from the fall of the autocracy to the imposition of Stalin's rule. Alexander Rabinowitch examines Petrograd in *Prelude to Revolution: The Petrograd Bolsheviks and the July 1917 Uprising* and *The Bolsheviks Come to Power.* For revolutionary Moscow in-depth see Diane Koenker, *Moscow Workers and the 1917 Revolution.* The front line troops come under lively scrutiny in Allan K. Wildman's two-volume *The End of the Russian Imperial Army.*

10. The beneficiaries of the revolution have been as popular a set of subjects as the revolution itself. The classic work on this subject is Leopold H. Haimson, *The Russian Marxists and the Origins of Bolshevism.*

11. For more on the civil war and its effects, see Diane Koenker, William G. Rosenberg, and Ronald Grigor Suny, eds., *Party, State and Society in the Russian Civil War: Explorations in Social History.*

12. Fitzpatrick, *Russian Revolution,* 64. The bureaucracy is treated extensively by Robert Service in *The Bolshevik Party in Revolution: A Study in Organizational Change, 1917–1923.*

13. For more on Moscow during the revolution, see Timothy J. Colton, *Moscow: Governing the Socialist Metropolis,* 71–151; for its demographic problems, see David L. Hoffmann, *Peasant Metropolis: Social Identities in Moscow, 1929–1941,* 12–31, esp. 25; for background, see Thurston, *Liberal City, Conservative State;* for the civil war, see Mauricio Borrero, *Hungry Moscow: Scarcity and Urban Society in the Russian Civil War, 1917–1921.*

14. Kurt Wiedenfeld, *The Remaking of Russia,* 85.

15. For more on the policy of NEP and Soviet society, see Sheila Fitzpatrick, Alexander Rabinowitch, and Richard Stites, eds., *Russia in the Era of NEP: Explorations in Soviet Society and Culture;* Lewis H. Siegelbaum, *Soviet State and Society between Revolutions, 1918–1929.* For more on the economics of NEP, see Alexander Erlich, *The Soviet Industrialization Debate, 1924–1928;* Alec Nove, *An Economic History of the U.S.S.R.*

16. See the chapter "Living with NEP" in Siegelbaum, *Soviet State and Society,* 135–87.

17. Diane P. Koenker vividly describes the many problems for women in the workforce in "Men against Women on the Shop Floor in Early Soviet Russia: Gender and Class in the Socialist Workplace," 1438–64; see also her detailed investigation of printer culture in *Republic of Labor: Russian Printers and Soviet Socialism, 1918–1930,* 194–207.

18. Elizabeth Wood, *The Baba and the Comrade: Gender and Politics in Revolutionary Russia,* 147–69.

19. Alan M. Ball, *Russia's Last Capitalists: The Nepmen, 1921–1929,* 15–16; for a lurid account of 1920s Moscow, see Lancelot Lawton, *The Russian Revolution, 1917–1926,* 278–99, 308–14.

20. Catriona Kelly and Vadim Volkov, "Directed Desires: *Kul'turnost'* and Consumption," in *Constructing Russian Culture,* ed. Kelly and Shepherd, 291–92; see also Katerina Clark's discussion of "Romantic Anticapitalism" in her *Petersburg, Crucible of Cultural Revolution,* 16–23.

21. For more on NEP-era culture, see Sheila Fitzpatrick, *The Cultural Front: Power and Culture in Revolutionary Russia;* Abbott Gleason, Peter Kenez, and Richard Stites, eds., *Bolshevik Culture: Experiment and Order in the Russian Revolution;* and Mally, *Culture of the Future.* For NEP-era Moscow in particular, see Colton, *Moscow,* 153–247.

22. Wood argues that economic recovery, concerns over NEP, and Trotsky's attention to the cultural front spurred discussion of these mundane questions after 1923; see *The Baba and the Comrade,* 195–97.

23. Mally, *Culture of the Future,* xviii. A new and burgeoning literature addresses the construction of daily life and behavior; see Bernstein, *The Dictatorship of Sex;* Gorsuch, *Youth in Revolutionary Russia;* Healey, *Homosexual Desire in Revolutionary Russia;* Naiman, *Sex in Public;* and Wood, *The Baba and the Comrade.* See also Oleg Kharkhordin, *The Collective and the Individual in Russia: A Study of Practices;* N. B. Lebina, *Povsednevnaia zhizn' sovetskogo goroda:*

Normy i anomalii, 1920–1930 gody; idem., *Rabochaia molodezh' Leningrada : Trud i sotsial'nyi oblik, 1921–1925 gody.*

24. In *Realistic Utopias: The Ideal Imaginary Societies of the Renaissance, 1516–1630* Miriam Eliav-Feldon argues for the supremacy of hygiene in utopian construction: "The most essential condition for the creation of a perfect community is the cleansing of filth and the banishment of illness. . . . If we were to put all our texts together, we should find that this subject probably occupies more space than any other" (31).

25. Joyce Oramel Hertzler, *The History of Utopian Thought,* 289.

26. René Dubos, *Mirage of Health: Utopias, Progress, and Biological Change,* 1–29.

27. A foreign contemporary of Ivan IV's *oprichniki* noted that they "sweep away" treason; see "Poslanie Ioganna Taube i Elerta Kruze," *Russkii istoricheskii zhurnal* 8 (1922), 38; cited in Maureen Perrie and Andrei Pavlov, *Ivan the Terrible,* 113.

28. Stephen Lessing Baehr outlines the utopian impulse in early Russian literature. While he does not specifically address hygiene, he notes the emphasis on iron and industrialization in the nineteenth century; see the epilogue in *The Paradise Myth in Eighteenth-Century Russia: Utopian Patterns in Early Secular Russian Literature and Culture,* 163–68.

29. Vincent Geoghegan, *Utopianism and Marxism,* 22–34.

30. Saint-Simon trumpeted the organic nature of society and the transformative powers of science. Fourier obsessively detailed the changes that his system would bring about and inspired phalansteries in Romania and Saint Petersburg. Owen, the most appreciated utopist by Marx and Engels, concentrated on the workers. See Frank E. Manuel and Fritzie P. Manuel, *Utopian Thought in the Western World,* 586–87, 595–96, 600–601, 644–48, 703–5.

31. Milka Bliznakov, "The Realization of Utopia: Western Technology and Soviet Avant-Garde Architecture," in *Reshaping Russian Architecture: Western Technology, Utopian Dreams,* ed. William C. Brumfield, 146–47.

32. Stites emphasizes the importance of these three authors in his discussion of popular, utopian, and literary influences during the revolutionary era. Here their hygiene prescriptions are highlighted. See *Revolutionary Dreams,* 26–27, 32–33.

33. Stites calls it "the most important radical novel in nineteenth century literature"; *Revolutionary Dreams,* 26.

34. See Stites, *Revolutionary Dreams,* 42. Katerina Clark addresses the emblematic hero, his progress, and his influence in *The Soviet Novel: History as Ritual,* 51, 56–60.

35. Wood, *The Baba and the Comrade,* 25.

36. John F. Kasson examines the novel in *Civilizing the Machine: Technology and Republican Values in America, 1776–1900,* 192–202.

37. Alexander Bogdanov, "Red Star," in *Red Star: The First Bolshevik Utopia,* ed. Loren R. Graham and Richard Stites, 30–140.

38. In the early 1920s Proletkul't fell into decline after being subordinated to the Commissariat of Enlightenment. See Mally, *Culture of the Future,* xix, 2–3, 193–228; see also Sheila Fitzpatrick, *The Commissariat of Enlightenment: Soviet Organization of Education and the Arts under Lunacharsky, October 1917–1921.*

39. Mally, *Culture of the Future,* 162–63.

40. The Central Institute of Hematology and Blood Transfusions was founded in 1926. See Stites, *Revolutionary Dreams,* 26–33; see also Bogdanov, "Red Star," 86. For an

account of Bogdanov's death, see Loren R. Graham, "Bogdanov's Inner Message," in Bogdanov, *Red Star,* 251–52.

41. Bogdanov, "Red Star," 34.

42. Elizabeth Wood points out the longstanding interest in private behavior as a public issue among Russian intellectuals; see *The Baba and the Comrade,* 21. Science, medicine, and mechanization were also important in the West's battle for cleanliness; see Joseph A. Amato, *Dust: A History of the Small and the Invisible,* 110–25.

43. Alexander Vucinich, *Social Thought in Tsarist Russia: The Quest for a General Science of Society, 1861–1917,* 7–12, 14, 233; and Loren R. Graham, *Science in Russia and the Soviet Union: A Short History,* 1–75.

44. Louise McReynolds and Cathy Popkin, "The Objective Eye and the Common Good," in *Constructing Russian Culture,* ed. Kelly and Shepherd, 66–71, 81–92.

45. Lewis H. Siegelbaum, "*Okhrana Truda:* Industrial Hygiene, Psychotechnics, and Industrialization in the USSR," in *Health and Society in Revolutionary Russia,* ed. Solomon and Hutchinson, 224–45; in more depth, see Graham, *Science in Russia,* 79–98.

46. Stephen E. Hanson, *Time and Revolution: Marxism and the Design of Soviet Institutions.*

47. Anson Rabinbach examines Taylorism as part of a general fascination with overcoming the body's limitations by mechanizing movement in *The Human Motor: Energy, Fatigue, and the Origins of Modernity,* 238–88.

48. Hanson, *Time and Revolution,* 97–99; Alan M. Ball, *Imagining America: Influence and Images in Twentieth-Century Russia,* 23–55.

49. On Fordism, see Lynne Attwood and Catriona Kelly, "Programs for Identity: The 'New Man' and the 'New Woman,'" in *Constructing Russian Culture,* ed. Kelly and Shepherd, 256. Alan M. Ball notes that while capitalist exploitation was condemned, American prosperity—as seen with the American Relief Administration (ARA), American popular literature, and Hollywood films—was envied; see "The Roots of Golden America in Early Soviet Russia," in *The Human Tradition in Modern Russia,* ed. William B. Husband, 51–64.

50. Alexei Gastev, poet and theorist, was central to the spread of NOT. See Kurt Johansson, *Aleksej Gastev: Proletarian Bard of the Machine Age,* 7, 10, 103. For more on Gastev and his uneasy reception, see Kendall E. Bailes, "Alexei Gastev and the Soviet Controversy over Taylorism, 1918–24," 373–94. For NOT cell numbers, see Toby Clark, "The 'New Man's' Body: A Motif in Early Soviet Culture," in *Art of the Soviets: Painting, Sculpture and Architecture in a One-Party State, 1917–1992,* ed. Mathew Cullerne Brown and Brandon Taylor, 37.

51. Naiman comments that NEP was "a type of vaccination"; *Sex in Public,* 263.

52. Clark notes the roots of these binary oppositions in her discussion of "Romantic Anticapitalism" among the intelligentsia before and after the revolution; *Petersburg, Crucible of Cultural Revolution,* 16–17.

53. As Mary Douglas argues in *Purity and Danger,* "Dirt is the by-product of a systematic ordering and classification of matter, in so far as ordering involves rejecting inappropriate elements" (36). In her introduction to *Utopias: Russian Modernist Texts, 1905–1940,* Catriona Kelly comments that with the onset of revolution "no work of art was now seen as politically neutral" (xx). The same could be said of even the seemingly most mundane daily actions.

54. Naiman, in *Sex in Public,* calls the civil war "a time of uncompromising—and thus comforting—purity" (5). This comfort in the past's strict delineation of revolutionary and counterrevolutionary behavior was poetically and pathetically portrayed in the longings of F. V. Gladkov's Polia Makova in the mid-1920s soap *Cement.* Polia reacted violently to the policies of NEP and was subsequently dropped from the party for her lack of understanding of political pragmatism. Lenin had noted in 1919 the difficulty of keeping "clean communist hands" when serious revolutionaries needed to work along with the "counter-revolutionary bourgeois co-operators"; "Achievement and Difficulties of the Soviet Government," in *Collected Works,* 29:73. For an account of *Cement,* see Clark, *The Soviet Novel,* 68–82.

55. Douglas, *Purity and Danger,* 95. George Vigarello studies the concept from a historical perspective in *Concepts of Cleanliness: Changing Attitudes in France since the Middle Ages.*

56. Lenin, "Speech on the Organization of a Farm Laborers Union," in *Collected Works,* 29:38.

57. Lenin, "Letter to American Workers" (1918), in *Collected Works,* 28:63.

58. Newspapers employed similarly descriptive epithets. See Jeffrey Brooks, *Thank You, Comrade Stalin! Soviet Public Culture from Revolution to Cold War,* 131–49. Marx had originally used this term for usurers and profit mongers. See, e.g., his *Capital* or *Theories of Surplus Value.*

59. Lenin, "Speech at a Meeting at the Former Michelson Works, August 30, 1918," in *Collected Works,* 28:91.

60. Lenin, "How to Organise Competition?" (1917), in *Collected Works,* 26:414.

61. Lenin, "The Itch" (1918), in *Collected Works,* 27:37; also *Polnoe sobranie sochinenii,* 35:361. The Russian *Chesotka* is usually translated as "The Itch," but it might also be rendered as "Scabies." Lenin also used "infection" to connote the spread of socialist thought, implying that the ideas spread rapidly and easily. See "Speech Delivered at a Non-Party Conference in Blagusha-Lefortovo District" (1920), in *Collected Works,* 30:350.

62. Figes and Kolonitskii, *Interpreting the Russian Revolution,* 154.

63. For example, Alexandra Kollontai used such visual cues to denote the bourgeois tendencies of Vasia's lover and his mistress in her *Love of Worker Bees.* In *Sex in Public* Naiman notes the use of fashion and jewelry as symptom of "ideological contamination" (183). Bernstein explores the further connections of NEP, prostitution, and gender in *The Dictatorship of Sex,* 67–68.

64. Halfin explores the difficulties of party purity and consequent anxiety over the hidden enemy in *Intimate Enemies,* 42–43.

65. By dredging up Oblomov, Lenin chided party operatives for their inactivity and also portrayed them as holdovers of the worst type. In I. A. Goncharov's novel *Oblomov* (1859) the titular hero is incapable of performing useful actions or making decisions. Goncharov's novel was seen as a critique of the superfluous aristocracy, which contributed nothing to Russia's progress.

66. Lenin, "Speech to a Meeting of the Communist Group at the All-Russian Congress of Metalworkers" (1922), in *Collected Works,* 33:223.

67. Kharkhordin provides a fascinating account of these "illnesses," with the emphasis on curing rather than cutting the offenders out of party membership; see *The Collective*

and the Individual in Russia, 36–40. Naiman points out the similar tendency to see NEP as debilitating; see *Sex in Public,* 173. Halfin provides a more detailed set of quotations from party debates on illness; see *Intimate Enemies,* 64–68.

68. Koenker, *Republic of Labor,* 105.

69. Trotsky warned against "cant—a disease that is dangerous and catching"; quoted in "How to Begin" (1923), in *Problems of Everyday Life,* 66. Gorsuch notes similar advice for youth who had contact with the infectious agents of the old order; see *Youth in Revolutionary Russia,* 29–34, 176.

70. According to Naiman, by the mid-1920s "the Soviet press argued with increasing frequency that the life of the social organism *depended* on the course assumed by the personal lives of its members" (*Sex in Public,* 92).

71. In his investigation, Kharkhordin comes to the conclusion that while the term had some connection to the church—it had been used to connote the recruitment of clergy for the army since the time of Catherine the Great—there was no evidence that the Marxists borrowed it directly; see *The Collective and the Individual in Russia,* 135. Nadya L. Peterson provides a fascinating interpretation of purge memoirs according to the inversion of cleanliness/filth in "Dirty Women: Cultural Connotations of Cleanliness in Soviet Russia," in *Russia, Women, Culture,* ed. Helena Goscilo and Beth Holmgren, 192–96.

72. With disunity, the party faithful saw the possibility of corruption, ulcers, rot, disease, and, of course, illness. See Kharkhordin, *The Collective and the Individual in Russia,* 138–39.

73. Deprivations also included denying access to health care. See Alexopoulos, *Stalin's Outcasts,* 1–3.

74. David G. Horn, *Social Bodies: Science, Reproduction, and Italian Modernity,* 19. The stress on the collective emerged in nineteenth-century Russia. See also David L. Hoffmann, "European Modernity and Soviet Socialism," in *Russian Modernity: Politics, Knowledge, Practices,* ed. David L. Hoffmann and Yanni Kotsonis, 253; Porter, *Health, Civilization, and the State,* 73–75. Foucault argues that it was not because societies were corporeal in nature that biological metaphors were so prominent but rather because the dichotomy of "healthy/ morbid" was so easily transferred to discussions of society; see *Birth of the Clinic,* 35–36.

75. Porter, *Health, Civilization, and the State,* 73–78. For a survey of three leading nineteenth-century ideologists of criminal degeneracy who used corporeal concepts in their diagnoses of society—Bénédict Augustin Morel of France, Cesare Lombroso of Italy, and Henry Maudsley of England—see Daniel Pick, *Faces of Degeneration: A European Disorder, c. 1848–c. 1918.*

76. Horn, *Social Bodies,* 28.

77. Robert Proctor, *The Nazi War on Cancer,* 46.

78. These corporeal constructions can also be seen in the social-engineering concepts of the "gardening state," where society is an organism that needs to be managed, purified, and maintained through the excision of the unfit and the molding of the remainder. Weiner uses the "gardening state" concept of sociologist Zygmunt Bauman to describe the biological and sociological aspects of the purification drives of the later Soviet period; *Making Sense of War,* 27–29, 191–235.

79. As B. S. Sigal put it, life was a physical and chemical process with no room for a "soul"; *Trud i zdorov'e rabochei molodezhi,* 5. N. A. Semashko, *Puti sovetskoi fizkul'tury,* 17. For a more thorough discussion of physiology and psychology, see Loren R. Graham, *Science and Philosophy in the Soviet Union,* 355–429.

80. James Riordan, "The Rise, Fall and Rebirth of Sporting Women in Russia and the USSR," 190.

81. In his introduction to *Language and Revolution* Halfin notes that "despite their almost proverbial emphasis on consciousness as a body-transcending force, [the communists] were also very interested in yoking the body to the tasks of socialism" (16).

82. Zetkin, *Reminiscences of Lenin,* 59.

83. Peterson, "Dirty Women," in *Russia, Women, Culture,* ed. Goscilo and Holmgren, 177.

84. Clark, "The 'New Man's' Body," in *Art of the Soviets,* ed. Brown and Taylor, 34.

85. For more on the diseases of the modern era, see Robert A. Nye, "Metaphors of Pathology in the *Belle Epoque:* The Rise of a Medical Model of Cultural Crisis," in his *Crime, Madness, and Politics in Modern France: The Medical Concept of National Decline,* 132–70.

86. Porter, *Health, Civilization, and the State,* 43.

87. Michael Hau, *The Cult of Health and Beauty in Germany: A Social History, 1890–1930,* 1.

88. Laura Goering details not just the interest in neurasthenia but a bleeding of the language of disease into cultural critiques; see her "'Russian Nervousness': Neurasthenia and National Identity in Nineteenth-Century Russia," 38.

89. Catriona Kelly connects the issues of masculinity, cold baths, the will, and national potency in "The Education of the Will: Advice Literature, *Zakal,* and Manliness in Early Twentieth-Century Russia," in *Russian Masculinities in History and Culture,* ed. Barbara Evans Clements, Rebecca Friedman, and Dan Healey, 131–51.

90. Kelly, *Refining Russia,* 251.

91. A. Zalesskaia, "Opyty rabot v nochnom sanatorii pri lechebno-proteznom institute," *Ezhenedel'nik MOZa* 4, no. 157 (28 January 1926): 59.

92. See Bernstein's lengthy discussions of neurasthenia in *The Dictatorship of Sex,* 73–99, esp. 82–89.

93. Susan Gross Solomon's investigation of social hygiene is discussed at length in succeeding chapters. For the present issue, see her "David and Goliath in Soviet Public Health: The Rivalry of Social Hygienists and Psychiatrists for Authority over the *bytovoi* Alcoholic," 254–75. Kenneth Pinnow's investigation of suicide in the 1920s reported attempts by medical professionals to define and diagnose problems as a means to gain authority; see his "Cutting and Counting: Forensic Medicine as a Science of Society in Bolshevik Russia, 1920–29," in *Russian Modernity,* ed. Hoffmann and Kotsonis, 115–37. On crime see Sharon Kowalsky, "Making Crime Soviet: Women, Deviance, and the Development of Criminology in Early Soviet Russia."

94. Alexopoulos, *Stalin's Outcasts,* 61.

95. Evgeny Steiner notes a focus on contrasting the dirty and organic with the transformative force of a "corrector" in pieces like *Topotun* and *Moidodyr;* see his *Stories for Little Comrades: Revolutionary Artists and the Making of Early Soviet Children's Books,* 98–99. In the story, the washbasin introduced himself as "Umyval'nikov nachal'nik i mochalok komandir!"

96. A. L. Mendel'son, *Gipnoz i vnushenie* (pub. 5,500); idem, *Ob ukreplenii pamiati* (pub. 10,000).

97. Mark Steinberg notes a similar tendency in Bogdanov, who, while head of Proletkul't, separated the "sociologically proletarian" from the "ideologically proletarian" in worker poetry; see *Proletarian Imagination: Self, Modernity, and the Sacred in Russia, 1910–1925,* 60.

98. Lenin, "Report at the Second All-Russia Trade Union Congress, January 20, 1919," in *Collected Works,* 28:424.

99. Gorsuch, *Youth in Revolutionary Russia,* 92. Kelly examines the genre of advice literature and its goals in "'The Personal Does Not Exist': Advising the Early Soviet Mass Reader, 1917–1953," in her *Refining Russia,* 230–311.

100. Naiman, *Sex in Public,* 46–47. Gorsuch argues that this interest in control may have come from a general fear of disorder throughout Europe in the postwar years; see *Youth in Revolutionary Russia,* 125. Peterson notes that a lack of physical cleanliness impeded mobility within the middle class and that cleanliness of body and environment was necessary for the ambitious; see "Dirty Women," in *Russia, Women, Culture,* ed. Goscilo and Holmgren, 190–91.

101. Kelly, *Refining Russia,* xxvi–xxvii; Hoffmann, *Stalinist Values,* 16–17.

102. In Soviet advice literature, modified behavior led to social stability. See Kelly, *Refining Russia,* 250–52.

103. For Europe, see Goubert, *The Conquest of Water,* 109. The photos compiled by V. N. Zanozin and E. A. Adamenko in *Blagotvoritel'nost' i miloserdie: Rubezh XIX–XX vekov* show the intersection of these concepts at the turn of the century: orphans are taught to dance (55), adults attend lectures (162), and nursery school children wash then dry themselves using individually numbered towels (238).

104. In *The Civilizing Process: Sociogenetic and Psychogenetic Investigations* Elias argues that the rise of manners in Europe worked toward the domestication of citizens. Kelly has studied the applicability of *The Civilizing Process* to Russia; see *Refining Russia,* xxv–xxxii.

105. Trotsky, "Not by Politics Alone," in *Problems of Everyday Life,* 18.

106. Steve Smith and Catriona Kelly, "Commercial Culture and Consumerism," in *Constructing Russian Culture,* ed. Kelly and Shepherd, 152–55.

107. Kelly notes the use of the informal second person singular in slogans, etc.; see *Refining Russia,* 255.

108. Michael S. Gorham, *Speaking in Soviet Tongues: Language Culture and the Politics of Voice in Revolutionary Russia,* 104–6.

109. Trotsky, "The Struggle for Cultured Speech" (1923), in *Bolshevik Visions: First Phase of the Cultural Revolution in Soviet Russia,* ed. William G. Rosenberg, 1:230–33.

110. According to Kelly, "Nothing was so trivial as to escape scrutiny and excoriation" (*Utopias,* xxi). See also Julie A. Cassiday, "Flash Floods, Bedbugs and Saunas: Social Hygiene in Maiakovskii's Theatrical Satires of the 1920s," 643–57.

111. Vladimir Mayakovsky, *Mystery-Bouffe,* 39–139, and *The Bedbug,* 141–96, in *The Complete Plays of Vladimir Mayakovsky.*

112. In the chapter "Colonial Perspectives: Representations and Realities of Rural Crime and Justice" Stephen P. Frank examines the ways in which assumptions about peasant backwardness colored complaints regarding peasant crime; see *Crime, Cultural Conflict,*

and Justice in Rural Russia, 1856–1914, 19–50. Cathy A. Frierson writes at length on the image of the peasantry, including a chapter entitled "The Gray Peasant: Unadorned and Besieged," in her *Peasant Icons: Representations of Rural People in Late Nineteenth-Century Russia*, 116–38. Similar diatribes against dirt as symbol of "peasant barbarousness" infected other European health discourse; see Goubert, *The Conquest of Water*, 110.

113. Kelly contemplates this signifier of civilization in *Refining Russia*, xxix. Aaron Retish reveals the ways in which rituals of citizenship were created in order to control the peasantry and direct revolutionary discourse; see "Creating Peasant Citizens: Rituals of Power, Rituals of Citizenship in Viatka Province, 1917," 47–67.

114. See, e.g., A. I. Akkerman, *Sud nad prostitutkoi i svodnitsei: Delo grazhd. Evdokimovoi po obvineniiu v soznatel'nom zarazhenii sifilisom i grazhd. Sviridovoi v svodnichestve i soobshchnichestve* (pub. 5,000). The Moskovskii otdel zdravookhranenia (hereafter MOZ) poster series entitled "V sele Gory zhili tri brata Martynovy" consisted of twenty posters that contrasted the ignorant peasant Vasilii and his travails with syphilis against the urbanite Peter, who was easily cured under the Soviet system of public health (pub. 10,000). Another six-poster series entitled "Agitatsiia sanprosveta MOZa za bor'bu s epidemicheskimi zabolevaniami" (pub. 7,000) played on the variation god versus science. Fedor, who was infected with typhus, went to the babka and died. His wife was saved at the hospital, and the rest of the village lived because of the health cell.

115. B. S. Sigal, *Venericheskie bolezni*, 41–42 (pub. 10,000; two printings in catalogue). A 1957 study upheld the contention that syphilis acquired by sharing objects was the chief means of transmission in the countryside; see L. A. Artamonova and A. A. Studnitsyn, "Bor'ba s venericheskimi i kozhnymi bolezniami," in *Okhrana narodnogo zdorov'ia v SSSR*, ed. M. D. Kovrigin, 166. Laura Engelstein finds similar biases in prerevolutionary diagnosis of syphilis in the countryside; see her chapter "Morality and the Wooden Spoon: Syphilis, Social Class, and Sexual Behavior" in her *The Keys to Happiness: Sex and the Search for Modernity in Fin-de-Siècle Russia*, 165–211.

116. Stephen Frank examines the medical-advice letters published in Dr. V. N. Voskresenskii's newspaper column from Riazan province, finding that the doctor manipulated requests and selectively addressed questions to maintain the stereotype; see "'Ask the Doctor!' Peasants and Medical-Sexual Advice in Riazan Province, 1925–1928," in *The Human Tradition in Modern Russia*, ed. Husband, 93–107.

117. Amato notes the metaphoric connotations of dust with the peasantry in *Dust*, 36–38.

118. For a well-contextualized account of science, enlightenment, and the intelligentsia in the late nineteenth century, see McReynolds and Popkin, "The Objective Eye and the Common Good," in *Constructing Russian Culture*, ed. Kelly and Shepherd, 81–92.

119. Peterson, "Dirty Women," in *Russia, Women, Culture*, ed. Goscilo and Holmgren, 188–89; Douglas, *Purity and Danger*, 2.

120. Jonathan Coopersmith, *The Electrification of Russia, 1880–1926*. Amato examines the importance of electrification in the fight against dust in *Dust*, 126–28.

121. For the equation of the feminine and the female peasant with filth in Russian culture, see Peterson, "Dirty Women," in *Russia, Women, Culture*, ed. Goscilo and Holmgren, 178–79, 188–90.

122. Robert Edelman, "Everybody's Got to Be Someplace: Organizing Space in the Russian Peasant House, 1880 to 1930," in *Russian Housing in the Modern Age: Design and Social History*, ed. William C. Brumfield and Blair A. Ruble, 7–24.

123. B. S. Ginzburg, *Sud nad mater'iu, podkinuvshei svoego rebenka: Delo gr. Tikhonovoi po obvineniiu ee: 1/v prestupno-nebrezhnom otnoshenii k svoemu rebenku, povlekshem za soboi riad tiazhelykh zabolevanii; 2/v ostavlenii rebenka na proizvol sud'by: Instsenirovka* (pub. 10,000).

124. See Akkerman's *Sud nad prostitutkoi i svodnitsei.*

125. Naiman notes that women were symbols of Russia's backwardness as well as a point of intervention; see *Sex in Public*, 27–45, 187.

126. Quoted in Zetkin, *Reminiscences of Lenin*, 68; also cited in Wood, *The Baba and the Comrade*, 38, and Naiman, *Sex in Public*, 187.

127. Zetkin, *Reminiscences of Lenin*, 51.

128. Wood, *The Baba and the Comrade*, 39; The uneasy relationship of the 1920s regime to women's emancipation and political participation emerged in debates over the celebration of International Women's Day; see Choi Chatterjee, *Celebrating Women: Gender, Festival Culture, and Bolshevik Ideology, 1910–1939*, 59–104.

129. The Soviet League of the Militant Godless, created in 1925, was the official organ for fighting religion; it claimed over five million members by the 1930s, more than the communist party; see Daniel Peris, *Storming the Heavens: The Soviet League of the Militant Godless*, 2. Islam was exposed to similarly derisive tirades; see Michaels, *Curative Powers*, 52–53. The church itself used the language of contagion to describe its relationship to religious dissidence in the late imperial period; see Daniel Beer, "The Medicalization of Religious Deviance in the Russian Orthodox Church (1880–1905)," 451–82.

130. I. D. Strashun, *Bor'ba za zdorov'e—bor'ba s religiei* (pub. 15,080).

131. Il'ia Davydovych Strashun (1892–1967) served as director of the Sanitary Enlightenment publishing house from 1921 to 1930 and helped found the Social Hygiene Museum in 1930; see Heinrich E. Schulz, Paul K. Urban, and Andrew I. Lebed, eds., *Who Was Who in the USSR*, 527.

132. Strashun, *Bor'ba za zdorov'e*, 4–10.

133. For syphilis spread through icons, see N. A. Semashko, *O svetlom i temnom v rabochem bytu*, 48 (pub. 10,000). For icons collecting dust in the home, see Zheleznyi, *Kak zhit', chtoby zdorovym byt'?*, 34–35.

134. While the party pointed to the wearing of a veil as causing medical problems, getting the medical community to argue the same was difficult; see Cavanaugh, "Backwardness and Biology," 250–51.

135. See, e.g., figure 6.7: "Down with Religious Holidays."

136. This may have links to Soviet attacks on saint cults and the fight between science and religion for what Richard Kieckhefer identifies as "charismatic power"; see *Magic in the Middle Ages.* For Soviet trials of religion, see Stites, *Revolutionary Dreams*, 108.

137. O. Stepanova, "Ot durmana k novomy bytu," *ZNB* 15 (August 1927): 11.

138. S. A. Gurevich, "Uchastie trudiashchikhsia v ozdorovlenii truda i byta tvorit sotsialisticheskuiu kul'turu," in *Ozdorovlenie truda i revoliutsiia byta: Sbornik trudov instituta MOZa po izucheniiu professional'nykh boleznei*, ed. MOZ, 72–73 (pub. 2,000).

139. Lebina, *Povsednevnaia zhizn'*, 205. Kelly notes the same tendency in etiquette manuals; see *Refining Russia*, 253.

140. Henri Béraud, *The Truth about Moscow: As Seen by a French Visitor*, 74.

141. In *Sex in Public* Naiman argues that utopia made the Soviets particularly concerned with eliminating history since "the past, when linked to the present, provides a conduit for contamination of the future" (155). The bourgeois bedbug of Maiakovskii makes a similar point.

142. In *Purity and Danger* Douglas argues that "in chasing dirt, in papering, decorating, tidying we are not governed by anxiety to escape disease, but are positively re-ordering our environment, making it conform to an idea" (2).

143. Naiman, *Sex in Public*, 5–6, 12–14.

144. Naiman discusses the problems of transmission of utopias into language as well as the reality of taking utopia into the NEP world; see *Sex in Public*, 13.

145. Clark argues that although *Cement* was the "prototypical Soviet novel" (69) it was still distinguished by a laxness of plot and lack of direction from above for the hero; see *The Soviet Novel*, 68–82.

146. Clark articulates this as a tension between interest in *bytie* and *byt'*; see her *Common Places: Mythologies of Everyday Life in Russia*, 29–33.

147. Clark opens her investigation of revolutionary purification with a discussion of the life of one family bent on complete purification of bourgeois detritus from their lives; see *Petersburg, Crucible of Cultural Revolution*, 1–3.

148. In "Leninism and Workers' Clubs" (1924) Trotsky argued that "indifference" to problems of everyday life and culture was just as bad as "fantasizing" about everyday life and falling into abstractions; see *Problems of Everyday Life*, 305.

149. Trotsky, "Attention to Trifles!," in *Problems of Everyday Life*, 74–75; this piece is reprinted in *The Military Writings of Leon Trotsky*, 4.

150. Ibid.

151. Ibid., 76.

152. Foucault, *Discipline and Punish*, 141. Pierre Bourdeiu identifies hygienic practices as a source of class and modern identity; see *Distinction: A Social Critique of the Judgment of Taste.*

153. Semashko, *O svetlom i temnom*, 44–45.

154. Trotsky, "How to Begin," in *Problems of Everyday Life*, 69. In "Tasks of Communist Education" (1923), Trotsky argued that although people were a product of their societies, the "revolutionist" could still agitate for a new life and would create the conditions for future, perfected citizens (107–8).

Chapter 2. The State: Diagnosing, Monitoring, and Disciplining

1. Although many socialist utopists hoped for a gradual, peaceful change in society, they often utilized force in matters of health, employing health police to investigate citizens. Renaissance utopists posited health inspectors to regulate life and ensure progress; see Eliav-Feldon, *Realistic Utopias*, 39.

2. The concept of *lichnost'*, which developed in post-Petrine Russia and was associated with Western ideas of individualism and self-assertion, was translated into the Russian context in a very different fashion because of the nineteenth-century intellectuals'

disgust with the bourgeois values of the merchant class and a commitment to the communal ideals of Christianity or socialism. The lower classes may have had even less hunger for the concept of individuality. For a detailed discussion of the evolution of the concept in Russia, see Derek Offord, "*Lichnost'*: Notions of Individual Identity," in *Constructing Russian Culture,* ed. Kelly and Shepherd, 13–15.

3. *Obshchestvennost',* denoting a collective view of society, was more popular with Russian thinkers than the individualistic notions of liberty that were strong in the West. See Catriona Kelly and Vadim Volkov, "*Obshchestvennost', Sobornost'*: Collective Identities," in *Constructing Russian Culture,* ed. Kelly and Shepherd, 26–27.

4. Kelly, *Utopias,* 3.

5. Porter, *Health, Civilization, and the State,* 24, 37–42.

6. According to Foucault's *History of Sexuality,* in the eighteenth century the concept of state power mutated as "governments perceived that they were not dealing simply with subjects, or even with a 'people,' but with a 'population'" (25).

7. Sweden and Germany instituted health police in the late eighteenth and early nineteenth centuries; see Porter, *Health, Civilization, and the State,* 46–49, 52–54, 97–100; Rosen, *A History of Public Health,* 110–14. On medicine and statistics, see Theodore M. Porter, *The Rise of Statistical Thinking, 1820–1900,* 17–19; Keith Michael Baker, *Condorcet: From Natural Philosophy to Social Mathematics.*

8. Foucault, *History of Sexuality,* 140.

9. Porter, *Health, Civilization, and the State,* 57–58. See also Dorrinda Outram, *The Body and the French Revolution: Sex, Class and Political Culture;* Dora Weiner, *The Citizen-Patient in Revolutionary and Imperial Paris.*

10. V. O Samoilov recounts Peter's nearly five-month stay in Amsterdam, where he had a special stone corridor built between his hotel and the lab; see *Istoriia Rossiiskoi meditsiny,* 27. For Leyden and Paris, see Sigerist, *Socialized Medicine,* 67.

11. On Peter's efforts to improve the infrastructure, see Samoilov, *Istoriia Rossiiskoi meditsiny,* 28–37; Gantt, *Russian Medicine,* 49–51. Medical innovations pervaded all of Peter's endeavors; for example, regulations governing the health of workers in maritime law were based on western European—especially French—examples; see Basil Haigh, "Design for a Medical Service: Peter the Great's Admiralty Regulations (1722)," 129–46; J. T. Alexander, "Medical Developments in Petrine Russia," 198–221.

12. Gantt, *Russian Medicine,* 50–51. For an overview of Peter's efforts to bring medical instruction and medical workers to Russia, see Lindsey Hughes, *Russia in the Age of Peter the Great,* 312–14.

13. Ransel details the pro-natalist policy changes of the Russian tsars, from strong prohibitions against infanticide to positive reinforcements for fertile families; see *Village Mothers,* 20.

14. For a detailed summary of Catherine's efforts, see Samoilov, *Istoriia Rossiiskoi meditsiny,* 50–71. For an account in English, see John T. Alexander, *Bubonic Plague in Early Modern Russia: Public Health and Urban Disaster,* 36–60.

15. Samoilov, *Istoriia Rossiiskoi meditsiny,* 59; Alexander, *Bubonic Plague in Early Modern Russia,* 36, 51.

16. Isabel de Madriaga, *Catherine the Great: A Short History,* 78, 105, 111.

17. Alexander, *Bubonic Plague in Early Modern Russia,* 55–57.

18. Kelly, *Refining Russia,* 8–12.

19. Hutchinson, *Politics and Public Health,* xvii. Nicholas I's reforms were prompted by cholera epidemics; see Roderik E. McGrew, *Russia and the Cholera, 1823–1832.*

20. Porter, *Health Civilization, and the State,* 67–69. The "social question" centered around the need to reform society in order to reform the individual; see Paul Rabinow, *French Modern: Norms and Forms of the Social Environment,* 10–11, 82–103.

21. Rosen, *A History of Public Health,* 199–214. See also S. Finer, *The Life and Times of Edwin Chadwick;* and R. A. Lewis, *Edwin Chadwick and the Public Health Movement.*

22. Rosen, *A History of Public Health,* 218. This legislation included the Public Health Act of 1848, although it was not renewed in 1855 (223).

23. Porter, *Health, Civilization, and the State,* 54; Porter, *The Rise of Statistical Thinking,* 40–70; James H. Cassedy, *American Medicine and Statistical Thinking, 1800–1860,* 207–29.

24. Porter, *Health, Civilization, and the State,* 101.

25. Hyde, *The Soviet Health Service,* 23; Porter, *Health, Civilization, and the State,* 101–2.

26. Suellen Hoy, *Chasing Dirt: The American Pursuit of Cleanliness,* 34–35; Porter, *Health, Civilization, and the State,* 89, 147–49; Porter, *The Greatest Benefit to Mankind,* 377–79; Jane Lewis, *The Politics of Motherhood: Child and Maternal Welfare in England, 1900–1939,* 11. More generally, see John Duffy, *The Sanitarians: A History of American Public Health;* David Armstrong, *The Political Anatomy of the Body.*

27. Hutchinson, *Politics and Public Health,* 19.

28. Patterson, "Typhus and Its Control," 365–67. In 1908, among half of the Russian recruits called up for military service, 30 percent were found unfit; see Hyde, *The Soviet Health Service,* 14.

29. Samuel C. Ramer, "The Zemstvo and Public Health," in *The Zemstvo in Russia: An Experiment in Local Self-Government,* ed. Terence Emmons and Wayne S. Vucinich, 279; Gantt, *Russian Medicine,* 87.

30. Hutchinson, *Politics and Public Health,* xviii.

31. Gantt, *Russian Medicine,* 81; Hyde, *The Soviet Health Service,* 33. Private charitable organizations seemed to enjoy some leeway and remained strong in the post-emancipation period; see Adele Lindenmeyr, *Poverty Is Not a Vice: Charity, Society, and the State in Imperial Russia.*

32. Frieden, *Russian Physicians,* 9–11; Gantt, *Russian Medicine,* 87. For more on the radical Pirogov society, see L. O. Kanevskii, E. I. Lotova, and Kh. I. Idel'chik, eds., *Osnovnye cherty razvitiia meditsiny v Rossii v period kapitalizma, 1861–1917;* Ramer, "The Zemstvo and Public Health," in *The Zemstvo in Russia,* ed. Emmons and Vucinich, 289.

33. Samoilov, *Istoriia Rossiiskoi meditsiny,* 140–86. For an account of the Twelfth International Congress of Doctors held in Moscow in August 1897, see 171–77.

34. Ramer, "The Zemstvo and Public Health," in *The Zemstvo in Russia,* ed. Emmons and Vucinich, 298; Hyde, *The Soviet Health Service,* 26. Hutchinson notes the general tendency of Russian medicine to glorify German medicine; see *Politics and Public Health,* 22.

35. Ramer, "The Zemstvo and Public Health," in *The Zemstvo in Russia,* ed. Emmons and Vucinich. 281, 298.

36. Frieden, *Russian Physicians,* 80.

37. Samoilov, *Istoriia Rossiiskoi meditsiny,* 129.

38. Joseph Bradley, "'Once You've Eaten Khitrov Soup You'll Never Leave!' Slum Renovation in Late Imperial Russia," 1.

39. McReynolds and Popkin, "The Objective Eye and the Common Good," in *Constructing Russian Culture,* ed. Kelly and Shepherd, 60–66.

40. Frieden, *Russian Physicians,* 1–5.

41. Not all Russian doctors agreed with *zemstvo* medical principles, which led to the splintering of the Pirogov society. See John F. Hutchinson, "'Who Killed Cock Robin?' An Inquiry into the Death of Zemstvo Medicine," in *Health and Society in Revolutionary Russia,* ed. Solomon and Hutchinson, 15–19.

42. Kaser, *Health Care in the Soviet Union and Eastern Europe,* 38.

43. N. A. Semashko, *Okhrana zdorov'ia rabochikh i rabotnits krest'ian i krest'ianok za desiat' let,* 5, 7.

44. Hutchinson, *Politics and Public Health,* 78. Hutchinson argues that, contrary to community physicians' claims, the problem was not too much government but not enough, and centralization would have aided reform; see 79, 95–103.

45. Rachel G. Fuchs, "France in a Comparative Perspective," in *Gender and the Politics of Social Reform in France, 1870–1914,* ed. Elinor A. Accampo, Rachel G. Fuchs, and Mary Lynn Stewart, 163.

46. Rosen, *A History of Public Health,* 350. In 1901–2 the British found 40 percent of all recruits unfit for the military; see Hyde, *The Soviet Health Service,* 56. For natalism, see Seth Koven and Sonya Michel, eds., *Mothers of a New World: Maternalist Politics and the Origins of Welfare States;* M. Ladd-Taylor, *Mother-Work: Women, Children, Welfare and the State, 1890–1930;* Gisela Bock and Pat Thane, eds., *Maternity and Gender Policy: Women and the Rise of the European Welfare States, 1880s–1950s;* Theda Skocpol, *Protecting Soldiers and Mothers: The Political Origins of Social Policy in the United States;* and Paul Weindling, *Health, Race and German Politics between National Unification and Nazism, 1870–1945.*

47. Fuchs, "France in a Comparative Perspective," in *Gender and the Politics of Social Reform in France,* ed. Accampo, Fuchs, and Stewart, 163.

48. For an in-depth discussion of Italian programs, see Horn, *Social Bodies.*

49. In 1901 doctors in St. Petersburg and Moscow started infant programs under the name "Drops of Milk." The 1911 Society to Fight Infant Death used lectures and other programs to encourage breast feeding; see R. M. Bravaia, *Okhrana materinstva i mladenchestva na zapade i v SSSR: Istoricheskii ocherk,* 186, 188 (hereafter *OMM na zapade i v SSSR*).

50. Michelle D. Denbeste-Barnett, "Earnestly Working to Improve Russia's Future, 1867–1905," 88–111.

51. McReynolds and Popkin, "The Objective Eye and the Common Good," in *Constructing Russian Culture,* ed. Kelly and Shepherd, 75.

52. Armstrong, *The Political Anatomy of the Body,* 10–14.

53. Porter, *Health, Civilization, and the State,* 57–60, 121–27. In Germany prior to World War I, socialists steadily expanded clinical care with educational support; see Weindling, *Health, Race and German Politics,* 180.

54. In *Discipline and Punish,* Foucault argues that in modern society "the body becomes a useful force only if it is both a productive body and a subjected body" (26). For more

on the concept, see M. Raeff, *The Well-Ordered Police State;* Bryan S. Turner, *The Body and Society: Explorations in Social Theory;* idem, *Regulating Bodies: Essays in Medical Sociology.*

55. Hutchinson, *Politics and Public Health,* 26.

56. Hyde, *The Soviet Health Service,* 22.

57. Social control was one of three methods of control (the other two being party and state), envisioned as the basis of the Soviet state in the 1920s; see E. A. Rees, *State Control in Soviet Russia: The Rise and Fall of the Workers' and Peasants' Inspectorate, 1920–1934,* 6–7.

58. Holquist, "Information," 427–48; idem, *Making War,* 206–40. In *Stalinist Values* Hoffmann concludes that the Soviet system of the 1930s was "distinguished by its virtually limitless interventionism and application of state violence" (13). As shown here, the health service of the 1920s had neither the power nor the resources for such tactics.

59. Wood extrapolates this argument from her examination of Trotsky in *The Baba and the Comrade,* 196–97.

60. Sigerist, *Socialized Medicine,* 24.

61. On 26 October 1917 the Medical-Sanitary Department of the Petrograd Military Revolutionary Committee was set up to meet the medical needs of the revolutionaries. Women served prominently as stretcher bearers. See Hutchinson, *Politics and Public Health,* 173–74; Hyde, *The Soviet Health Service,* 31. For the early Petrograd organization, see Christopher Williams, "Soviet Public Health: A Case Study of Leningrad, 1917–1932."

62. N. Bukharin and E. Preobrazhensky, *The ABC of Communism: A Popular Explanation of the Program of the Communist Party of Russia,* 365–66.

63. This was a variation on social hygiene and ideas of preventative medicine espoused by the Pirogov society; see Kaser, *Health Care in the Soviet Union and Eastern Europe,* 38.

64. Schulz, Urban, and Lebed, eds., *Who Was Who in the USSR,* 497. Semashko reemerged during the 1940s trial of Nina Kliueva and Grigorii Roskin, the husband-and-wife team who sought a biotherapy for cancer; see Nikolai Krementsov, *The Cure: The Story of Cancer and Politics from the Annals of the Cold War,* 109–26.

65. In *Okhrana zdorov'ia* Semashko noted that the only things that forced the old regime to look at worker health were "epidemics and the workers' movement" (3). Semashko further stated that the party program codified social hygiene by advocating "the carrying out of widespread cleansing and sanitary measures with the goal of preventing the spread of disease" (15).

66. Hutchinson, *Politics and Public Health,* 193.

67. For example, Z. P. Solov'ev and A. N. Sysin were Pirogov physicians who embraced the revolution and the Bolsheviks in 1917. Although many were initially hostile, they eventually came to work with the regime. In 1922 the Pirogov group was dissolved. See Hutchinson, *Politics and Public Health,* 168–82; Vinogradov, Ashurkov, and Kurashov, "Osnovnye tempy razvitiia sovetskogo zdravookhraneniia," in *Okhrana narodnogo zdorov'ia v SSSR,* ed. Kovrigin, 34–35.

68. Susan Gross Solomon, "Social Hygiene and Soviet Public Health," in *Health and Society in Revolutionary Russia,* ed. Solomon and Hutchinson, 178–79, 191; George Steinmetz, *Regulating the Social: The Welfare State and Local Politics in Imperial Germany,* 198.

69. On Soviet eugenics, see Mark B. Adams, "Eugenics as Social Medicine in Revolutionary Russia: Prophets, Patrons, and the Dialectics of Discipline-Building," in *Health and Society in Revolutionary Russia,* ed. Solomon and Hutchinson, 200–223.

70. Solomon, "Social Hygiene and Soviet Public Health," in *Health and Society in Revolutionary Russia,* ed. Solomon and Hutchinson, 175–77, 181–83, 189–93.

71. Neil B. Weissman, "Origins of Soviet Health Administration: Narkomzdrav, 1918–1928," in *Health and Society in Revolutionary Russia,* ed. Solomon and Hutchinson, 97. For a thumbnail biography of Semashko, see Sigerist, *Medicine and Health,* 29. For a longer appreciation in Russian see E. D. Ashurkov et. al., eds., *N. A. Semashko: Izbrannye zdravookhraneniia,* 5–49. For Semashko's thoughts, see N. A. Semashko, *Health Protection in the U.S.S.R.*; idem, "The Tasks of Public Health in Soviet Russia" (1919); idem, "Work of People's Commissariat of Health" (1920). These are available in English in *Bolshevik Visions,* ed. Rosenberg, 1:130–32, 139–45.

72. Weissman, "Origins of Soviet Health Administration," in *Health and Society in Revolutionary Russia,* ed. Solomon and Hutchinson, 101–2. For a personal account of the early Medical Sanitary Department of the Petrograd Military Revolutionary Committee, which preceded Narkomzdrav, see M. I. Barsukov, *The Organization of Hygiene and Sanitation Services in the USSR.* In March 1918 the Soviet government and the main medical institutions moved to Moscow; see Hyde, *The Soviet Health Service,* 38. For more on the organization of the department, see A. Ia. Gutkin and Z. G. Frenkel, eds., *Zdravookhranenie v sovetskoi Rossii za X let, 1917–1927.* In English see Sigerist, *Medicine and Health,* 24; Hutchinson, *Politics and Public Health,* 191–95; and Hyde, *The Soviet Health Service,* 34–39.

73. I. Strashun, "Desiat' let bor'by proletariata za zdorov'e," in *Desiat' let oktiabria i sovetskaia meditsina,* ed. Semashko, 33. For a list of the major epidemics from 1886 to 1923, see E. M. Ivanov, *40 let deiatel'nosti Moskovskoi sanitarnoi organizatsii, 1883–1923,* 14; Gantt, *Russian Medicine,* 140–44, 162; Hyde, *The Soviet Health Service,* 48–49, 89. Starting in 1921, the ARA sent nearly three hundred Americans over for a two-year relief mission. For more on the ARA, see Bertrand M. Patenaude, *The Big Show in Bololand: The American Relief Expedition to Soviet Russia in the Famine of 1921,* xi; and the chapter entitled "The Citizen's Hunger," in Aaron Retish's dissertation "Peasant Identities in Russia's Turmoil: Status, Gender, and Ethnicity in Viatka Province, 1914–1921." Epidemic disease in the early camp system was particularly devastating; see Mary Shaeffer Conroy, "Health Care in Prisons, Labour and Concentration Camps in Early Soviet Russia, 1918–1921," 1257–74.

74. D. B. Gorfin, "Osnovnye etapy razvitiia sovetskogo zakonodatel'stva o sanitarnykh organakh," in *Annaly istorii meditsiny: Sbornik trudov,* ed. M. I. Barsukov, 48.

75. H. G. Wells, *Russia in the Shadows,* 29–30.

76. Conroy, *The Soviet Pharmaceutical Business,* 47–148.

77. Cholera, passed by fecal contamination of water or food, is characterized by cramping, vomiting, and severe diarrhea. Epidemic typhus is spread by the louse, murine typhus by rat fleas, and scrub typhus by mites. Although each of these types existed within Russia, health authorities concentrated on the louse as the primary vector of infection. Headaches, chills, fever, confusion, rashes, vomiting, and sensitivity to light all characterize typhus infection, which can result in death. For public health efforts to combat urban disease, see Porter, *Health, Civilization, and the State,* 79–81.

78. Gantt, *Russian Medicine,* 140.

79. Patterson, "Typhus and Its Control," 373.

80. Weissman, "Origins of Soviet Health Administration," in *Health and Society in Revolutionary Russia,* ed. Solomon and Hutchinson, 102; Patterson, "Typhus and Its Control," 361.

81. Patterson derived these figures from A. Sysin, "Epidemii v Rossii v 1914–22 godakh," *Vrachebnaia gazeta* 10–11 (1927): 265–69; and L. A. Tarasevich, "Epidemii poslednikh let v Rossii," *Obshchestvennyi vrach* 1 (1922): 43–50, cited by Patterson in "Typhus and Its Control," 376.

82. Hyde, *The Soviet Health Service,* 15–16.

83. Lenin, "Report of the All-Russia Central Executive Committee and the Council of People's Commissars, December 5," in *Collected Works,* 30:228; cited in Vinogradov, Ashurkov, and Kurashov, "Osnovnye tempy razvitiia sovetskogo zdravookhraneniia," in *Okhrana narodnogo zdorov'ia v SSSR,* ed. Kovrigin, 43.

84. Patterson, "Typhus and Its Control," 379–80.

85. K. F. Flerov, *Sypnoi tif i bor'ba s nim* (Moscow: Narkomzdrav, 1919), 17–18, 44–50; cited in Patterson, "Typhus and Its Control," 380.

86. N. Semashko, "Politika v dele zdravookhraneniia za desiat' let," in *Desiat' let oktiabria i sovetskaia meditsina,* ed. Semashko, 3.

87. Semashko, *Osnovy sovetskoi meditsiny,* 25. Hutchinson translates *ozdorovlenie* as "healthifying." Here the term is translated as "sanitation" such as the KOTiB; see Hutchinson, *Politics and Public Health,* xv.

88. Semashko, *Osnovy sovetskoi meditsiny,* 14.

89. Solomon, "Social Hygiene and Soviet Public Health," in *Health and Society in Revolutionary Russia,* ed. Solomon and Hutchinson, 175.

90. For district-by-district dispensary numbers in Moscow, see MOZ, *Spravochnik dispanserizirovannykh predpriiatii g. Moskvy na 1-e Oktiabria 1926 g.*

91. L. S. Bogolepova, "Sanitarnoe prosveshchenie i samodeiatel'nost' naseleniia," in *Okhrana narodnogo zdorov'ia v SSSR,* ed. Kovrigin, 580.

92. Bogolepova, *Ezhenedel'nik MOZa* 1 (1926), 34–35, quoted in *Zdravookhranenie v sovetskoi Rossii za X let (1917–1927),* ed. Gutkin and Frenkel, 17.

93. Foucault, *Discipline and Punish,* 189–91.

94. A. M. Merkov, "V. I. Lenin i statistika," in *Zdorov'e naseleniia i metody ego izucheniia (izbrannye proizvedeniia),* 18.

95. Hyde, *The Soviet Health Service,* 95.

96. The first Moscow tuberculosis dispensary appeared in 1918 in Zamoskvorech'e district. The first vendispensary appeared in 1921, with a center to study the method founded in 1923. See Iarovinskii, *Zdravookhranenie Moskvy, 1581–2000, gg,* 96.

97. Rosen, *A History of Public Health,* 148–49.

98. For an examination of the Foucauldian nature of the dispensary and harnessing the medical "gaze" to the needs of state control, see Armstrong, *The Political Anatomy of the Body,* 7–13; and Cassedy, *American Medicine,* 207–29.

99. Porter, *Health, Civilization, and the State,* 60–61.

100. Kaser, *Health Care in the Soviet Union and Eastern Europe,* 38; Alexander, *Bubonic Plague in Early Modern Russia,* 31, 32.

101. A. I. Lapina and S. V. Massino, "Bor'ba s tuberkulezom," in *Okhrana narodnogo zdorov'ia v SSSR,* ed. Kovrigin, 157.

102. Hyde, *The Soviet Health Service,* 96. The first dispensaries looked toward tuberculosis cures. By 1921 fifteen had been established; see Weissman, "Origins of Soviet Health Administration," in *Health and Society in Revolutionary Russia,* ed. Solomon and Hutchinson, 107. However, by 1925 223 tuberculosis dispensaries peppered the RSFSR; see Hyde, *The Soviet Health Service,* 95–96.

103. Strashun, "Desiat' let bor'by proletariata za zdorov'e," in *Desiat' let oktiabria i sovetskaia meditsina,* ed. Semashko, 59.

104. For more detailed information on these inspections, see *Trud i zdorov'e rabochikh,* the multivolume work edited by Ia. Iu. Kats.

105. In 1927 Moscow there were fifty-four hospitals for psychiatric and general illnesses that served 258,983 people over the course of 1925–26. House calls (*pomoshch' na domu*), reserved for the very ill, claimed seventy-six establishments that had 636,828 visits in 1925–26. These were joined by 287 dispensaries for general care (*ambulatorii*), thirteen specialized tuberculosis dispensaries, and five dispensaries for venereal disease. They reported 17,015,718 visitors in 1925–26. *Ambulatoriia* in the Russian setup were distinguished from specialized dispensaries, but in worldwide public health the general term "dispensary" was used for this type of care; see *Vsia Moskva 1928,* 39.

106. MOZ, *Materialy o deiatel'nosti lechebno-profilakticheskikh uchrezhdenii MOZa za 1926/7 goda po dannym statisticheskogo otdeleniia MOZa,* 27.

107. The exact number was 629,726 for 1925–26; see *Vsia Moskva 1928,* 39.

108. Ia. Iu. Kats, *Mediko-sanitarnaia organizatsiia Moskvy i Moskovskoi gub. i novaia ekonomicheskaia politika,* 10, 18–19.

109. Porter, *Health, Civilization, and the State,* 178–79; Armstrong, *The Political Anatomy of the Body,* 13–16.

110. Rosen, *A History of Public Health,* 357.

111. The first decree nationalizing former palaces and spas was signed by Lenin in 1919. In 1920 Crimean resorts were nationalized. The House of Leisure originated in 1920. In 1923 Narkomzdrav founded a department to oversee them, and in 1926 the Central Institute of Kurortology and Physiotherapy of Narkomzdrav USSR was established to investigate therapeutic techniques; see Hyde, *The Soviet Health Service,* 68, 72–73, 84.

112. G. S. Eremenko, D. G. Oppengeim, and G. N. Pospelova, "Kurorty, sanatorii, i doma otdykha," in *Okhrana narodnogo zdorov'ia v SSSR,* ed. Kovrigin, 271–75.

113. L. Nemchenko, ed. *Social Insurance in the Soviet Union,* 39.

114. MOZ, *Kratkii obzor sostoianiia zdravookhraneniia v Moskve i guberniiakh,* 26 (pub. 5,100). In 1920 Moscow Houses of Leisure served 240 people, in 1921 7,213, and in 1923 17,010. In 1925 46.3 percent of the patrons were women and 53.7 percent were men. Of these, 60.3 percent were over thirty; see Fedynskaia, "O domakh otdykha," *ZNB* 1 (January 1926): 2–3; MOZ, *Kratkii obzor sostoianiia,* 26; *Vsia Moskva 1928,* 39.

115. British Trade Union Delegation, *Russia Today,* 157; Wells, *Russia in the Shadows,* 128–31.

116. Weissman, "Origins of Soviet Health Administration," in *Health and Society in Revolutionary Russia,* ed. Solomon and Hutchinson, 109. After 1924 expansion into the

countryside, preventative medicine, and sanitation programs were undermined by untrained personnel and lack of medicine. Attempts to economize in 1926 did not improve Narkomzdrav's budgets; see Christopher M. Davis, "Economics of Soviet Public Health, 1928–1932: Development Strategy, Resource Constraints, and Health Plans," in *Health and Society in Revolutionary Russia,* ed. Solomon and Hutchinson, 148–51.

117. Weissman, "Origins of Soviet Health Administration," in *Health and Society in Revolutionary Russia,* ed. Solomon and Hutchinson, 107–10.

118. Sally Ewing provides an account of the political battles between Narkomzdrav and Narkomtrud (the Commissariat of Labor) over the funding and distribution of medical care, as well as the prerevolutionary origins of the insurance system; see "The Science and Politics of Soviet Insurance Medicine," in *Health and Society in Revolutionary Russia,* ed. Solomon and Hutchinson, 69–96; see also Gantt, *Russian Medicine,* 176; Christopher M. Davis, *Economic Problems of the RSFSR Health System, 1921–1930,* 15.

119. Ewing, "The Science and Politics of Soviet Insurance Medicine," in *Health and Society in Revolutionary Russia,* ed. Solomon and Hutchinson, 79.

120. Nemchenko, ed., *Social Insurance in the Soviet Union,* 6.

121. Sigerist, *Socialized Medicine,* 89. The Soviet population in 1926 was 147 million, of which nearly 18 percent were urban and 82 percent rural; see G. F. Konstantinov, *Zdravookhranenie v SSSR (Statisticheskii spravochnik),* 15.

122. Narkomtrud and Narkomzdrav were important in these determinations during the 1920s. By the 1930s Narkomtrud prevailed in its fight for class-based medicine over physician-directed, patient-centered programs; see Ewing, "The Science and Politics of Soviet Insurance Medicine," in *Health and Society in Revolutionary Russia,* ed. Solomon and Hutchinson, 70–71.

123. Davis, *Economic Problems of the RSFSR Health System,* 19, 32. By the late 1920s the *lishentsy,* outcast groups with perceived ties to capitalism, were denied citizenship and dropped from medical care as well as housing, employment, and education; see Alexopoulos, *Stalin's Outcasts, 1926–1936,* 3.

124. Gantt, *Russian Medicine,* 10–19. Hutchinson notes that a constant complaint of medical professionals was rude treatment by the population at large; see Hutchinson, *Politics and Public Health,* 25; Samuel C. Ramer, "Feldshers and Rural Health Care in the Early Soviet Period," in *Health and Society in Revolutionary Russia,* ed. Solomon and Hutchinson, 122–25.

125. Jeanette E. Tuve, *The First Russian Women Physicians,* 4–9. Denbeste-Barnett argues that the radical movement's emphasis on female education and poor attitude toward medicine in Russia opened the field to women; see "Earnestly Working to Improve Russia's Future, 1867–1905," 25–58. Although physicians had been unable to organize prior to the revolution, the threat of Bolshevism united them; see Hutchinson, *Politics and Public Health,* 182.

126. Weissman, "Origins of Soviet Health Administration," in *Health and Society in Revolutionary Russia,* ed. Solomon and Hutchinson, 109; Hutchinson, *Politics and Public Health,* 114–15; Sigerist, *Socialized Medicine,* 53.

127. Naiman, "Discourse Made Flesh," in *Language and Revolution,* ed. Halfin, 292.

128. Samoilov, *Istoriia Rossiiskoi meditsiny,* 183.

129. Field, *Soviet Socialized Medicine;* statistics from R. A. Reynolds, "Doctors in Soviet Russia," *Nation,* September 24, 1930, 317, cited in Tuve, *The First Russian Women Physicians,* 123. For the recruitment process, see Denbeste-Barnett, "Earnestly Working to Improve Russia's Future, 1867–1905," 59–87.

130. Doctors were casualties of the war, civil strife, and were victims of epidemic disease. They were also part of the general flight of intellectuals after the revolution; for the statistics, see Weissman, "Origins of Soviet Health Administration," in *Health and Society in Revolutionary Russia,* ed. Solomon and Hutchinson, 106.

131. Statistics from Norton T. Dodge, *Women in the Soviet Economy,* 112, cited in Tuve, *The First Russian Women Physicians,* 123.

132. Hyde, *The Soviet Health Service,* 98.

133. Rosen marvels at the breadth of Soviet public health education in comparison to the rest of the world; see *A History of Public Health,* 403.

134. Z. Solov'ev, "Zdravookhranenie i oborona strany sovetov," in *Desiat' let oktiabria i sovetskaia meditsina,* ed. Semashko, 16. For the theory of sanitary enlightenment see I. Shtrum, *Sovetskaia vlast' i sanitarnoe prosveshchenie.* Bogolepova, "Sanitarnoe prosveshchenie i samodeiatel'nost' naseleniia," in *Okhrana narodnogo zdorov'ia v SSSR,* ed. Kovrigin, 579.

135. Strashun, "K s"ezdu," *Sanitarnoe prosveshchenie* 1 (1924), 2. The second meeting took place in Leningrad in 1924 and was attended by eighty delegates; see Bogolepova, "Sanitarnoe prosveshchenie i samodeiatel'nost' naseleniia," in *Okhrana narodnogo zdorov'ia v SSSR,* ed. Kovrigin, 581.

136. Lynne Attwood, *Creating the New Soviet Woman: Women's Magazines as Engineers of Female Identity, 1922–53,* 2; Denise Gestaldo, "Is Health Education Good for You? Re-thinking Health Education through the Concept of Bio-power," in *Foucault, Health and Medicine,* ed. Alan Peterson and Robin Burton, 114–15.

137. Bogolepova, "Sanitarnoe prosveshchenie i samodeiatel'nost' naseleniia," in *Okhrana narodnogo zdorov'ia v SSSR,* ed. Kovrigin, 579. In Moscow sanitary enlightenment began energetically with cholera inoculation drives; see Iarovinskii, *Zdravookhranenie Moskvy, 1581–2000, gg,* 83.

138. Patterson, "Typhus and Its Control," 380. In 1920 Petrograd saw a week devoted to cleaning up trash near water stations, as well as a week for the *bania* and its cleanup; see Botvinnik, "Kratkaia istoriia razvitiia obshchestvennykh nachal v zdravookhranenii Leningrada," in *Obshchestvennye nachala v sovetskom zdravookhranenii,* ed. S. Ia. Freidmin, 37. Much of the energy for these campaigns was supplied by the Commission for the Fight for Cleanliness, which was established by Sovnarkom (Soviet of People's Commissars) on 28 January 1919. Organizers claimed that by 1923 they had eradicated epidemic disease; see V. M. Zhdanov and Iu. D. Lebedev, "Sanitarno-epidemiologicheskii deiatel'nosti," in *Okhrana narodnogo zdorov'ia v SSSR,* ed. Kovrigin, 93–96.

139. For lectures, see Narkomzdrav, *Otchet narodnogo komissariata zdravookhraneniia k 8-mu s"ezdu sovetov,* 26; quoted in Weissman, "Origins of Soviet Health Administration," in *Health and Society in Revolutionary Russia,* ed. Solomon and Hutchinson, 107. According to Z. P. Solov'ev, "Deiatel'nost' glavnogo voenno-sanitarnogo upravleniia," 1922 numbered 6,000 listeners who could have attended 1,000 events and 1923 six million for 120,000 lectures; reprinted in B. D. Petrov, ed., *S. P. Solov'ev: Izbrannye proizvedeniia,* 411.

140. The account gave the 1921 numbers as 620 in Moscow and 222 throughout the province, though the provincial data was "incomplete"; see Kats, *Mediko-sanitarnaia organizatsiia Moskvy,* 11.

141. Z. Solov'ev, "Zdravookhranenie i oborona strany sovetov," in *Desiat' let oktiabria i sovetskaia meditsina,* ed. Semashko, 17.

142. T. F. Makarova, "Meditsinskaia pechat'," in *Okhrana narodnogo zdorov'ia v SSSR,* ed. Kovrigin, 481–84. The situation of the printing presses was generally abysmal after 1917. Although the presses had no hope of reaching the entire population or even the literate segment, the Bolsheviks pushed to revitalize publications generally, starting with military education and moving outward; see Stephen White, *The Bolshevik Poster,* 19, 39–41. For a dramatic account of the problems of publishing in the early years of the revolution, see Robert A. McGuire, *Red Virgin Soil: Soviet Literature in the 1920s,* 4–10.

143. Makarova, "Meditsinskaia pechat'," in *Okhrana narodnogo zdorov'ia v SSSR,* ed. Kovrigin, 485.

144. The natal press numbers cover 1923–29 and private press numbers cover 1919–29; see Strashun, "Desiat' let bor'by proletariata za zdorov'e," in *Desiat' let oktiabria i sovetskaia meditsina,* ed. Semashko, 75.

145. L. O. Kanevskii and I. S. Sokolov, "25 let sovetskogo sanitarnogo prosveshcheniia," *Gigiena i zdorov'e* 11–12 (1942): 57.

146. Bernstein, *The Dictatorship of Sex,* 8–10, 16.

147. Kelly, *Refining Russia,* 248–49.

148. Urban dwellers were more likely to be literate than rural people. Men were more likely than women to read. See M. O. Veselov, *15-let: Bor'ba za pogolovnuiu gramatnost' v Moskovskoi oblasti,* 3. For union-by-union reports, see V. A. Kumanev, *Sotsializm i vsenarodnaia gramotnost': Likvidatsiia massovoi negramotnosti v SSSR,* 161. In the 1920s union-wide literacy campaigns supported change for political reasons; see Charles E. Clark, *Uprooting Otherness: The Literacy Campaign in NEP-Era Russia;* V. L. Soskin, *Sovetskaia massovaia kul'tura: U istokov, 1917–1927 gg.,* 40–64. Military units had their own campaigns; see Mark von Hagen, *Soldiers in the Proletarian Dictatorship: The Red Army and the Soviet Socialist State, 1917–1930,* 89–114.

149. Victoria E. Bonnell, *Iconography of Power: Soviet Political Posters under Lenin and Stalin,* 3. Stephen White surveys the history of poster art from the revolution to collapse in "The Art of the Political Poster," in *Russian Cultural Studies: An Introduction,* ed. Catriona Kelly and David Shepherd, 154–55. White deals extensively with the early period of poster production in *The Bolshevik Poster,* where he discusses the stenciled ROSTA (Russian Telegraph Agency) windows; see 101–4, 109–12.

150. The move away from lengthy explanations toward simple rules is a popular tendency. John C. Burnham studies the United States advertising techniques that overwhelmed the transmission of scientific fact; see *How Superstition Won and Science Lost: Popularizing Science and Health in the United States,* 62–65.

151. *Lubok,* or block prints, were popular at the turn of the century. Icons, long a staple of religious practice, also influenced artists; see White, *The Bolshevik Poster,* 1–7.

152. Kelly, *Refining Russia,* 256.

153. In *Refining Russia* Kelly identifies a similar problem in detailing an author's background and makes the compelling case that authors of etiquette manuals should be seen

not as typical of the entire population but rather as a "type" possessing common motivations in the production of books, such as a "a highly characteristic mission of the Russian intelligentsia, and educated elite more generally, to *vospityvat' narod* (educate the people)" (xliii).

154. Porter, *Health, Civilization, and the State,* 55; Rosen, *A History of Public Health,* 180–81.

155. Georgina D. Feldberg, *Disease and Class: Tuberculosis and the Shaping of Modern North American Society,* 123; Michael E. Teller, *The Tuberculosis Movement: A Public Health Campaign in the Progressive Era,* 21.

156. Rosen, *A History of Public Health,* 395, 401–2; Teller, *The Tuberculosis Movement,* 49.

157. Teller, *The Tuberculosis Movement,* 58–63.

158. Burnham, *How Superstition Won and Science Lost,* 58–59.

159. Gantt, *Russian Medicine,* 169.

160. John Dewey, *Impressions of Soviet Russia and the Revolutionary World: Mexico—China—Turkey,* 53–54.

161. Theodore Dreiser, *Dreiser Looks at Russia,* 91–92.

162. Ramer, "The Zemstvo and Public Health," in *The Zemstvo in Russia,* ed. Emmons and Vucinich, 304–5.

163. Bogolepova, "Sanitarnoe prosveshchenie i samodeiatel'nost' naseleniia," in *Okhrana narodnogo zdorov'ia v SSSR,* ed. Kovrigin, 577–78.

164. Sally West notes the condescending, didactic approach to workers in prerevolutionary advertising in "The Material Promised Land: Advertising's Modern Agenda in Late Imperial Russia," 350–54.

165. Quoted in Ella Winter, *Red Virtue,* 51. This passage also appears in Gorsuch, *Youth in Revolutionary Russia,* 9, where I first came across it.

166. Hoffmann, *Stalinist Values,* 45–54. The year 1918 saw the first exhibitions. In 1919 the first museum exhibition, trains with propaganda posters, and lectures reached several thousand people a month; Petrograd opened museums in the same year; see Botvinnik, "Kratkaia istoriia," in *Obshchestvennye nachala v sovetskom zdravookhranenii,* ed. Freidmin, 36. District exhibitions also opened at the same time, including the House of Sanitary Enlightenment for Rogozhsko-Simonovskii district; see Iarovinskii, *Zdravookhranenie Moskvy, 1581–2000, gg.,* 91. One foreigner's description of such an exhibition dwelled upon the setting's grandeur and its possible effect on visitors as much as on the propaganda; see R. F. McWilliams and Margaret McWilliams, *Russia in Nineteen Twenty-Six,* 60–61.

167. Lynn Mally, *Revolutionary Acts: Amateur Theater in the Soviet State, 1917–1938,* 6–9, 42. For prerevolutionary theater, see Louise McReynolds, *Russia at Play: Leisure Activities at the End of the Tsarist Era,* 14–44.

168. A. Dzinbikovskaia et al., comps., *Konchilos' schast'e: Sanitarnyi lubok v 2-kh kartinakh* (pub. 2000); see also V. Zhitomirskii and A. Ostrovskii, *Sem' zaraz ub'em zaraz: Sanitarnyi lubok v 2-kh kartinakh,* 11–16.

169. The actors wore blue workers' blouses. Mally outlines many types of *agitsud* (agricultural trials), including medical; see *Revolutionary Acts,* 61–73; see also Richard Stites, *Russian Popular Culture: Entertainment and Society since 1900,* 51. For striking photos of the group, see František Deák, "'Blue Blouse' (1923–1928)," 35–46.

170. Propaganda extolled many techniques, among which agitation—the use of an

idea to generate dissatisfaction—roused people to action. In the case of hygiene-related agitation, these plays often combined political activism, prescriptions for hygienic living, and even the exploitation of women in the workforce in a single play. Theoretical distinctions often broke down in practice; see Frank Ellis, "The Media as Social Engineer: The Creation of Homo Sovieticus, 1921–1953: Theoretical Background," in *Russian Cultural Studies,* ed. Kelly and Shepherd, 198.

171. Contemporary accounts considered them most effective; see Julie A. Cassiday, *The Enemy on Trial: Early Soviet Courts on Stage and Screen,* 52–53, 60–64, 80.

172. M. Frenkel noted that these plays were popular—in particular *Konchilos' schast'e*—because they didn't require the same concentration as lectures; see "Vnimanie k sanpostanovkam!" *Sanitarnoe prosveshchenie* 2 (1924): 7–8. For the Moscow case that inspired the misrepresentation of a mock sanitary trial as a real trial, see the play by the husband-and-wife team L. A. Vasilesvkaia and L. M. Vasilevskii, *Sud nad samogonshchikami, delo Karpova Tikhona i ego zheny Agaf'i po obvineniiu v izgotovlenii i tainoi torgovle samogonkoi,* vi. See also Stites, *Russian Popular Culture,* 51; Cassiday, *The Enemy on Trial,* 69–70.

173. Gorsuch, *Youth in Revolutionary Russia,* 61.

174. Bogolepova, "Sanitarnoe prosveshchenie i samodeiatel'nost' naseleniia," in *Okhrana narodnogo zdorov'ia v SSSR,* ed. Kovrigin, 585.

175. Mally, *Revolutionary Acts,* 83–90.

176. Stites, *Russian Popular Culture,* 28.

177. Bogolepova, "Sanitarnoe prosveshchenie i samodeiatel'nost naseleniia," in *Okhrana narodnogo zdorov'ia v SSSR,* ed. Kovrigin, 580. For more on the question of popular cinema as either entertainment or enlightenment, see Denise J. Youngblood, *Movies for the Masses: Popular Cinema and Soviet Society in the 1920s,* 35–49.

178. Other titles included *Osobniak golubinykh, Dispanser—trud i byt, Tuberkulez—zaraznaia bolezn' and "Pervaia pomoshch'.* For more on this subject, see Strashun, "Desiat' let bor'by proletariata za zdorov'e," in *Desiat' let oktiabria i sovetskaia meditsina,* ed. Semashko, 75.

179. Quoted in Youngblood, *Movies for the Masses,* 158. See also Alexander Wicksteed, *Life under the Soviets,* 119.

180. According to Lebina, nearly 50 percent of attendees preferred "revolutionary" themes; see *Povsednevnaia zhizn',* 247.

181. Strashun, "Desiat' let bor'by proletariata za zdorov'e," in *Desiat' let oktiabria i sovetskaia meditsina,* ed. Semashko, 72. The 1928 guide to Moscow specified two health museums—the general Health Museum of Narkomzdrav (with three divisions) and the Exhibition on Women's Health. See *Vsia Moskva 1928,* 281; Bogolepova, "Sanitarnoe prosveshchenie i samodeiatel'nost naseleniia," in *Okhrana narodnogo zdorov'ia v SSSR,* ed. Kovrigin, 579; Botvinnik, "Kratkaia istoriia," in *Obshchestvennye nachala v sovetskom zdravookhranenii,* ed. Freidmin, 36.

182. Samuel Northrup Harper, *Civic Training in Soviet Russia,* 210–21.

183. Kats, *Mediko-sanitarnaia organizatsiia Moskvy,* 11.

184. Strashun, "Desiat' let bor'by proletariata za zdorov'e," in *Desiat' let oktiabria i sovetskaia meditsina,* ed. Semashko, 72. Leningrad also had a hygiene museum with thirteen different departments. It greeted nearly thirty thousand patrons in just four months of 1921; see Leningradskii meditsinskii zhurnal, *Putevoditel' po muzeiu zdravookhraneniia Leningradskogo obzdravotdela,* 35.

185. Botvinnik, "Kratkaia istoriia," in *Obshchestvennye nachala v sovetskom zdravookhranenii,* ed. Freidmin, 36.

186. The cabinet of medical oddities, exemplified in Russia by Peter the Great's *kunstkamera,* was an earlier example of this, but it was primarily intended for medical practitioners. See Anthony Anemone, "The Monsters of Peter the Great: The Culture of the St. Petersburg Kunstkamera in the Eighteenth Century," 583–602. These later health exhibitions were intended for viewing by patients and the public; see Teller, *The Tuberculosis Movement,* 60–63; Rosen, *A History of Public Health,* 393, 400; Katherine McCuaig, *The Weariness, the Fever, and the Fret: The Campaign against Tuberculosis in Canada, 1900–1950,* 34.

187. Traveling exhibitions made stops throughout rural areas. Corner exhibitions took advantage of more urban settings, with displays set up at busy intersections; see TsMAM f. 1474, op. 2, d. 17, l. 6.

188. Porter, *Health, Civilization, and the State,* 46; Porter, *The Rise of Statistical Thinking,* 40–70. For military and population management, see Hoffmann, "European Modernity," in *Russian Modernity,* ed. Hoffmann and Kotsonis, 252; Fuchs, "France in a Comparative Perspective," in *Gender and the Politics of Social Reform in France,* ed. Accampo, Fuchs, and Stewart, 163; Feldberg, *Disease and Class,* 12; Cassedy, *American Medicine,* ix, 178, 191, 207–29; and Armstrong, *The Political Anatomy of the Body,* 42–53.

189. Hoffmann, "European Modernity," in *Russian Modernity,* ed. Hoffman and Kotsonis, 252–53; Pinnow, "Cutting and Counting," in *Russian Modernity,* ed. Hoffmann and Kotsonis, 115.

190. Vl. Zaitsev, *Trud i byt rabochikh podrostkov,* 295–354.

191. Porter, *The Rise of Statistical Thinking,* 40–70; Cassedy, *American Medicine,* 191, 207–29.

192. According to Liza Kagan, writing in 1926, 62.9 percent of women were illiterate; see *Put' k obshchestvennoi rabote,* 18. Numbers were much lower for the general population, though the number of literate members in younger groups (12–14, 15–19) was increasing; see Soskin, *Sovetskaia massovaia kul'tura,* 58.

193. Wood, *The Baba and the Comrade,* 15.

194. S. Kal'manson, and D. Bekariukov, *Beregi svoe zdorov'e! Sanitarnaia pamiatka dlia rabochikh podrostkov,* 4 (pub. 10,000). D. D. Bekariukov was another holdover from the Pirogov Commission for the Spread of Hygienic Knowledge to the People. From 1917 to 1927 he headed the Moscow Bureau of School Sanitation and wrote over sixty books; see Schulz, Urban, and Lebed, eds., *Who Was Who in the USSR,* 56.

195. Public participation (*obshchestvennost'*) is discussed in Hutchinson, *Politics and Public Health,* 28; Bogolepova, "Sanitarnoe prosveshchenie i samodeiatel'nost naseleniia," in *Okhrana narodnogo zdorov'ia v SSSR,* ed. Kovrigin, 579–81; Hyde, *The Soviet Health Service,* 31.

196. McReynolds and Popkin, "The Objective Eye and the Common Good," in *Constructing Russian Culture,* ed. Kelly and Shepherd, 64–65.

197. In theory the cell was headed by a member of the KOTiB and usually had a doctor involved; see Botvinnik, "Kratkaia istoriia," in *Obshchestvennye nachala v sovetskom zdravookhranenii,* ed. Freidmin, 40–41.

198. Gutkin and Frenkel, eds., *Zdravookhranenie v sovetskoi Rossii za X let, 1917–1927,* 52. For Moscow see Iarovinskii, *Zdravookhranenie Moskvy, 1581–2000,* gg, 95.

199. Bogolepova, "Sanitarnoe prosveshchenie i samodeiatel'nost' naseleniia," in *Okhrana narodnogo zdorov'ia v SSSR*, ed. Kovrigin, 580.

200. At first devoted to tuberculosis, like the similarly tagged early dispensary, the health cells eventually broadened their mission and began treating all social diseases; see A. K. Bogomolov, *Dostizheniia sovetskoi meditsiny*, 26. See also *Material k dokladu otdela zdravookhraneniia na plenume Moskovskogo soveta RK i KD 27 Oktiabria 1925 g.*, 7; I. Geizer, *Ozdorovlenie truda i byta: Itogi deiatel'nosti MOZ za period c 1/x—1924 po 1/yii—1925 g.*, 23. A 1928 report claimed 3,652 people in 9,000 (general rather than tuberculosis) cells; see D. Gorfin, "10 let sovetskoi meditsiny i konkursy na luchshuiu sektsiiu zdravookhraneniia i luchshii vrachebnyi uchastok," *Voprosy zdravookhranenia* 4 (1928): 18.

201. Gorsuch argues that although the Komosomol attracted less than 10 percent of eligible youth in the mid-1920s, this was a result of lack of access in rural areas; see *Youth in Revolutionary Russia*, 12–15, 42, 188. Some Moscow factories had 80 percent involvement; see V. A. Diagilev, *Istoriia Moskvy*, 6:303.

202. Attwood and Kelly, "Programs for Identity," in *Constructing Russian Culture*, ed. Kelly and Shepherd, 256–64.

203. Harper, *Civic Training*, 77.

Chapter 3. The City: Instruction, Regulation, and Isolation

1. The first House of Leisure in Moscow was set up in Serebrianii bor later that year, and others soon followed. In May 1921 Lenin signed a decree turning this piecemeal practice into policy. See I. I. Kozlov, ed., *Zdravnitsy profsoiuzov SSSR: Kurorty, sanatorii, pansionaty i doma otdykha*, 4.

2. Bourgeois housing in the city was also confiscated, see A. Vainshtein, *Doma otdykha i sanatorii dlia zastrakhovannykh*, 15–16 (pub. 5,000).

3. British Trade Union Delegation, *Russia Today*, 157, 205–8.

4. Foucault, *Discipline and Punish*, 150. He notes that in addition to creating docile bodies through spatial and temporal separation, it was important to "assure the quality of the time used" (172).

5. Writing in the early 1930s, one Westerner observed of Soviet *otdykh*, "Most of the activities designated by the word in Russia are about as restful or reposeful as a Rugby International." Alexander Wicksteed, *My Russian Neighbors: Recollections of Ten Years in Soviet Moscow*, 205.

6. I. Gel'man, *Trud, utomlenie i otdykh*, 6 (pub. 10,000). For a detailed discussion of the hygiene of labor, see Siegelbaum, "*Okhrana Truda*," in *Health and Society in Revolutionary Russia*, ed. Solomon and Hutchinson, 224–45.

7. Izrail' Grigor'evich Gel'man (1881–1937) worked as a toxicologist, hygienist, professor, and clinician. Beginning in 1923 he was employed at the housing sanitation department of Narkomzdrav. Engels's emphasis on labor and riches was based on the connection between labor and health in utopian literature; see Eliav-Feldon, *Realistic Utopias*, 42.

8. Gel'man, *Trud*, 6, 8.

9. N. A. Semashko, *Kak otdykhat' letom*, 3 (pub. 10,000).

10. Sigal, *Trud i zdorov'e*, 37.

11. Bogdanov, *Red Star,* 68. Of course, there was a sexual dimension to this mechanical attraction, which the guide attributed to the operator having excess "enthusiasm" and the attraction of "powerful sensations."

12. Those in dangerous professions were promised a month-long vacation annually. See Semashko, *Kak otdykhat' letom,* 5; Vainshtein, *Doma otdykha i sanatorii,* 3. For leisure legislation, see A. F. Danilevich, *Rabochee vremia i otdykh.*

13. A. G. Kagan, *Rabochaia molodezh' na otdykhe,* 7 (pub. 5,000).

14. L. M. Vasilevskii, *Gigiena propagandista (Agitatora, lektora, prepodavatelia),* 9 (pub. 10,000).

15. Kagan, *Rabochaia molodezh',* 7.

16. Semashko, *Kak otdykhat' letom,* 5. See also the anonymous work *Gigiena i zdorov'e rabochego i ego sem'i,* 23 (pub. 4,000). Purposeful leisure figured in previous utopias; see Eliav-Feldon, *Realistic Utopias,* 42–43.

17. Kagan, *Rabochaia molodezh',* 9.

18. Gel'man, *Trud,* 34–35.

19. Kagan, *Rabochaia molodezh',* 9.

20. V. Gorinevskii, "Podvizhnye igry (s biologicheskoi tochki zreniia)," 5–21; quoted in *Igry i razvlecheniia: Sbornik statei,* ed. V. G. Marts, 7, 15 (pub. 5,000).

21. Gel'man, *Trud,* 37. The italics are perhaps meant to underscore the slogan-like rhythms of these words.

22. L. M. Vasilevskii, *Gigiena propagandista,* 18–19.

23. Kagan, *Rabochaia molodezh',* 10. Italics in original.

24. The Soviets depicted bourgeois leisure as decadent; see Bernstein, *Dictatorship of Sex,* 151–58. The bourgeoisie also grappled with leisure as wasted time. In *Leisure Settings: Bourgeois Culture, Medicine, and the Spa in Modern France,* Douglas Peter Mackaman notes that nineteenth-century spa medicine was packaged to allow the socially awkward French bourgeoisie to find a comfortable way to rest that was "impermeable to waste, indecency, excess, sloth, and the other social attributes the still forming bourgeoisie took to be antithetical to the dual guises of productivity and respectability" (6). Though not in deference to bourgeois sentiments, similar considerations over packaging leisure framed Soviet debates.

25. Semashko, *O svetlom i temnom,* 14–17.

26. Vainshtein, *Doma otdykha i sanatorii,* 9; Al. Mil'chakov, *Komsomol v bor'be za kul'turnyi byt,* 18–32 (pub. 10,000).

27. A. Lipets, "Voprosy byta v klube," *Klub* 7, no. 14 (July 1926): 35.

28. Stites, *Russian Popular Culture,* 18; Thurston, *Liberal City, Conservative State,* 133.

29. British Trade Union Delegation, *Russia Today,* 172.

30. Anon., "Untitled," *Rabochii klub* 1 (1925): 1. For the 1920s, see John Hatch, "Hangouts and Hangovers: State, Class and Culture in Moscow's Workers' Club Movement, 1925–1928," 98; idem, "The Politics of Mass Culture: Workers, Communists, and the Proletcult in the Development of Workers' Clubs, 1921–1925," 119–48. For the 1930s, see Lewis H. Siegelbaum, "The Shaping of Soviet Workers' Leisure: Workers' Clubs and Palaces of Culture in the 1930s."

31. A. Oborin, *O rabote profsoiuzov v gorode i v derevne,* 35. For club activities, see M. Leizerov, *Chto ty mozhesh' delat' v klube* (pub. 5,000); idem, *O rabochem klube.* According to V. F. Pletnev, the club was also a *vospitatel'* (educator); *Rabochii klub: Printsipy i metody raboty,* 15.

32. L. Kagan, *Rabota gorodskoi iacheiki VLKSM sredi devushek,* 50 (pub. 5,000).

33. Strashun, "Sanitarnoe prosveshchenie v rabochem klube," in *Sanitarnoe prosveshchenie v rabochem klube (Tsikl lektsii-dokladov i illiustrativnykh vecherov),* 7 (pub. 10,000).

34. On club evenings, see S. Dolinskii, "Metodika: Klubnaia vecherinka," *Klub* 3, no. 10 (March 1926): 12–22; on physical culture, see R. Roman and Veprinskii, *Rabochii, idi v klub! Materialy dlia zhivoi gazety* (pub. 10,000).

35. GARF f. 7952, op. 3, d. 226, l. 40 Trotsky outlined the many ways in which workers' clubs served as a base for education; see "Leninism and Workers' Clubs," in *Problems of Everyday Life,* 288–322.

36. A. Trunin, "Lektsionnaia rabota v klubakh," *Rabochii klub* 1 (1925): 23–24.

37. N. Semashko, "Bor'ba s khuliganstvom i nedostatki klubnoi raboty," *Klub* 9 (September 1926): 3–5.

38. Obozrenie, "Nashi kruzhki," *Rupor: Ezhemesiachnyi zhurnal kluba soiuza sovrabotnikov* 3–4 (March–April, 1924): 27.

39. I. Potemkin, "O kruzhkakh po bytu v rabochikh klubakh," *Klub* 5 (October 1925): 29–30.

40. V. Zorin, "Rabochii klub i pionery," *Klub* 1 (June 1925): 55.

41. V. M. Zlobina and B. S. Shcheprov, "Profsoiuzy v period vosstanovleniia narodnogo khoziaistva (1921–1925 gody)," in *Profsoiuzy Moskvy: Ocherki istorii,* ed. T. M. Dernitsyn et al., 178. Although the numbers were strong, some worried that they were competitive rather than healthful circles; see Kostriukov, "Gotov'tes' k konkursu," *ZNB* 10 (August 1925): 24.

42. GARF f. 5451, op. 11, d. 467, l. 4–5.

43. GARF f. 7952, op 3, d. 233(1), l. 4.

44. GARF f. A-2313, op. 1, d. 134, l. 5.

45. Thurston, *Liberal City, Conservative State,* 135.

46. GARF f. A-2313, op. 1, d. 134, l. 5.

47. Zlobina and Shcheprov, "Profsoiuzy v period vosstanovleniia," in *Profsoiuzy Moskvy,* ed. Dernitsyn et al., 17.

48. Gel'man, *Trud,* 36.

49. TsGAODM f. 634, op. 1, d. 7, l. 1. 212.

50. Thurston, *Liberal City, Conservative State,* 134.

51. Vl. Kholodkovskii, *Moskovskie parki kul'tury i otdykha,* 13.

52. A. Mol'kov, *Gosudarstvennyi institut sotsial'noi gigieny Narkomzdrava, 1919–1924,* 11 (pub. 1,000). Of the 1,194 excursions held in 1927, 732 examined questions of social behavior, 84 explored health care issues, 103 analyzed scientific questions, and 275 focused on economic themes; see GARF f. 5451, op. 11, d 479, l. 30. The excursion bureau conducted 3,612 tours of the city for 4,743 visitors, as well as governmental instructional tours for 6,446 people; see GARF f. 5451, op. 11, d. 479, l. 2. Koenker reports that activists worried that workers preferred the theater and other noncommunal pursuits to the healthful excursion; see *Republic of Labor,* 105.

53. The club struggled with overcrowding even as it was held up as a refuge from the crowded home. In the ideal Soviet society the home would only serve as a place to sleep. Life and leisure would be collective. See Anatole Kopp, *Town and Revolution: Soviet*

Architecture and City Planning, 1917–1935, 116; Hatch, "Hangouts and Hangovers," 100. Trotsky lamented the low club attendance; see "Leninism and Workers' Clubs," in *Problems of Everyday Life,* 299.

54. M. Zel'manov, "K voprosu vovlecheniia vzroslogo rabochego v klub (v poriadke diskussii)," *Klub* 3 (August 1925): 7.

55. Oborin, *O rabote profsoiuzov v gorode i v derevne,* 55. Komsomol men described young women as backward because they attended sewing circles and did less important club work. Thus, even if women attended the club, the sniping did not end; see Gorsuch, *Youth in Revolutionary Russia,* 102.

56. V. Kirov, "Biudzhet vremeni rabochego i klub," *Klub* 5 (October 1925): 61.

57. N. Semashko, "Bor'ba s khuliganstvom."

58. Lebina, *Rabochaia molodezh',* 122.

59. Oborin, *O rabote profsoiuzov,* 35. This concept was repeated in a Moscow poster entitled "Khoroshii klub—vernyi put' bor'by s p'ianstvom" (Moscow: Mosgublit, n.d.) (pub. 20,000). Russian State Library collection.

60. V. Zamoskvoretskii, "O bor'be s khuliganstvom," *Klub* 5 (October 1925): 64–69.

61. Trotsky, "Leninism and Workers' Clubs," in *Problems of Everyday Life,* 303. See A. F. Rodin, "Nauchnoe razvlechenie," in *Igry i razvlecheniia,* ed. Marts, 51; M. Zel'manov, "K voprosu vovlecheniia vzroslogo rabochego v klub (v poriadke diskussii)," *Klub* 3 (August 1925): 6–7.

62. Kagan, *Rabota gorodskoi iacheiki VLKSM,* 52–53.

63. M. Leizerov, *Krasnye ugolki,* 4, 17 (pub. 20,000; at least three reprints recorded).

64. GARF f. A-406, op. 7, d. 97, l. 20.

65. GARF f. 5451, op. 11, d. 467, l. 4.

66. René Fülüp-Miller, *The Mind and Face of Bolshevism: An Examination of Cultural Life in Soviet Russia,* 196.

67. Semashko, *Kak otdykhat' letom,* 8.

68. For prerevolutionary leisure—including taverns, gaming clubs, and dances—see introduction to *The Russian Worker: Life and Labor under the Tsarist Regime,* ed. Victoria Bonnell, 24–28.

69. AMO f. 66, op. 13, d. 7, l. 88; see, e.g., figure 6.7 in the present study.

70. Semashko, "Bor'ba s khuliganstvom," 4.

71. I. Potemkin, "O kruzhkakh po bytu v rabochikh klubakh," *Klub* 5 (October 1925): 30.

72. Koenker, *Republic of Labor,* 283–84.

73. There were 428 such incidents in 1923, 763 in 1924, 1,661 in 1925, and 4,438 during the first three quarters of 1926; see Gr. Avlov, *Sud nad khuliganami,* 37 (pub. 4,000).

74. Koenker, *Republic of Labor,* 283–85.

75. L. Zakharin vented the anxieties of the era when he stated: "In recent times the pages of newspapers and journals have been full of messages on the rise of hooliganism, scandals, and fights, and the flood of alcoholics." "Bor'ba za poriadok v klube," *Kul'turnyi front: Dvukhnedel'nyi zhurnal kul'traboty profsoiuzov* 2 (20 January 1926): 16.

76. See Stites, "Utopia in Space: City and Building," in *Revolutionary Dreams,* 190–204; Attwood, *Creating the New Soviet Woman,* 74; Horn, *Social Bodies,* 95.

77. Steinberg, *Proletarian Imagination*, 8. Bliznakov quotes Boris I. Arvatov's "The Materialized Utopia"—in particular its calls for "towns in the air; towns of glass and asbestos; towns on springs"—in her essay "The Realization of Utopia," in *Reshaping Russian Architecture*, ed. Brumfield, 145. El Lissitzky discussed at length the look and necessity of a new city in *Russia: An Architecture for World Revolution*, 27–71; as does N. A. Miliutin in *Sotsgorod*, 44–129.

78. S. I. Lebedev, "Ulitsa i gigiena," *Zhurnal Moskovskogo kommunal'nogo khoziaistva* 9–10 (May 1927): 38–39. This disquiet with the city formed a part of American views too; see James J. Kopp, "Cosimo Noto's *The Ideal City* (1903): New Orleans as Medical Utopia," *Utopian Studies* 1, no. 2 (1990): 122.

79. Kal'manson and Bekariukov, *Beregi svoe zdorov'e!*, 3.

80. Goering notes the prerevolutionary conflation of "urban" with "diseased" in her discussion of neurasthenia; see "'Russian Nervousness': Neurasthenia and National Identity in Nineteenth-Century Russia," 42.

81. Rudnitzkii, "Dopustimo li polovoe legkomyslie?," *ZNB* 3 (February 1926): 8–9.

82. S. I. Lebedev, "Ulitsa i gigiena," 38–39.

83. For the dangers of the city as reflected in worker fiction and poetry, see Steinberg, *Proletarian Imagination*, 199–207. For the connection of the street to criminality, chaos, and disease, see Gorsuch, *Youth in Revolutionary Russia*, 139–43, 148–60.

84. Steve Smith and Catriona Kelly, "Commercial Culture and Consumerism," in *Constructing Russian Culture*, ed. Kelly and Shepherd, 113–30, 136–39.

85. For 1920s Moscow cabarets and salacious goings-on, see William J. Chase, *Workers, Society and the Soviet State: Labor and Life in Moscow, 1918–1929*, 201–3.

86. Akkerman, *Sud nad prostitutkoi i svodnitsei*.

87. Sigal, *Venericheskie bolezni*, 41–42.

88. For a humorous take on this situation, see Rubanovskii, *Za knigu ili v pivnuiu?*

89. Laura L. Phillips, *Bolsheviks and the Bottle: Drink and Worker Culture in St. Petersburg, 1900–1929*, 72–95; Kathy S. Transchel, *Under the Influence: Working-Class Drinking, Temperance, and Cultural Revolution in Russia, 1895–1932*, 123–144; and S. A. Smith, "Masculinity in Transition: Peasant Migrants to Late-Imperial St. Petersburg," in *Russian Masculinities in History and Culture*, ed. Clements, Evans, Friedman, and Healey, 94–112.

90. Boris Andreev, *Sud nad negramotnym* (pub. 5,000).

91. I. V. Rebel'skii, *Instsenirovannye sudy (Kak ikh organizovyvat')*, 59.

92. N. Plamanov, "Kak my izzhili khuliganstvo (Klub pishchevikov im. Vorovskogo)," *Kul'turnyi front* 9 (1926): 36.

93. V. Altman, "Ob uchastii iunsektsii v bor'be s p'ianstvom," *Klub* 1 (January 1926): 16–20.

94. Drinking was conceived of as male-oriented leisure in Russia; see Transchel, *Under the Influence*, 24–27. For outside Russia, see Kathy Peiss, *Cheap Amusements: Working Women and Leisure in Turn-of-the-Century New York*, 17.

95. For a detailed discussion of the dangers of dancing, see Gorsuch, *Youth in Revolutionary Russia*, 120–25; for its popularity, see Stites, *Russian Popular Culture*, 21, 49; Koenker, *Republic of Labor*, 104. In the West dancing was favored by women; see Peiss, *Cheap Amusements*, 88–114.

96. L. M. Vasilevskii, *Gigiena molodoi devushki,* 33 (pub. 20,000).

97. TsAODM f. 634, op. 1, d. 7, l. 88.

98. TsAODM f. 634, op. 1, d. 81, l. 1.

99. Koenker, *Republic of Labor,* 104–5.

100. Lebina, *Povsednevnaia zhizn' sovetskogo goroda,* 235–55.

101. Gorsuch, *Youth in Revolutionary Russia,* 188.

102. Referrals to the night sanatorium could be obtained through the dispensary doctor, KOTiB, or the commission of the night sanatorium. See A. Zalesskaia, "Opyty rabot v nochnom sanatorii pri lechebno-proteznom institute," *Ezhenedel'nik MOZa* 4, no. 157 (28 January 1926): 58. Foucault refers to "enclosure" as the first step toward "disciplinary monotony"; see *Discipline and Punish,* 141.

103. Focusing on tuberculosis, N. Fridman argued that prerevolutionary Russia did have institutions for tuberculosis but no night sanatoriums per se; see "Nochnoi sanatorii kak odno iz vspomogatel'nykh uchrezhdenii dispansera dlia tuberkuleznykh bol'nykh," *Izvetsiia Narkomzdrava* 2–3 (1923): 13. For the American and German examples, see Teller, *The Tuberculosis Movement,* 80–81.

104. Barbara Bates, *Bargaining for Life: A Social History of Tuberculosis, 1876–1938,* 275.

105. Fridman, "Nochnoi sanatorii," 13.

106. Botvinnik, "Kratkaia istoriia razvitiia obshchestvennykh nachala v zdravookhranenii Leningrada," in *Obshchestvennye nachala v sovetskom zdravookhranenii,* ed. Freidmin, 39.

107. MOZ, *Materialy o deiatel'nosti lechebno-profilakticheskikh uchrezhdenii MOZa,* 6.

108. Vainshtein, *Doma otdykha i sanatorii,* 33–34.

109. Kapengut, "Rabochie o nochnom sanatorii," *ZNB* 3 (February 1927): 15.

110. Vainshtein, *Doma otdykha i sanatorii,* 35.

111. I. Geizer, "Na ploshchadke dlia tuberkuleznykh detei," *ZNB* 4–5 (May 1925): 13–14.

112. V. Protopopov, "Ploshchadka distsipliniruet rabochikh," *ZNB* 4–5 (1925): 15. See also "Na ploshchadke," 13–14.

113. Vainshtein, *Doma otdykha i sanatorii,* 35. See also Fridman, "Nochnoi sanatorii,"13; Haines, *Health Work in Soviet Russia,* 107.

114. Fridman, "Nochnoi sanatorii," 13; Haines, *Health Work in Soviet Russia,* 107.

115. B. B. Kagan, "Programma dlia raboty po sanprosvesheniiu v nochnykh sanatoriiakh," *Ezhenedel'nik MOZa* 31, no. 185 (5 August 1926): 444–45.

116. Fridman, "Nochnoi sanatorii," 14.

117. Haines, *Health Work in Soviet Russia,* 107.

118. E. Shestakova, "Rabochie v nochnykh sanatoriiakh," *ZNB* 3 (February 1926): 8.

119. Geizer, "Na ploshchadke," 14.

120. Kapengut, "Rabochie o nochnom sanatorii," 15.

121. A. Lipets, "Voprosy byta v klube," *Klub* 7, no. 14 (July 1926): 34–37.

122. Fedynskaia, "O domakh otdykha," *ZNB* 1 (January 1926): 2–3.

123. Steinberg presents a glowing vision of the countryside; see his *Proletarian Imagination,* 210–20.

124. For a brief history of the two systems, see Vainshtein, *Doma otdykha i sanatorii,* 52–55.

125. Vainshtein, *Doma otdykha i sanatorii,* 31–32. For the policy on sanatoriums, spas, and Houses of Leisure, see Narkomzdrav, *Kurorty SSSR: Spravochnik;* N. A. Semashko, *Chto takoe kurort i kak na nikh lechit'sia;* and Moskovskii Sovet RK i KD, Sektsiia domov otdykha MOZ, *Doma otdykha: Sbornik statei i materialov (1920–1923 gg.)* (pub. 3,000).

126. B. M. Khromov and A. V. Sveshnikov, *Zdravookhranenie Leningrada: Kratkii istoricheskii ocherk,* 63; Hyde, *The Soviet Health Service,* 68–69; Samoilov, *Istoriia Rossiiskoi meditsiny,* 183.

127. Hyde, *The Soviet Health Service,* 72.

128. Milka Bliznakov, "Soviet Housing during the Experimental Years, 1918 to 1933," in *Russian Housing in the Modern Age,* ed. Brumfield and Blair, 85.

129. Hyde, *The Soviet Health Service,* 71.

130. The House of Leisure system began construction during 1920–21. Under NEP it experienced great need and a weakening, but it recovered in 1924 when new funding was discovered in the form of the social insurance fund; see Vainshtein, *Doma otdykha i sanatorii,* 24–27.

131. MOZ, *Kratkii obzor sostoianiia zdravookhraneniia v Moskve,* 26.

132. MOZ, *Zdravookhranenie v Moskve i Moskovskoi gubernii,* 12. The same source reported twenty-seven sanatoriums in 1924–25 and 12,962 people served.

133. Fedynskaia, "O domakh otdykha," 2–3; MOZ, *Kratkii obzor sostoianiia,* 26. Selection favored workers and party members, as Anton Karlgren suggested in *Bolshevist Russia,* 192–94.

134. Vainshtein, *Doma otdykha i sanatorii,* 38.

135. Fedynskaia, "O domakh otdykha," 2–3.

136. Vainshtein, *Doma otdykha i sanatorii,* 2. The same quotation is cited by Fedynskaia, "O domakh otdykha," 2–3.

137. Stepan, "Kak otdykhaiut i lechatsia Moskovskie rabochie," *ZNB* 3 (February 1927): 8.

138. Garevskii, "Kul'turnaia rabota v domakh otdykha," *ZNB* 12–13 (June 1926), 6.

139. In *Discipline and Punish* Foucault refers to this as "infra-penalty" deployed at the level "the laws had left empty" (178). Along with the spatial separation of the body (enclosure), Foucault articulates the use of the regimen (timetable) in the creation of docile bodies; see 141–43, 149–51, 178.

140. Konstorum, "Nashi sanatorii i doma otdykha," *ZNB* 6 (June 1925): 1.

141. Koumiss therapy, involving the drinking of fermented mare's milk, was just one of the available cures. For descriptions of each (air baths, mineral-water cures, wine cures, and food therapy), see L. Gl. Gol'dfail' and I. D. Iakhnin, *Kurorty, sanatorii i doma otdykha SSSR, 1928,* 13, 458–70. See also Konstorum, "Nashi sanatorii," 1; in English see Hyde, *The Soviet Health Service,* 73–75.

142. Vainshtein, *Doma otdykha i sanatorii,* 44.

143. Konstorum, "Nashi sanatorii," 2.

144. Quoted in A. Berliand, "Tret'e soveshchanie po sanitarnomu prosveshcheniiu (Sektsiia sanprosveshcheniia IX-go s"ezda sanitarnykh vrachei, bakteriologov, i epidemiologov)," *Sanitarnoe prosveshchenie,* ed. I. D. Strashun and A. O. Edel'shtein, 5.

145. Vainshtein, *Doma otdykha i sanatorii,* 13; Kagan, *Rabochaia molodezh',* 11; Fedynskaia, "O domakh otdykha," 2.

146. "Kurort' na domu" (Kiev: Naukova Dumka, n.d.), Russian State Library collection.

147. Fedynskaia, "O domakh otdykha," 3; see also E. O. Kabo, *Ocherki rabochego byta: Opyt monograficheskogo issledovaniia*, 56–57.

148. Vainshtein, *Doma otdykha i sanatorii*, 19. American sanatoriums taught patients to manage disease outside the sanatorium and battle its spread with spittoons, etc. See Feldberg, *Disease and Class*, 91.

149. Lenin, "Letter to N. A. Semashko, 13-9-1921," in *Collected Works*, 45:298–99.

150. G-berg, "Dom otdykha-shkola novogo byta," *ZNB* 11 (August 1925): 14.

151. Konstorum, "Nashi sanatorii," 1.

152. Anon., "Odobrili rabotu domov otdykha i sanatoriev," *ZNB* 6 (March 1926): 9.

153. In her *Republic of Labor* Koenker refers to several stories of the union press that showed how "rest home stays . . . invited dreams of dalliance" (275).

154. Anon. "P'ianstvu i khuliganstvu ne dolzhno byt' mesta v domakh otdykha," *ZNB* 12–13 (June 1926): 12.

155. Ibid.; Nemudrov, "Tam, gde zhili monakhi (Dom otdykha MOZa v Zvenigorode imeni A. I. Rykova)," *ZNB* 7 (June 1925): 11.

156. Wall newspapers were short publications from health cells, red corners, or other small groups publicizing stories of interest to those in the factory, club, school, or building that the group represented. K-ch, "O chem nam pishut," *ZNB* 16 (August 1926): 19.

157. Anon., "P'ianstvu i khuliganstvu ne dolzhno byt'," 12.

158. *Buza* is an alcoholic beverage made from millet, buckwheat, or barley; see Garevskii, "Kul'turnaia rabota," 6.

159. AMO f. 2129, op 1, d. 386, l. 40.

160. AMO f. 2129, op. 1, d. 386, l. 32. Other telegrams reiterated this point; see 1. 46, 56.

161. AMO f. 2129, op. 1, d. 386, l. 35. See also 1. 54.

162. AMO f. 2129, op. 1, d. 386, l. 56. See also 1. 75.

163. G-berg, "Dom otdykha-shkola novogo byta," 14.

164. Konstorum, "Nashi sanatorii," 3.

165. Ibid.

166. Nemudrov, "Tam, gde zhili monakhi," 11.

167. Andr-va, "Doma otdykha—Shkola novogo byta: V dome otdykha im. Sverdlova," *ZNB* 3 (May 1925): 15.

168. British Trade Union Delegation, *Russia Today*, 157.

169. Anne O'Hare McCormick, *The Hammer and the Scythe: Communist Russia Enters the Second Decade*, 221.

170. Wells, *Russia in the Shadows*, 128–31.

171. Kholodkovskii, *Moskovskie parki kul'tury i otdykha*, 8.

172. Except for the Ivanovo-Vosnesenskii, Uralskaia, and Sibirskii krai regions, no other areas even approached double digits; see Gol'dfail' and Iakhin, *Kurorty, sanatorii i doma otdykha SSSR, 1928*, 405–38. For the 1970s, see Kovlov, *Zdravnitsy*, 3–4.

Chapter 4. The Home: Housekeeping, Social Duty, and Public Concern

1. The *zhenotdel* was the women's section of the party, which organized women's political work; see Wood, *The Baba and the Comrade*, 68–98.

2. The Soviet youth groups were broken down according to age: Octobrists (1–9), Pioneers (9–14), and Komsomol (14–23).

3. *Nash byt: Agit-byt-buffonada v 2-kh kartinakh, Rabochii klub* 1 (January 1925): 50–51. *Rabochii klub* was the national publication of Proletkult beginning in 1924. See Mally, *Revolutionary Acts;* Cassiday, *The Enemy on Trial.*

4. This is a classic example of what Wood points to as Soviet society's trouble in answering the pressing question: "Who makes the soup?" *The Baba and the Comrade,* 201–3.

5. For general discussions of this trend, see Attwood, *Creating the New Soviet Woman,* 4–11; and Wood, *The Baba and the Comrade,* 198–203; see also A. Kollontai, "The Family and the Communist State" (1918), 67–76, and L. Trotsky, "From the Old Family to the New" (1923), 76–83, both in *Bolshevik Visions,* ed. Rosenberg, 1:67–83.

6. Victor Buchli, *An Archaeology of Socialism,* 2, 25.

7. A special "Week for Sanitizing Homes," planned for the summer of 1921, promised to focus on "the meaning of the house for health," how to keep a healthy home, the politics of housing, and infectious diseases; see the planning circular issued by the Sanitary Enlightenment Committee of the Department of Health in GARF f. A-2313, op. 1, d. 12a, l. 10.

8. See Wendy Goldman, "The Origins of the Bolshevik Vision: Love Unfettered, Women Free," in her *Women, the State and Revolution: Soviet Family Policy and Social Life, 1917–1936,* 1–58; Wood, *The Baba and the Comrade,* 26–30.

9. Igal Halfin details the animosity of Bolsheviks toward traditional families as anti-collectivist, patriarchal, and exploitative; see "Intimacy in an Ideological Key: The Communist Case of the 1920s and 1930s," in *Language and Revolution,* ed. Halfin, 185–213.

10. For the history of the *zhenotdel,* see Wood, *The Baba and the Comrade,* 194–203. For a discussion of A. Kollontai, the *zhentodel* leader and theorist for women's emancipation, see Barbara Evans Clements, *Bolshevik Feminist: The Life of Aleksandra Kollontai.*

11. In the United States, domestic advice manuals resonated with the message of Christianity as well as political citizenship in the nineteenth and twentieth centuries; see Sarah A. Leavitt, *From Catharine Beecher to Martha Stewart: A Cultural History of Domestic Advice,* 22–24.

12. Chernyshevskii, *What Is to Be Done?,* 383.

13. Robert Eugene Johnson, *Peasant and Proletarian: The Working Class of Moscow in the Late Nineteenth Century,* 85–86.

14. Tyler Stovall, *The Rise of the Paris Red Belt;* Helmut Gruber, *Red Vienna: Working-Class Culture, 1919–1934,* 46.

15. For the origins of these ideas and their fate in the 1930s, see Victor Buchli, "The Narkomfin Communal House and the Material Culture of Socialism," in his *An Archaeology of Socialism,* 63–76.

16. Bliznakov, "Soviet Housing," in *Russian Housing in the Modern Age,* ed. Brumfield and Ruble, 86–108.

17. Some pamphlets went into minute detail on minor points of home maintenance. For example, M. P. Dubianskaia stated that the optimal temperature for the organism was 18 degrees Celsius and then filled out forty-six more riveting pages on proper heating; see *Gigiena zhilishch: Ob otoplenii pechami* (pub. 10,000).

18. N. Semashko, *Sotsial'nye prichiny bolezni*, 20 (pub. 3,000).

19. A. A. Ashikhmin, *Sotsial'nye bolezni i zhilishche*, vol. 3 of *Biblioteka Sanpredstavitelia 2-aia seriia broshiur (Komissiia sanitarnykh predstavitelei)*, ed. Z. G. Frenkel, 12 (pub. 6,000); idem, *Bolezn' i byt: Bor'ba s sotsial'nymi bolezniami* (pub. 5,000). It should be noted that all such commentary focused on "the modern man" even though women carried out these tasks.

20. For a discussion of public health and housing, see Enid Gauldie, *Cruel Habitations: A History of Working-Class Housing, 1780–1918*.

21. Chase, *Workers, Society and the Soviet State*, 188.

22. A. Mol'kov, *Materialy dlia besed o podderzhanii chistoty v zhilishche*, 4 (pub. 25,000).

23. Stites notes that artists either mocked or utilized religion in 1920s imagery; see *Russian Popular Culture*, 54.

24. "Kipiatok" and "Pechi," Institute of Sanitary Culture (Moscow: Mosgublit, 1927) (pub. 300). Russian State Library collection.

25. V. G. Khlopin's work on the foundations of hygiene began with information on air and dust and then moved on to water, sewers, housing, and clothing; see *Osnovy Gigieny*.

26. A. A. Ashikhmin, *Vozdukh nashikh zhilishch* vyp 3. *Komissiia Sanitarnykh predstavitelei*, ed. G. I. Demob, 5–11, 12–18, 18–20 (pub. 5,000); idem, *Bolezni i byt*, 14.

27. N. A. Semashko, *Nauka o zdorov'e obshchestva (Sotsial'naia gigiena)*, 20 (pub. 10,000).

28. A. Mol'kov, comp., *Zdorovoe zhilishche: Programma populiarnoi lektsii*, 9 (pub. 5,000).

29. For Russia, see Elizabeth Andrews Hachten, "Science in the Service of Society: Bacteriology, Medicine, and Hygiene in Russia, 1855–1907," 4, 340. This conflicted, slow transfer to germ theory was typical. For the American case, see Nancy Tomes, *The Gospel of Germs: Men, Women and the Microbe in American Life*; Katherine Ott, *Fevered Lives: Tuberculosis in American Culture Since 1870*, 37–38, 54.

30. "Chashche provetrivai komnatu," Gorod i derevnia, 1926–29 (pub. 2,000) and "Zakryvai bedro dlia musora, ne dyshi zarazoi," Gorod i derevnia, 1926–29 (pub. 2,000). Russian State Library collection.

31. V. Sukharev, *Rabochii, beregi svoe zdorov'e: K ozdorovleniiu rabochei sem'i*, 5 (pub. 10,000); Kal'manson and Bekariukov, *Beregi svoe zdorov'e!*, 13.

32. Semashko, *Nauka o zdorov'e obshchestva*, 20; N. A. Semashko, *Vvedenie v sotsial'nuiu gigienu*, 21.

33. One sanitary doctor claimed the following improvements over a period of two months: 14 better air; 3 transoms; 114 exterminations; 41 tidied up; 2 whitewashed walls; 34 added wallpaper; 1 moved food preparation out of living quarters; 2 moved clothes washing; 4 acquired single towels; 2 added trash cans; 4 added spittoons; 4 changed apts. See Bogatyrev, "Khronika dispanserizatsii," *Ezhenedel'nik MOZa* 34, no. 5 (26 August–2 September 1926): 497–98.

34. Douglas, *Purity and Danger*, 2. For another consideration of the meaning of dust in modern life, see Amato, *Dust*.

35. Tomes, *The Gospel of Germs*, 166–68.

36. Proctor, *The Nazi War on Cancer*, 104–5. Dust can retain dried sputum, which can spread chronic pulmonary tuberculosis for months or even years. Chronic pulmonary tuberculosis is the deadliest form of the disease and is responsible for 90 percent of

deaths. See Teller, *The Tuberculosis Movement*, 2, 18; McCuaig, *The Weariness, the Fever, and the Fret*, 11.

37. Ashikhmin, *Sotsial'nye bolezni i zhilishche*, 14.

38. Kal'manson and Bekariukov, *Beregi svoe zdorov'e!*, 13.

39. Ashikhmin, *Vozdukh nashikh zhilishch*, 21.

40. Similar calls for simple home decor appeared in American texts; see Tomes, *The Gospel of Germs*, 144.

41. At the bottom the poster emphasized that tchotchkes took up the space for air in the apartment. Other issues relating to collectibles are discussed by Buchli, *An Archaeology of Socialism*, 43–45.

42. Boym, *Common Places*, 35–38.

43. The poster "Kak soderzhat' zhilishche" was unfortunately too large and far too detailed to adequately reproduce here. Among its long list of rules, it advised wiping shoes before entering the home (Narodnyi komissariat truda, 1921), Russian State Library collection.

44. Kal'manson and Bekariukov, *Beregi svoe zdorov'e!*, 14.

45. V. P. Kalashnikov, *Pamiatka: Domovym sanpredstaviteliam (O gigiene zhilishch)*, 54.

46. Ibid.

47. TsMAM f. 2315, op. 1, d. 36, l. 323.

48. See recommendation 18 in figure 4.1.

49. Kal'manson and Bekariukov, *Beregi svoe zdorov'e!*, 14, 38.

50. One sanitation doctor reported many improvements, including adding 4 spittoons. See Bogatyrev, "Khronika dispanserizatsii," 497–98.

51. Kal'manson and Bekariukov, *Beregi svoe zdorov'e!*, 14.

52. McCuaig, *The Weariness, the Fever, and the Fret*, 10, 100.

53. Teller, *The Tuberculosis Movement*, 22.

54. Spitting was associated with tuberculosis; see David S. Barnes, *The Making of a Social Disease: Tuberculosis in Nineteenth-Century France*, 75. Others spread the idea that the condemnation of spitting went beyond contagion concerns; see Ott, *Fevered Lives*, 117, 118. John F. Kasson discusses the vulgarity of spitting outside the context of health in *Rudeness and Civility: Manners in Nineteenth-Century Urban America*, 125.

55. McCuaig, *The Weariness, the Fever, and the Fret*, 100; Teller, *The Tuberculosis Movement*, 70.

56. See the multiple slogans in Mol'kov, *Materialy dlia besed*, 10; see also the arguments of Kalashnikov, *Pamiatka*, 30.

57. Kal'manson and Bekariukov, *Beregi svoe zdorov'e!*, 12–13.

58. A. A. Sadov, *Zaraznye bolezni i byt*, 11 (pub. 10,000). Ashikhmin, *Bolezn' i byt*, 15.

59. Buchli, *An Archaeology of Socialism*, 52.

60. For an in-depth discussion of "lifestyle" syphilis, see Engelstein, *The Keys to Happiness*; for syphilis and kitchens, see Kal'manson and Bekariukov, *Beregi svoe zdorov'e!*, 16–19; for the nonvenereal theory in the American context, see Tomes, *The Gospel of Germs*, 107–8.

61. Kal'manson and Bekariukov recommended a distance of least a verst (about two-thirds of an English mile) for the trash heap; *Beregi svoe zdorov'e!*, 16. For more on this topic, see Sadov, *Zaraznye bolezni i byt*, 24; M. P. Dubianskaia, *Borites' s mukhami, klopami, komarami,*

vshami: Domashnie nasekomye—Nashi vragi, 16, 42. For the United States, see Tomes, *The Gospel of Germs,* 9.

62. L. M. Vasilevskii, *Gigiena pionera,* 31 (pub. 20,000).

63. Sadov, *Zaraznye bolezni i byt,* 27.

64. Ruth Schwartz Cowan points out the ways in which technological innovations actually increased work for middle- and upper-class women; see *More Work for Mother: The Ironies of Household Technology from the Open Hearth to the Microwave,* 65.

65. Wood, *The Baba and the Comrade,* 3, 194.

66. Bonnell, *Iconography of Power,* 78.

67. Kagan, *Put' k obshchestvennoi rabote,* 11–12. Another source estimated that in 1924 twenty thousand women were involved in social work in Moscow and the region; see Diagilev, *Istoriia Moskvy,* 6:303.

68. Wood, *The Baba and the Comrade,* 63.

69. Semashko, *Okhrana zdorov'ia rabochikh i rabotnits,* 37.

70. Jeffrey Brooks notes that in 1920s *Pravda* biographies for contests often appeared and served as a sphere for identity creation; see "Revolutionary Lives: Public Identities in *Pravda* during the 1920s," in *New Directions in Soviet History,* ed. Stephen White, 29. For more examples, see Zdravkor A-va, "Delegatka za rabotoi"; Andreeva, "Delegatka za rabotoi"; and E-ova, "Nashi rabotnitsy-delegatki"—all in *ZNB* 3 (May 1925), 7; or the group Rabotnitsa Grushicheva, "Kipit rabota" and "Aktivno rabotaet"; Popova, "God raboty"; Rabkor Efremovskii, "Boretsia s podkidyvaniem"; and Shlykova "Ukrepim nashu respubliku"—all in *ZNB* 4–5 (March 1926): 6; or L. L., "Delegatka Zhukova" and "Nashi delegatki"; Koroleva, "Bor'ba s prostitutsiei"; Chlen sektsii Kh., "Opravdali doverie izbiratel'nits"; Krumgart, "Delegatka za rabotoi"; G., "Vydvizhenka za rabotoi"; and Kharitonova, "Domashniaia khoziaika na obshchestvennoi rabote"—all in *ZNB* 17–18 (September 1926): 5. Lastly, see L. Polkovnikova, "Smotr nashemu aktivu" and "Na razlichnykh uchastkakh sovetskoi raboty," *ZNB* 16 (August 1927): 8.

71. Delegatka N. Gradusova, "Chetyre goda," *ZNB* 16 (August 1927): 8.

72. In *Common Places* Boym argues that these public tales resembled "a premodern potlatch, when the members of a rival tribe burn their furniture as a public sacrifice so that the neighbor will be obliged to burn more" (36).

73. Kagan, *Put' k obshchestvennoi rabote,* 9.

74. Ibid. Wood notes that the question of daily life involved implementation of equality and the relationship of party members with their spouses; see *The Baba and the Comrade,* 198.

75. Kagan, *Put' k obshchestvennoi rabote,* 10.

76. Ibid. Corporal punishment was considered out of vogue by the Soviets; see the treatment of the orphan Sirotin in the anonymous pamphlet *Agitsud nad prestupnikami* (pub. 300).

77. Kagan, *Put' k obshchestvennoi rabote,* 10.

78. G., "Vydvizhenka za rabotoi," *ZNB* 17–18 (September 1926): 5. The term *vydvizhenka* referred to upwardly mobile women.

79. Boris Andreev, *Sud nad starym bytom: Stsenarii dlia rabochikh klubov ko dniu rabotnitsy 8-go Marta (s metodicheskimi ukazaniiami).*

80. Boris Andreev, *Tretii front: Stseny iz sovremennogo rabochego byta v trekh deistviiakh,* 22 (pub. 7,000).

81. R. Gramova, "Vot gde temnota," *Kommunisticheskii trud* 278 (24 February 1921): 4.

82. "O chem pishut," *Kommunisticheskii trud* 354 (2 June 1921): 3.

83. The play appeared in Rebel'skii, *Instsenirovannye sudy,* 55–83.

84. Wood, *The Baba and the Comrade,* 14, 23.

85. N. Krupskaia, "Chto znachit byt' Lenintsem," in *Azbuka komsomol'tsa,* ed. A. Slepkov, 37–75.

86. Naiman links ambivalence toward the family and turn-of-the-century millenarianism. Dislike for children and family grew out of a discomfort with arousal and led to left-revolutionary depictions of "free love," which involved little love-making. Naiman further argues that the misogynist aspects of this discomfort with sexuality—women being distinctive for possessing larger sex organs, which supposedly overruled their intellect—were associated with both undifferentiated, uncontrolled, constant arousal and the particularly selfish, isolating bond between mother and child; see *Sex in Public,* 27–78.

87. Attwood, *Creating the New Soviet Woman,* 9.

88. See the article by Svet', "Rabochim nado pomoch' svoim zhenam'," *Rabotnitsa* 13 (1925), 17; cited in Attwood, *Creating the New Soviet Woman,* 34.

89. Lynn Mally examines the play in "Performing the New Woman: The Komsomolka as Actress and Image in Soviet Youth Theater."

90. S. Smidrovich, *Rabotnitsa i novyi byt,* 15 (pub. 15,000).

91. Wood, *The Baba and the Comrade,* 200–203.

92. See the posters "Chashche provetrivai komnatu" and "Zakryvai bedro." Hoy examines housework in the United States during the nineteenth and twentieth centuries and argues that chores traditionally assigned to women on farms remained theirs in the city; see *Chasing Dirt,* 98.

93. F. Niurina, "Rabota kluba s zhenami rabochikh," *Klub* 5 (October 1925): 55–63. Wood highlights comparable debates and notes how women, especially nonparty wives, were accused of domestic backwardness; see *The Baba and the Comrade,* 203–8.

94. R.D., *Sud nad domashnei khoziaikoi.*

95. L. Vasias, "Sestra sotsial'noi pomoshchi-organizator novogo byta," *ZNB* 9 (May 1927): 5. See also this chapter's opening play, *Nash byt,* 44–51; Naiman, *Sex in Public,* 88.

96. Rykova, "Zdravookhranenie v Zamraione: Doklad tov. Rykovoi na plenume sektsii zdravookhraneniia Mossoveta," *Ezhenedel'nik MOZa* (25 March–1 April 1926): 218.

97. Vasilevskii, *Gigiena pionera,* 23–24. N. N. Iordanskii advised acquainting children with hygiene from the first meeting at school; see *Sanitarno-gigienicheskaia rabota shkoly* (pub. 3,000).

98. Zheleznyi, *Kak zhit', chtoby zdorovym byt'?,* 34.

99. Kagan, *Put' k obshchestvennoi rabote,* 31.

100. O. Spandar'ian, *Pochemu Varia otdala svoikh detei v pionery,* 27 (pub. 10,000).

101. I. Mil'man, "Bortsy za zdorovyi byt," *ZNB* 13–14 (1927): 16. Catriona Kelly expands upon the idea of children as revolutionaries of daily life, noting the ways in which this also resulted in control of the children; see "Shaping the 'Future Race': Regulating the Daily Life of Children in Early Soviet Russia," in *Everyday Life in Early Soviet Russia: Taking the Revolution Inside,* ed. Christina Kiaer and Eric Naiman, 256–81.

102. *Za novyi byt v nashei smene: Prezidium konferentsii zdraviacheek shkol Baumanskogo raiona,* 7 (pub. 1,000).

103. S. Kozakevich, "Kto prav?," *ZNB* 4–5 (1925): 15.

104. "Vospominaniia o V. I. Lenine" (Molodaia gvardiia, 1955), 114; quoted in E. D. Ashurkov, "Leninskie printsipy sovetskogo zdravookhraneniia," in Institut organizatsii zdravookhraneniia i istorii meditsiny im. N. A. Semashko, *Leninskie idei ob okhrane zdorov'ia naroda,* 11.

105. Zheleznyi, *Kak zhit', chtoby zdorovym byt'?,* 34–35.

106. Ia. Iu. Kats, *Sistema i metody dispanserizatsii,* 42. For similar activities in Leningrad, see I. Strashun, "Desiat' let bor'by proletariata za zdorov'e," in *Desiat' let oktiabria i sovetskaia meditsina,* ed. Semashko, 78–79.

107. A 1928 report put health cell involvement at twenty-seven thousand but claimed an additional five hundred special "school" health cells with around ten thousand children, totalling thirty-seven thousand—probably an inflated estimate. See D. Gorfin, "10 let sovetskoi meditsiny i konkursy na luchshuiu sektsiiu zdravookhraneniia i luchshii vrachebnyi uchastok," *Voprosy zdravookhranenia* 4 (1928): 18; Bogomolov, *Dostizheniia sovetskoi meditsiny,* 26. See also *Material k dokladu otdela zdravookhraneniia,* 7; Geizer, *Ozdorovlenie truda i byta,* 23. In the mid-1920s, eighty-five hundred health cells patrolled and inspected Moscow; see Bogomolov, *Dostizheniia sovetskoi meditsiny,* 26.

108. Moskovskii sovet, *Material k dokladu otdela zdravookhraneniia,* 7.

109. V. Terlikova, "Pobol'she vnimaniia zdraviacheikam," *ZNB* 9 (May 1927): 3.

110. Gantt, *Russian Medicine,* 170.

111. Bogatyrev, "Khronika Dispanserizatsii," 497–98.

112. TsGAMO f. 2129, op. 1, d. 97, l. 1.

113. TsGAMO f. 2129, op. 1, d. 97, l. 17–18.

114. TsGAMO f. 2129, op. 1, d. 97, l. 33.

115. TsGAMO f. 2129, op. 1, d. 97, l. 20. In the case of an alcoholic thrown out of the building for "incurable" alcoholism, the court made the decision, see TsGAMO f. 2129, op. 1, d. 97, l. 17.

116. Kats, *Sistema i metody dispanserizatsii,* 44.

117. TsGAMO f. 2129, op. 1, d. 97, l. 2.

118. TsGAMO f. 2129, op. 1, d. 97, l. 30.

119. Kats, *Sistema i metody dispanserizatsii,* 43.

120. V. Stoianovskaia, "Chto dolzhen znat' i delat' chlen zdraviacheiki po tuberkulezu," *Gigiena i zdorov'e rabochei i krest'ianskoi sem'i* 14 (July 1926): 5.

121. Klin, "Veselye nravy," *ZNB* 7 (April 1926): 13.

122. Rul'neva, "Nuzhna zdraviacheika," *ZNB* 3 (February 1926): 15.

123. Zdravkor T-va, "Zdraviacheika na strazhe," *ZNB* 3 (May 1925): 16.

124. Zdravkor tipografii im. Dunaeva-Tumanova, "Obshchezhitie studentov," *ZNB* 3 (May 1925): 15.

125. Rabochii O., "Kak byt'?," *ZNB* 3 (February 1926): 14.

126. Zdravkor tipografii im. Dunaeva O. Bitkova, "Zdraviacheika ne spit," *ZNB* 3 (May 1925): 17.

127. Leavitt, *From Catharine Beecher to Martha Stewart,* 80–87.

128. Stoianovskaia, "Chto dolzhen znat' i delat'," 5.

129. V. A. Obukh, ed., and A. K. Bogomolov, comp., *Zdravookhranenie v Moskve (Dispanserizatsiia rabochego naseleniia)*, 45.

130. Ibid., 27.

131. This report also boasted 87 centers, with 181 doctors and 120 fel'dshers; see MOZ, *Kratkii obzor sostoianiia zdravookhraneniia v Moskve i guberniiakh*, 30.

132. V. A. Obukh, "Uchraspred MOZa," 2 (January 1924); quoted in Ia. Kats, *Sistema i metody dispanserizatsii*, 4.

133. I. Stoklitskii, "Iz-pod vlasti durmana—k trudu (Rogozhsko-Simonovskii Narkodispanser)," *ZNB* 8–9 (May 1926): 12.

134. The chronological inception of medical inspection was as follows: Belgium (1895), England (1898), the Netherlands (1903), Baden (1906), Bavaria (1909), Italy (1912), Austria (1919), Prussia (1921), Saxony (1921), France (1942); see Rosen, *A History of Public Health*, 374, 425; Teller, *The Tuberculosis Movement*, 74; Duffy, *The Sanitarians*, 208; Reinhard Sieder, "Housing Policy, Social Welfare, and Daily Life in 'Red Vienna,' 1919–34"; Gruber, *Red Vienna*, 66.

135. Bates, *Bargaining for Life*, 113. The British only set up special training in 1919; see Rosen, *A History of Public Health*, 377. Tomes notes that U.S. inspectors complained about conditions more than ignorance; see *The Gospel of Germs*, 188–95.

136. Kabo, *Ocherki rabochego byta*, 29–32.

137. Ibid., 35–38.

138. For Moscow province in 1921, official government inspectors (*zhilishchno-sanitarnye inspektory*) numbered fifteen, with forty-two controllers and eighteen inspectors; see Kats, *Mediko-sanitarnaia organizatsiia Moskvy*, 8. For additional groups, see V. F. Ivanov, "Opyt obsledovaniia byta dispanserizirovannykh rabochikh v Chistoprudnom ob"edinenii," *Ezhenedel'nik MOZa* 17, no. 170 (29 April 1926): 286. In Moscow in 1928, 4,500 people worked for seventy-two KOTiB in addition to the 27,000 involved in the 9,000 health cells of the city; see Gorfin, "10 let," 18.

139. P-va, "Delegatki za rabotoi (Khamovnicheskii raion)," *ZNB* 17–18 (September 1926): 3.

140. Kats, *Sistema i metody dispanserizatsii*, 22. In 1926 Moscow's population totaled 2,026,000; see Bliznakov, "Soviet Housing," in *Russian Housing in the Modern Age*, ed. Brumfield and Ruble, 107.

141. Freidmin, *Obshchestvennye nachala*, 34.

142. Weissman, "Origins of Soviet Health Administration," in *Health and Society in Revolutionary Russia*, ed. Solomon and Hutchinson, 106.

143. Halle, *Woman in Soviet Russia*, 360–61.

144. Béraud, *The Truth about Moscow*, 157–60. A similarly scathing portrayal can be found in John Wynne Hird, *Under Czar and Soviet: My Thirty Years in Russia*, 257–65.

145. Attwood and Kelly, "Programs for Identity," in *Constructing Russian Culture*, ed. Kelly and Shepherd, 264–67.

146. Joseph Bradley, *Muzhik and Muscovite: Urbanization in Late Imperial Russia*, 41, 196.

147. Johnson, *Peasant and Proletarian*, 84; Thurston, *Liberal City, Conservative State*, 18–19; Koenker, *Moscow Workers*, 54–55.

148. Bliznakov, "Soviet Housing," in *Russian Housing in the Modern Age,* ed. Brumfield and Ruble, 107.

149. William Craft Brumfield, "Building for Comfort and Profit: The New Apartment House," in *Russian Housing in the Modern Age,* ed. Brumfield and Ruble, 79.

150. Wiedenfeld, *The Remaking of Russia,* 86.

151. By 1921 half the population of Moscow had taken up "reclaimed" houses of the bourgeoisie, but they were of poor quality. See Chase, *Workers, Society and the Soviet State,* 27–28, 74; Colton, *Moscow,* 158–64. For anecdotal accounts of apartments, see the chapter "How Moscow Keeps House" in Anna Louise Strong's *The First Time in History: Two Years in Russia's New Life (August, 1921 to December, 1923),* 134–53; Marguerite E. Harrison, *Marooned in Moscow: The Story of an American Woman Imprisoned in Russia,* 94–97; and the chapter "In the Homes of the People," in Lancelot Lawton's *The Russian Revolution,* 315–26. Kabo described the general discomfort in *Ocherki rabochego byta,* 90; see also Vladimir Paperny, "Men, Women and the Living Space," in *Russian Housing in the Modern Age,* ed. Brumfield and Ruble, 157; Lebina, *Povsednevnaia zhizn',* 182–84; Bliznakov, "Soviet Housing," in *Russian Housing in the Modern Age,* ed. Brumfield and Ruble, 85. Boym details the often odd results of these separations; see *Common Places,* 124–30; see also Koenker, *Republic of Labor,* 178–80.

152. Ivanov, "Opyt obsledovaniia byta," 286. The 1923 all-union health survey of worker youth found that among urban youth 77.8 percent lived in private apartments, 10 percent in barracks, and 12.2 percent in house communes. Of these, the number living with only one other person was 8.7 percent, two people 24 percent, three people 20.8 percent, four people 13.8 percent, five people 10.1 percent, and six or more people 22.6 percent; see Zaitsev, *Trud i byt rabochikh podrostkov,* 31–32.

153. Ivanov, "Opyt obsledovaniia byta," 287.

154. Chase attributes the decreased death rate to better sewer services and water provision; see *Workers, Society and the Soviet State,* 78. Colton also credits infrastructure improvements with increased health, though he does acknowledge the support of hygiene education and dispensaries; see *Moscow,* 171.

155. Sukharev, *Rabochii, beregi svoe zdorov'e,* 12.

156. Karlgren, *Bolshevist Russia,* 197. A decidedly unsympathetic viewer, he detailed problems of Soviet citizens in the 1920s.

157. Kabo, *Ocherki rabochego byta,* 51, 54, 59. Domestic manuals in the United States often attempted to provide "low-cost" alternatives (e.g., furniture made from boxes); see Leavitt, *From Catharine Beecher to Martha Stewart,* 91–96.

158. These magic water taps appeared particularly odd in light of propaganda posters warning of the problem of faucet theft; see "Sledi za umyval'nikom" (pub. 14,000), Russian State Library collection.

159. For an anecdotal account of plumbing and hot-water problems, see Harrison, *Marooned in Moscow,* 49, 107; Sukharev, *Rabochii, beregi svoe zdorov'e,* 11. Similar advice appeared in the United States; see Tomes, *The Gospel of Germs,* 144.

160. Anon., "Tribuna chitatelei: Kto obratit vnimanie?," *Kommunisticheskii trud* 276 (February 1921): 3.

161. Hoy gives these estimates for the American case, here used to illustrate a possible workload; see *Chasing Dirt,* 158.

162. Béraud, *The Truth about Moscow,* 42.

163. Jessica Smith, *Woman in Soviet Russia,* 146.

164. I. I. Fainshmidt, N. S. Morozovskii, and L. D. Ul'ianov, *Sotsial'no-gigienicheskie usloviia i tuberkulez v Ukrainskom sele,* 225–28.

165. Chase, *Workers, Society and the Soviet State,* 196.

166. Kalashnikov, *Pamiatka,* 31.

167. Bravaia, *OMM na zapade i v SSSR,* 68–69; and B. S. Ginzburg, *Okhrana materinstva i mladenchestva,* 18.

168. Semashko, *Nauka o zdorov'e obshchestva,* 17.

169. The measurements were given as 80, 1, 5, and 7 arshin, the latter being equivalent to twenty-eight inches or seventy-one centimeters. See Semashko, *Nauka o zdorov'e obshchestva,* 78–79. Semashko recommended 28.8 square meters of well-ventilated space per person with a sunny .5 square meters of window for every 2.5 to 3.5 square meters of space; see *Vvedenie v sotsial'nuiu gigienu,* 20.

170. Ivanov, "Opyt obsledovaniia byta," 287.

171. Zaitsev, *Trud i byt rabochikh podrostkov,* 33.

172. A. A. Sakhnovskaia, *Chesotka i bor'ba s neiu,* 16 (pub. 13,000).

173. E. G. Bibanova, *Kak gotovit' iz rebenka v vozraste do 3-kh let budushchego stroitelia novoi zhizni,* 61.

174. Ashikhmin, *Sotsial'nye bolezni,* 23. American authors blamed poor domestic situations for the appeal of the pub; see Leavitt, *From Catharine Beecher to Martha Stewart,* 24–25. French sanitarians blamed crowding for pushing adults into the pub.

175. Barnes, *The Making of a Social Disease,* 128.

176. Ashikhmin, *Sotsial'nye bolezni,* 19.

177. Olga Matich, "Remaking the Bed: Utopia in Daily Life," in *Laboratory of Dreams: The Russian Avant-Garde and Cultural Experiment,* ed. John E. Bowlt and Olga Matich, 59–78.

178. Jeffrey Brooks reports that in obituaries of great men published in *Pravda,* information on family or home appeared in only 7 percent of the 495 cases. These omissions would seem to reflect the perceived insignificance of these elements in relation to power; see "Revolutionary Lives," in *New Directions in Soviet History,* ed. White, 34–35.

179. Il'ianskii and Lapin, "Beregi zdorov'e—i nikakikh gvozdei!," *ZNB* 4–5 (1925): 10.

180. Quoted in Zetkin, *Reminiscences of Lenin,* 68.

181. Semashko, *Nauka o zdorov'e obshchestva,* 20.

182. Rebecca Spagnolo, "When Private Home Meets Public Workplace: Service, Space, and the Urban Domestic in 1920s Russia," in *Everyday Life in Early Soviet Russia,* ed. Kiaer and Naiman, 230–55.

183. V. Kirov, "Biudzhet vremeni rabochego i klub," *Klub* 5 (October 1925): 61.

184. Susan M. Kingsbury and Mildred Fairchild, *Factory, Family, and Woman in the Soviet Union,* 249–50.

185. Kagan saw overburdening as purely a woman's problem. He insisted that women needed to organize tasks more scientifically and work together to form communal organizations and thus help themselves. Supposedly one woman could do 143 pounds of laundry in eight hours in a communal laundry; see *Put' k obshestvennoi rabote,* 24–25.

186. The oft-quoted comment by Lenin is actually not as quixotic as it is usually

presented. In the 1917 article "Can the Bolsheviks Retain State Power?" he stated, "We are not utopians. We know that an unskilled labourer or a cook cannot immediately get on with the job of state administration." The inclusion of "immediately" does indicate, however, that it seemed likely; see *Collected Works,* 26:113.

Chapter 5. The Family: Maternity, Birth, and Parenthood

1. Haines, *Health Work in Soviet Russia,* 165–69.

2. Hoffmann demonstrates how Stalin's pro-natalist policies were built upon this European base rather than on traditional values. See the chapter "Stalinist Family Values," in his *Stalinist Values,* 88–117.

3. This intersection of gendered practitioners and women's issues was evident in Russia before the revolution; see Denbeste-Barnett, "Earnestly Working to Improve Russia's Future," 88–111. Jane Lewis explores the relationship between female practitioners and powerful men in "Women and Late-Nineteenth-Century Social Work," in *Regulating Womanhood: Historical Essays on Marriage, Motherhood and Sexuality,* ed. Carol Smart, 78–99; see also Ann Oakley, *The Captured Womb: A History of the Medical Care of Pregnant Women.*

4. For more on state intrusion through natalism, see the introduction to *Mothers of a New World,* ed. Koven and Michel, 1–42. From 1874 to 1919 the French promulgated the state's control over women's bodies through protective labor legislation; see Elinor Accampo, "Gender, Social Policy, and the Formation of the Third Republic," in *Gender and the Politics of Social Reform in France,* ed. Accampo, Fuchs, and Stewart, 9–13.

5. In the United States the Children's Bureau provided free instruction to mothers; see Molly Ladd-Taylor, *Raising a Baby the Government Way: Mothers' Letters to the Children's Bureau, 1915–1932;* see also Kriste Lindenmeyer, *"A Right to Childhood": The U.S. Children's Bureau and Child Welfare, 1912–1946.* In *OMM na zapade i v SSSR,* R. M. Bravaia noted that Germany had 360 consultations in 1910 and 2,600 by 1920. Infant deaths decreased from 15.1 per 100 in 1913 to 14.5 in 1919 (97–98). England had 1,700 centers by 1918, with 700 in private hands. These centers, which taught breast-feeding and housekeeping, claimed a drop in infant deaths from 12.8 percent in 1901–910 to 10 percent in 1911–20 (100); for U.S. programs, see 101. For a general overview of natalist programs throughout Europe, see *Mothers of a New World,* ed. Koven and Michel; Porter, *Health, Civilization, and the State,* 168–73; and Rosen, *A History of Public Health,* 264–71. The Swiss pioneered the eight-week leave in 1877. In 1878 Germans offered three weeks. Neither country, however, included benefits and pay. In 1883 Germany and Austria-Hungary offered three weeks paid leave. By 1900 the United Kingdom, Portugal, Norway, Holland, and Belgium all had unpaid leave; see Fuchs, "France in a Comparative Perspective," in *Gender and the Politics of Social Reform,* ed. Accampo, Fuchs, and Stewart, 166. For Vienna, see Sieder, "Housing Policy, Social Welfare, and Family Life in 'Red Vienna'," 35–48; Horn, *Social Bodies,* 92. Porter, *Health, Civilization, and the State,* 174–75. For a book-length study focusing on Britain and France, see Susan Pedersen, *Family, Dependence, and the Origins of the Welfare State: Britain and France, 1914–1945.*

6. Bravaia, *OMM na zapade i v SSSR,* 147. On Catherine the Great and the influence of "French ideas," see 150–52.

7. Kelly, *Refining Russia,* 9; Ransel, *Village Mothers,* 20–21.

8. For a discussion of the problems with these rather impressionistic statistics, and their more careful production over time, see Ransel, *Village Mothers*, 20–22, 26–30, 32–38. See also Samuel C. Ramer, "Childbirth and Culture: Midwifery in the Nineteenth-Century Russian Countryside," in *The Family in Imperial Russia: New Lines of Historical Research*, ed. David L. Ransel, 218–35.

9. In 1901 doctors in St. Petersburg and Moscow started infant programs under the name "Drops of Milk." The society used lectures and other programs to encourage breast-feeding; see Bravaia, *OMM na zapade i v SSSR*, 186, 188.

10. O. P. Nogina, *Tridtsat' let okhrany materi i rebenka v SSSR*, 30 (English: *Mother and Child Care in the USSR*); Bravaia, *OMM na zapade i v SSSR*, 189.

11. Bravaia, *OMM na zapade i v SSSR*, 84–85; Wood, *The Baba and the Comrade*, 108–10.

12. Wood, *The Baba and the Comrade*, 29.

13. R.D., *Sud nad domashnei khoziaikoi*, 6. In *Sex in Public* Naiman refers to the mid-1920s—especially 1926—as the height of the Komsomol effort "to colonize 'private life'" (109).

14. OMM was at first part of the Commissariat of Social Security and then transferred in March 1920 to Narkomzdrav. On this transfer, see Bravaia, *OMM na zapade i v SSSR*, 206; Hyde, *The Soviet Health Service*, 52. For Semashko's founding principles, see "Protection of Mother, Baby, and Child in Russia" (1921), in *Bolshevik Visions*, ed. Rosenberg, 1:149–50.

15. O. P. Nogina, "Okhrana materi i rebenka v S.S.S.R.," *ZNB* 7 (June 1925): 1.

16. For the distribution of the book, see GARF f. A-482 op. 1 d. 556, l. 85. For comparative natalist policies, see "Problema OMM na zapade i v sovetskoi Rossii," in Ginzburg, *Okhrana materinstva i mladenchestva*, 6–44.

17. Stepan, "Okhrana materi i rebenka (Na plenume sektsii)," *ZNB* 17–18 (1925): 8.

18. Reformers argued for safe, legal abortions to cut down on complications resulting from illegal abortions; see Strashun, "Desiat' let bor'by," in *Desiat' let oktiabria*, ed. Semashko, 65; Gutkin and Frenkel, eds., *Zdravookhranenie v sovetskoi Rossii*, 45–46. Restrictions made it difficult to abort, though private clinics were more accessible. For abortion policies and their limitations, see Goldman, *Women, State and Revolution*, 254–95. For health and abortion issues, see Bernstein, *The Dictatorship of Sex*, 167–71.

19. Haines, *Health Work in Soviet Russia*, 51; Elizabeth Waters, "Child-Care Posters and the Modernization of Motherhood," 65; idem, "Teaching Mothercraft in Post-Revolutionary Russia," 29–56. Elizabeth Waters's two articles explore the topic of motherhood and propaganda in depth with excellent illustrations. David L. Ransel carefully details the slow progress of these programs into the countryside; see his *Village Mothers*, 43–79.

20. Waters, "Teaching Mothercraft," 30. A nineteen-poster series from OMM of MOZ featured general advice, from breast-feeding and cleansing to specific ideas about feeding according to the clock and literacy. One poster was entitled "Learn to Read—The Children of Literate Mothers Die Less Frequently" (Moscow: OMM, n.d.) (pub.20,000), Russian State Library collection.

21. A. Gens, "Pechatnaia propaganda idei okhrany materinstva i mladenchestva," *Okhrana materinstva i mladenchestva* 11 (1927), 54; Waters, "Teaching Mothercraft," 31.

22. A. N. Antonov, *Sanitarno-prosvetitel'naia rabota po OMM*, 5. or the consultation, see

A. N. Rakhmanov, "Konsul'tatsiia dlia beremennykh i rodil'nits, kak osnova okhrany materinstva i mladenchestva," *Okhrana materinstva i mladenchestva* 1 (1926): 16–20.

23. Waters, "Teaching Mothercraft," 32, 35–36. For a discussion of the fight against female illiteracy, see Clark, *Uprooting Otherness*, 96–116.

24. Bogolepova, "Sanitarnoe prosveshchenie i samodeiatel'nost naseleniia," in *Okhrana narodnogo zdorov'ia v SSSR*, ed. Kovrigin, 580.

25. The All-Russia exhibition for OMM started in 1919 and toured for only two years before burning down; see Antonov, *Sanitarno-prosvetitel'naia rabota*, 25–26; see also N. I. Langova, comp., *Vystavka "OMM."* B. S. Ginzburg included discussion to accompany a poster collection in the village in *Populiarnye besedy po OMM (v pomoshch' izbachu): Prilozhenie k khudozhestvennoi vystavke-lubku po OMM*. For reproductions of an OMM poster display touching on breast-feeding, cleanliness, alcohol, etc., see "Vystavka po okhrane materinstva vo dvortse truda," *Iskusstvo i promyshlennost'* 2 (February–March 1924): 47–52.

26. GARF f. A-482, op. 1, d. 556, l. 85.

27. GARF f. A-482, op. 1, d. 156, l. 27.

28. GARF f. A-482, op. 1, d. 556, l. 85. These figures are suspect. Organizers were fighting a hard battle for scarce resources and undoubtedly inflated figures. This makes the limited numbers reported seem even more modest.

29. Haines, *Health Work in Soviet Russia*, 65.

30. G., "Tam, gde boriutsia s zhenskoi besprizornost'iu," *ZNB* 15 (August 1927): 5; Ransel, *Village Mothers*, 48.

31. In 1927 the average stay was sixty-one days, according to *Materialy o deiatel'nosti lechebno-profilakticheskikh uchrezhdeni MOZa za 1926/27 goda*, 7; see also E. A. Vasich, "Doma materi i rebenka," in *Okhrana materinstva i mladenchestva v Moskve i Moskovskoi gubernii: Illiustrirovannyi sbornik*, ed. Moskovskii komitet nedeli OMM, 30 (hereafter *OMM v Moskve*).

32. A. Balander, "Dom grudnogo rebenka," in *OMM v Moskve*, ed. Moskovskii komitet nedeli OMM, 40.

33. See Melenevskaia, *Okhrana materinstva i mladenchestva: "Obshchestvennoe vospitanie v rannem vozraste,"* 11. For a long list of do's and don'ts, see *OMM v Moskve*, 1. Waters explores the imposition of scientific care in greater depth, noting the centrality of medical professionals, rest, hygiene, breast-feeding, etc.; see "Teaching Mothercraft," 30, 37–42. Paula Michaels argues that in 1930s Central Asia attention to "biomedicine" versus "ethnomedicine" was evidence of an attempt to take control of the home and infiltrate it with Soviet thought; see *Curative Powers*, 52–54.

34. Langova, *Vystavka "OMM,"* 10.

35. Ibid., 4, 10.

36. Ransel, *Village Mothers*, 22, 31. Annmarie Adams points out that from about 1870 on in England, formula was said to be better than mother's milk; see *Architecture in the Family Way*, 127.

37. Ginzburg, *Sud nad materiu, podkinuvshei svoego rebenka*, 42. For similar sentiments see B. Sigal, *Kak vyrastit' zdorovogo rebenka;* see also A. Antonov, *Ot chego byvaiut letnie ponosy i kak uberech' ot nikh rebenka*, 4–5.

38. "Vystavka po okhrane materinstva vo dvortse truda," 51; M. Sh., *Rodil'nitsa i ee rebenok*, 15–16, 20. For more on the *soska* see David L. Ransel, *Mothers of Misery: Child Abandonment in Russia*, 270–71; idem, *Village Mothers*, 30–32.

39. Ransel, *Mothers of Misery,* 269–271.

40. V. V. Spaskii, "Why Do So Many Infants Die in Russia? The Outcome of Early Feeding with Kasha or the *Soska*" (pub. 50,000), Russian State Library collection.

41. Sigal, *Kak vyrastit' zdorovogo rebenka,* 15.

42. Antonov, *Sanitarno-prosvetitel'nyi patronazh,* 4.

43. V. V. Spaskii, "What Saves Russia from Massive Infant Deaths?" The Fact that Ninety-two Mothers Out of a Hundred Breast-Feed" (pub. 50,000), Russian State Library collection.

44. A. N. Antonov, *Kak uberech' rebenka ot Angliiskoi bolezni.*

45. For the language of, and investigations into, women's reproduction, see Hoffmann, *Stalinist Values,* 110–11.

46. For the expert testimony in the B. S. Ginzburg agitational trial, see *Sud nad vrachom meduchastka,* 49.

47. I. S. Katsenel'son, *Sovety materiam,* 17; see also Langova, *Vystavka "OMM,"* 17.

48. *ZNB* 15 (August 1927).

49. B. S. Sigal, *Sud nad mater'iu, vinovnoi v plokhom ukhode za det'mi, povlekshem za soboi smert' rebenka,* 9.

50. R. K., "Prichiny krika rebenka," in *Mat' i ditia: Sbornik dlia materi,* ed. Moskovskii podotdel OMM, 32–34.

51. I. Geizer, "Ugolok materi i rebenka," *ZNB* 14–15 (July 1926): 5.

52. Haines, *Health Work in Soviet Russia,* 170.

53. Sigal, *Sud nad mater'iu, vinovnoi v plokhom ukhode,* 8.

54. Ibid.

55. T. Verezhnikov, "Ozdorovlenie byta," *ZNB* 17–18 (December 1925): 17–18; see also Waters, "Child-Care Posters," 90.

56. This is similar to Western treatment; see Ludmilla Jordanova, *Sexual Visions: Images of Gender in Science and Medicine between the Eighteenth and Twentieth Centuries,* 31.

57. Haines, *Health Work in Soviet Russia,* 61.

58. Wood, *The Baba and the Comrade,* 23.

59. Melenevskaia, *Okhrana materinstva i mladenchestva,* 8.

60. O. P. Nogina, *Organizatsiia i rabota iaslei: Rukovodstvo dlia zaveduiushchikh iasliami i meditsinskogo personala iaslei i iaslei-sadov,* 8; Goldman addresses the many problems in *Women, State and Revolution,* 59–100.

61. MOZ, *Kratkii obzor sostoianiia zdravookhraneniia v Moskve,* 23; Nogina, *Tridtsat' let okhrany materi,* 24; idem, "V bor'be za novyi byt," *ZNB* 2 (April 1925): 11; Ransel, *Village Mothers,* 51.

62. Kagan, *Put' k obshchestvennoi rabote,* 30.

63. For a rundown of youth-oriented institutions, see Strashun, "Desiat' let bor'by," in *Desiat' let oktiabria i sovetskaia meditsina,* ed. Semashko, 68. In 1926 the breakdown was as follows: ambulatories (75), inspection cabinets (14), doctors for the health of children and youth (1,162, of which 74 were doctor-instructors), institutions for physically weak children (71), sanatoriums (90); see also 29, 69. In Soviet Central Asia during the Stalin era, the doctor cut a similarly heroic figure; see Michaels, *Curative Powers,* 59–64.

64. Chlen Soveta, "Konkurs na luchshuiu mat' i rebenka na Khamovnikakh," *ZNB* 11–12 (June 1927): 12.

65. S. D., "Konkurs na luchshego rebenka v Moskve," in *Mat' i ditia,* ed. Moskovskii podotdel OMM, 37. Soviet doctors pointed out that such contests had started in the United States and Britain; see Waters, "Teaching Mothercraft," 36. Contests also figured in other areas of production, such as the printing industry; see Koenker, *Republic of Labor,* 128.

66. Chlen soveta, "Konkurs na luchshuiu mat' i rebenka," 12.

67. Only one depiction of a doctor bordered on the negative. In Ginzburg's *Sud nad vrachom meduchastka* the doctor was charged, but as the trial played out, each woman was personally blamed for her infant's death and for following the midwife instead of the doctor. The court acknowledged that the doctor was hampered by uncooperative local officials and poor material conditions. Brooks describes a different yet still connected state figure—the party—as a surrogate father figure; see *Thank You, Comrade Stalin!,* 25.

68. R. D., *Sud nad domashnei khoziaikoi;* see also L. A. Vasilevskaia and L. M. Vasilevskii, *Sud nad akusherkoi Lopukhinoi, sovershivshei operatsiiu aborta, sledstviem chego iavilas' smert' zhenshchiny, i instsenirovannyi pokazatel'nyi sud.*

69. N. K. Mitropol'skii, *Doloi babok! Doloi oshibki i sueveriia pri rozhdenii i vospitanii detei;* see also Ransel, *Village Mothers,* 48–52.

70. Mitropol'skii, *Doloi babok!,* 7–8, 16. For additional anti-midwife propaganda see, G. I. Lebedeva, ed., *Znakharsha: Skaz.* Anti-practitioner propaganda also targeted males who followed traditional practice, although they were usually not associated with natal medicine or the city; see A. A. Khrustalev, *Znakhar' i doktor;* Leonid Subbotin, *Znakhar'-obmanshchik i babkina loshad': Komediia v 3 deistviiakh;* Ginzburg, "Problema," in his *Okhrana materinstva i mladenchestva,* 21; and figure 5.6.

71. The poster "Because of the Help of Midwives" contrasted a dirty, scrawny, hunched-over, elderly midwife in a cluttered interior with a white-suited, upright, healthy nurse in a hospital of spartan metal beds; see "Ot pomoshchi babok," box 261, folder entitled "Child Birth," in Alan Mason Chesney Medical Archives, National Library of Medicine, Bethesda, Md. See also the midwife in figure 5.6; Ginzburg, "Problema," in his *Okhrana materinstva i mladenchestva,* 8, 23; the posters in "Vystavka po okhrana materinstva vo dvortse truda," 51; and Bernstein, *The Dictatorship of Sex,* 125–27.

72. Interestingly, while Lopukhina was described as an *akushera* (obstetrician), this title was discredited at the trial and she was treated as a midwife. Lopukhina's name alluded to its literal meaning (*lopukh*), a type of prickly-leaved herb and also the name of Peter the Great's tradition-bound first wife, Evdokia Lopukhina. Vasilevskaia and Vasilevskii, *Sud nad akusherkoi Lopukhinoi,* 6.

73. B. Sigal, *Sud nad mater'iu, vinovnoi v rasprostranenii skarlatiny,* 12, 43. See Irina Petrovna's behavior in Ginzburg's *Sud nad materiu, podkinuvshei svoego rebenka,* 34.

74. Vasilevskaia and Vasilevskii, *Sud nad akusherkoi,* 6; Waters, "Child-Care Posters," 65. For holy water, spirits, and prayers see Sigal, *Sud nad mater'iu, vinovnoi v rasprostranenii skarlatiny,* 18–19; for herbs, see 7. For a picture of the log, see Mitropol'skii, *Doloi babok!,* 21.

75. Sigal, *Sud nad mater'iu, vinovnoi v rasprostranenii skarlatiny;* see also Mitropolskii, *Doloi babok!,* 22–27.

76. "Buranova," or "new Borax." See E. B. Demidovich, *Stat'ia 155 ugolovnogo kodeksa RSFSR: Sud nad gr. Kiselevym po obvineniiu v zarazhenii tripperom.*

77. Ibid. See also Ginzburg, *Sud nad materiu.*

78. "Nikogda ne davai rebenku zhevki" and "Ne khodi k babkam," box 261, folder entitled "Public Health Posters Maternal / Child Health Series #12," in Alan Mason Chesney Medical Archives, National Library of Medicine, Bethesda, Md.

79. Mitropolskii, *Doloi babok!*, 9.

80. Traditional remedies were often symbolic—a rod to beat away disease or a knife to cut the pain out of giving birth—but the midwife might also use mercury for syphilis or ergot for abortions: see Gantt, *Russian Medicine*, 18; Vasilevskaia and Vasilevskii, *Sud nad akusherkoi*, 9; Mitropol'skii, *Doloi babok!*, 10. In the West medical professionals similarly attacked midwives; see Judith Walzer Leavitt, *Brought to Bed: Childbearing in America, 1750–1950*.

81. Ransel reports the experiences of nurses attached to mobile dispensaries in the countryside and the suspicion and mistrust they encountered from the population; see *Village Mothers*, 52–56.

82. N. Semashko, "Predisloviia," in *Sputnik po okhrane materinstva i mladenchestva*, 3.

83. Bravaia, *OMM na zapade i v SSSR*, 210.

84. Ibid., 100. American nurse inspectors appeared in 1908 in New York City to inspect families for their children's health. The program expanded rapidly. See Duffy, *The Sanitarians*, 208.

85. Rakhmanov, "Konsultatsii dlia zhenshchin," in *Trudov III v sesoiuznogo soveshchaniia po okhmatmladu*; quoted in Bravaia, *OMM na zapade i v SSSR*, 213.

86. A. N. Khanevskii, "Desiat' let iasel'noi raboty v g. Moskve," in *Okhrana materinstva i mladenchestva: Sbornik statei*, ed. O. P. Nogina and S. O. Dulitskii, 73 (hereafter *OMM: Sbornik statei*).

87. Bravaia, *OMM na zapade i v SSSR*, 220; Bogolepova, "Sanitarnoe prosveshchenie i samodeiatel'nost naseleniia," in *Okhrana narodnogo zdorov'ia v SSSR*, ed. Kovrigin, 585; Gorsuch, *Youth in Revolutionary Russia*, 102.

88. Kabo, *Ocherki rabochego byta*, 50.

89. I. L. Fel'dman, "Srednii personal v uchrezhdeniiakh Moskovskogo p/otdela OMM," in *OMM: Sbornik statei*, ed. Nogina and Dulitskii, 156. For other complaints involving incompetence and inaction, see E. Konius, "Sanitarno-prosvetitel'naia rabota sestry i akursherki," *Okhrana materinstva i mladenchestva* 2 (1927): 26–31.

90. Antonov, *Sanitarno-prosvetitel'nyi patronazh*, 22; S. O. Dulitskii, "Konsul'tatsii dlia grudnykh detei za 1918–1928 gg.," in *OMM: Sbornik statei*, ed. Nogina and Dulitskii, 16.

91. S.D-i, "Konsul'tatsiia dlia grudnykh detei, no. 27," *ZNB* 7 (June 1925): 2.

92. Khanevskii, "Desiat' let iasel'noi raboty v g. Moskve," in *OMM: Sbornik statei*, ed. Nogina and Dulitskii, 72–73. See also O. Nogina, "K trekhdnevniku okhrany materinstva i mladenchestva," *ZNB* 4–5 (March 1927): 1; A. I. Lagutiaeva, "Novyi byt i sestra-vospitatel'nitsa," *Okhrana materinstva i mladenchestva* 1 (1926): 38–41.

93. Shiffer, "Sestra konsul'tatsii," *ZNB* 4–5 (March 1927): 10. For more on the qualifications of nurses, see Lagutiaeva, "Novyi byt i sestra-vospitatl'nitsa," 38–41.

94. A decline from 50 to 19 percent for feeding, from 72 to 37 percent for diapering, from 59 to 42 percent for bathing, from 42 to 17 percent for sense organs, and from 63 to 59 percent for the *soska*. Women held on to the *soska* determinedly; see Antonov, *Sanitarno-prosvetitel'nyi patronazh*, 41.

95. Ibid., 7, 22.

96. P. Dorokhov, *Vspleski: Rasskazy "Novaia Moskva,"* 16. For a list of these added burdens in the American context, see Tomes, *The Gospel of Germs.*

97. L. Vasias, "Sestra sotsial'noi pomoshchi-organizator novogo byta," *ZNB* 9 (May 1927): 5.

98. E. A. Vasich, "Doma materi i rebenka," in *OMM v Moskve,* ed. Moskovskii komitet nedeli OMM, 30.

99. L. Kubasov, "O dome otdykha dlia materei s det'mi," *ZNB* 1–2 (January 1927): 6.

100. Ibid.

101. Geizer, "Ugolok materi i rebenka," 5; see also AMO f. 2129, op. 1, d. 185, l. 2.

102. M. Amshinskii, "V sanatorii im. Karla Libknekhta," *ZNB* 1–2 (January 1927): 13.

103. T. Dobrova, "O rabote nochnogo sanatoriia pri lechebno-proteznom institute," *Ezhenedel'nik MOZa* 4 (28 January 1926): 62.

104. V. Diushen wrote of the opposition between traditional motherhood/family and socialism; see Goldman, *Women, State, and Revolution,* 9–11; Naiman, *Sex in Public,* 190. See also Bernstein, *The Dictatorship of Sex,* 41–72, 135–82.

105. Melenevskaia, *Okhrana materinstva i mladenchestva,* 5.

106. Dorokhov, *Vspleski,* 22.

107. Nogina, "K trekhdnevniku," 1. By 1926 authorities claimed that 80 percent of Moscow infants were under medical supervision; see V. P. Lebedeva and G. N. Speranskii, eds., *Kniga materi (Kak vyrastit' zdorovogo i krepkogo rebenka i sokhranit' svoe zdorov'e),* 11; cited in Waters, "Teaching Mothercraft," 50.

108. Wood, *The Baba and the Comrade,* 161. Semashko, *O svetlom i temnom,* admits the numbers were "still very low" in 1928 (25); see also Nogina, *Organizatsiia i rabota iaslei,* 8.

109. MOZ, *Materialy o deiatel'nosti lechebno-profilakticheskikh uchrezhdenii MOZa,* 6. For figures on the RSFSR and USSR for the 1920s, see Bravaia, *OMM na zapade i v SSSR,* 208. Moscow ante-natal clinics served 63,155 children and mothers in 1920; by 1927 that figure had increased almost tenfold; see S. O. Dulitskii, "Konsul'tatsii dlia grudnykh detei za 1918–1928," in *OMM: Sbornik statei,* ed. Nogina and Dulitskii, 26.

110. *Tsentral'noe statisticheskoe upravlenie, Narodnoe khoziaistvo soiuza SSR v tsifrakh,* 41.

111. MOZ, *Materialy o deiatel'nosti,* 6; Bravaia, *OMM na zapade i v SSSR,* 208.

112. MOZ, *Materialy o deiatel'nosti,* 6–7; Waters, "Teaching Mothercraft," 30. Women of Central Asia were targeted during the Stalin period, and here, too, the state claimed significant inroads; see Michaels, *Curative Powers,* 129–52.

113. M. Ikan, "Itogi i perspektivy," *ZNB* 15 (August 1927): 2; see also O. Nogina, "Desiat' let okhrany materinstva i mladenchestva," *ZNB* 19–20 (October 1927): 24.

114. P. G., "V konsul'tatsii No. 2," *ZNB* 7–8 (April 1927): 8.

115. Waters, "Teaching Mothercraft," 49–50.

116. Again, these statistics are suspect. Standards for measuring infant deaths and live births have been in flux in Russia as long as statistics have been gathered. In the desperate battle for limited resources in the 1920s, organizers faced a conundrum. To overstate their success might result in a drop in their allocations, with authorities deeming the problem solved. Conversely, understating their success would open the program to

charges of ineffectiveness. The numbers give a rough indication of perceived change; see Nogina, "K trekhdnevniku," 1.

117. This set the stage for the more invasive policies of the 1930s, which further subjugated the family to the state. Although Stalinist family policy has often been depicted as a retreat, Hoffmann argues that the changes of the 1930s were part of the encroachment of state authority characteristic of modern states worldwide; see *Stalinist Values,* 88–117.

118. Nogina, "Desiat' let okhrany materinstva i mladenchestva v Moskve," 7.

119. Hyde, *The Soviet Health Service,* 54.

120. V. P. Lebedeva, "Okhrana materinstva i mladenchestva na puti k kommunizmu," in *OMM v Moskve,* ed. Moskovskii komitet nedeli OMM, 4–5.

Chapter 6. The Body: Hygiene, Modernity, and Mentality

1. Clark, "The 'New Man's' Body," in *Art of the Soviets,* ed. Brown and Taylor, 36. Stites evokes the machine dream in *Revolutionary Dreams,* 149–55. For Europe, see Orvar Lofgren, "Rational and Sensitive: Changing Attitudes to Time, Nature, and the Home," in *Culture Builders: A Historical Anthropology of Middle-Class Life,* ed. Jonas Frykman and Orvar Lofgren, 20, 31.

2. In the late 1920s Gastev referred to Ford as a prophet alongside Marx; see Hanson, *Time and Revolution,* 124.

3. Johansson, *Aleksej Gastev,* 7, 10, 103. For NOT cell numbers, see Clark, "The 'New Man's' Body," in *Art of the Soviets,* ed. Brown and Taylor, 37. As a sign of his popularity, Gastev's *Poetry of the Worker's Blow* was Proletkul't's first publication; see Naiman, *Sex in Public,* 65.

4. Slava Gerovitch, "Love-Hate for Man-Machine Metaphors in Soviet Physiology: From Pavlov to Physiological Cybernetics," 544. By the late 1920s the automaton aroused no controversy; see Clark, "The 'New Man's' Body," in *Art of the Soviets,* ed. Brown and Taylor, 23; Johansson, *Aleksej Gastev,* 7, 103; and Rolf Hellebust, "Aleksei Gastev and the Metallization of the Revolutionary Body," 507–8, and his *Flesh to Metal: Soviet Literature and the Alchemy of Revolution;* see also Hanson, *Time and Revolution,* 125.

5. A. Gastev, *Kak nado rabotat': Prakticheskoe vvedenie v nauku organizatsii truda,* 5.

6. Clark, "The 'New Man's' Body," in *Art of the Soviets,* ed. Brown and Taylor, 37; Gerovitch, "Love-Hate for Man-Machine Metaphors," 344.

7. Gastev, *Kak nado rabotat',* 5.

8. Stites, *Revolutionary Dreams,* 48; Sigal, *Trud i zdorov'e,* 1. For a contemporary technical physiology textbook that adapted machine metaphors, see P. G. Arkhipov, D. N. Lukashevich, and I. V. Sazhin, eds., *Sputnik lektora: Konspekty lektzii po anatomii i fiziologii cheloveka.* See also G. Bosse, *Chelovek—zavod;* Muramevich, *Kak zhivet i rabotaet chelovecheskoe telo* (both recommended by "E.S." in the files of VTsSPS GARF f. 5451, op. 9, d. 496, l. 140).

9. GARF, f. A-7954, op. 1, d. 72, l. 119. For similar comments, see Gel'man, *Trud,* 8.

10. A. Gastev, *Iunost', idi!,* 17. Kelly explores multiple schedules for youth in "Shaping the 'Future Race,'" in *Everyday Life in Early Soviet Russia,* ed. Kiaer and Naiman, 258–61.

11. Gastev's schedule called for less sleep than the oft-quoted 8-8-8 formula; see Gastev, *Iunost', idi!,* 17.

12. Kasson, *Rudeness and Civility,* 195.

13. Monastic conventions and church prohibitions had long stressed simplicity of diet. As Enlightenment impulses entered the country, simplicity was stressed even more. In her instructions to her grandchildren Catherine the Great advocated a simple, plain diet, with snacks between meals to consist only of bread; see Madriaga, *Catherine the Great,* 108; Chernyshevskii, *What Is to Be Done?,* 273, 279, 281.

14. Harmke Kamminga and Andrew Cunningham, "Introduction: The Science and Culture of Nutrition, 1840–1940," in *The Science and Culture of Nutrition, 1840–1940,* ed. Harmke Kamminga and Andrew Cunningham, 8, 10; see also Teller, *The Tuberculosis Movement,* 102–3.

15. Eliav-Feldon refers to Andrew Boorde and Luigi Cornaro, also noting that many utopias followed this theme; see *Realistic Utopias,* 42. For the nineteenth century, see the chapter "The Government of the Body: Medical Regimens and the Rationalization of Diet," in Turner, *Regulating Bodies,* 177–95; Weindling, *Health, Race, and German Politics,* 155; and Harvey A. Levinston, *Revolution at the Table: The Transformation of the American Diet,* 87–92.

16. Naiman, *Sex in Public,* 208. He also teases out the meaning of food in other works; see *Sex in Public,* 208–49.

17. The E.S. article "Obshche-obrazovatel'nye kruzhki v rabochikh klubakh" contained in the files of VTsSPS recommended a set of lectures for the worker club on nutrition that acquainted workers with the "preliminary processing of fuel (food) before being received into the blood and compared the apparatus of the machine with the apparatus of the human." GARF f. 5451, op. 9, d. 496, l. 12. See the dietary poster "Chelovek—zhivaia mashina" (Moscow: Narkomzdrav, 1927; pub. 5,000), Russian State Library collection. On chewing, see Vasilevskii, *Gigiena pionera,* 28. See also Kal'manson and Bekariukov, *Beregi svoe zdorov'e!,* 15. Thorough chewing, or Fletcherizing, gained prominence in the United States at the turn of the century; see Levinston, *Revolution at the Table,* 87–92. On pregnancy and food, see A. Antonov, *Pamiatka materi,* 5.

18. Semashko, *Nauka o zdorov'e obshchestva,* 13.

19. Zheleznyi, *Kak zhit', chtoby zdorovym byt'?,* 22.

20. Burnham, *How Superstition Won and Science Lost,* 60.

21. Semashko, *Nauka o zdorov'e obshchestva,* 14.

22. A. N. Ginodman and E. I. Iurovskaia, "K piatiletiiu raboty dietstolovykh v Moskve," in *Piat' let raboty dietstolovykh,* ed. MOZ, 1–2. Although modest, the number of such cafeterias rose steadily: 1924 (10); 1924–25 (24); 1925–26 (26); 1926–27 (27); 1927–28 (27); 1928–29 (27); B. E. Dobrusina, "Vozniknovenie i etapy razvitiia dietolecheniia v Moskve," in *Piat' let raboty dietstolovykh,* ed. MOZ, 4 (pub. 3,000).

23. "Rabota dietostolovoi profilaktoriia imeni Shumskoi (Dolozheno na konferentsii v institute im. V. A. Obukha)," *Ezhenedel'nik MOZa* 3, no. 156 (1926): 40–41.

24. Chernyshevskii, *What Is to Be Done?,* 371; Bellamy, *Looking Backward.*

25. See Mauricio Borrero, "Communal Dining and State Cafeterias in Moscow and Petrograd, 1917–1921," in *Food in Russian History and Culture,* ed. Musya Glants and Joyce Toomre, 162–76; see also Smith, *Woman in Soviet Russia,* 189–95.

26. In 1921 twenty-four doctors and forty-two assistants engaged in this type of work; see Kats, *Mediko-sanitarnaia organizatsiia Moskvy,* 8. For other problems, see Borrero, *Hungry Moscow,* 168–69, 173; Smith, *Woman in Soviet Russia,* 189–95.

27. Koenker, *Moscow Workers,* 56.

28. Naiman, *Sex in Public,* 210–15.

29. Zaitsev, *Trud i byt rabochikh podrostkov,* 30.

30. For the popular use of military metaphors, see Brooks, *Thank You, Comrade Stalin!,* 22–25; Frank Ellis, "The Media as Social Engineer: The Creation of Homo Sovieticus, 1921–1953: Theoretical Background," in *Russian Cultural Studies,* ed. Kelly and Shepherd, 199.

31. Zheleznyi, *Kak zhit', chtoby zdorovym byt'?,* 3.

32. Il'ianskii and Lapin, "Beregi zdorov'e—i nikakikh gvozdei!," *ZNB* 4–5 (1925): 10.

33. N. Semashko, *Sotsial'nye bolezni,* 16 (pub. 3,000). For similar reference to the body as fortress, see Semashko, *Sotsial'nye bolezni i bor'ba s nimi,* 12 (pub. 15,000).

34. On Europe, see Rosen, *A History of Public Health,* 77. On Russian monasticism and bodily management, see the life of St. Sergius in *Medieval Russia's Epics, Chronicles, and Tales,* ed. Serge A. Zenkovsky, 262–90. In the late nineteenth and early twentieth centuries Germany's "life reform movement" recommended a disciplined body to achieve health in the face of increasing societal fears of man's estrangement from the natural; see Hau, *The Cult of Health and Beauty in Germany,* 1–3; Porter, *Health, Civilization, and the State,* 55.

35. Stites explores the cult of time management; see *Revolutionary Dreams,* 155–59.

36. Zheleznyi, *Kak zhit', chtoby zdorovym byt'?,* 5–6.

37. Sukharev, *Rabochii, beregi svoe zdorov'e,* 17–22.

38. M. Dubianskaia, "Lichnaia gigiena: Nochnoi otdykh," *Gigiena i zdorov'e rabochei sem'i* 9 (May 1926): 11.

39. Kal'manson and Bekariukov, *Beregi svoe zdorov'e!,* 28.

40. Zheleznyi, *Kak zhit', chtoby zdorovym byt'?,* 6–7; see also Vasilevskii, *Gigiena pionera,* 24.

41. Here Zheleznyi strayed slightly from the schedule for adults, recommending nine hours of sleep for Pioneers; *Kak zhit', chtoby zdorovym byt'?,* 6–7.

42. Kelly, "Shaping the 'Future Race,'" in *Everyday Life in Early Soviet Russia,* ed. Kiaer and Naiman, 261–64.

43. Iu. N. Vonzblein, *Put' k zdorov'iu,* 9 (pub. 10,000); see also Vasilevskii, *Gigiena Pionera,* 24; Kal'manson and Bekariukov, *Beregi svoe zdorov'e!,* 7; Vasilevskii, *Gigiena propagandista.*

44. Mary Lynn Stewart, *For Health and Beauty: Physical Culture for Frenchwomen, 1880s–1930s,* 65.

45. Sukharev, *Rabochii, beregi svoe zdorov'e,* 9.

46. This was a prerevolutionary concept; see Kelly, "The Education of the Will," in *Russian Masculinities in History and Culture,* ed. Clements, Friedman, and Healey, 131–51.

47. On lice, see, Sukharev, *Rabochii, beregi svoe zdorov'e,* 10; see also Sakhnovskaia, *Chesotka i bor'ba s neiu.*

48. Kal'manson and Bekariukov, *Beregi svoe zdorov'e!,* 7.

49. Ibid. The humorous *Ne myt'em tak katan'em: Komediia v trekh aktakh piati kartinakh* (Moscow: Glabpolitprosvet TsK VLKSM, 1926) recounted how to wash.

50. During one campaign half of Moscow's population supposedly participated; see Semashko, *Okhrana zdorov'ia rabochikh i rabotnits krest'ian i krest'ianok,* 19; N. Dzhumaliev, *V. I. Lenin i okhrana zdorov'ia trudiashchikhsia,* 57.

51. Sukharev, *Rabochii, beregi svoe zdorov'e,* 10.

52. A. Mol'kov, ed., *Sanitarnoe prosveshchenie: V shkole i cherez shkolu,* 33–34.

53. Ibid. See also Kal'manson and Bekariukov, *Beregi svoe zdorov'e!*, 20–21.

54. Kal'manson and Bekariukov, *Beregi svoe zdorov'e!*, 11.

55. See Mol'kov, *Sanitarnoe prosveshchenie*, 32; Kal'manson and Bekariukov, *Beregi svoe zdorov'e!*, 9–10; Sukharev, *Rabochii, beregi svoe zdorov'e*, 9; and "Moskovskii profaktiv o rabote MOZa," *ZNB* 11–12 (June 1927): 4.

56. M. D., "Posle piati," *ZNB* 7–8 (April 1927): 18; Kal'manson and Bekariukov, *Beregi svoe zdorov'e!*, 10. Sukharev carried similar instructions on motions and directions for brushing; see *Rabochii, beregi svoe zdorov'e*, 9. A 1921 six-poster series by Gosizdat emphasized "Deti! Beregite zuby!" (pub. 50,000), Russian State Library collection.

57. Mol'kov, *Sanitarnoe prosveshchenie*, 32.

58. For a discussion of pregnant women's teeth, see Antonov, *Pamiatka materi*, 5.

59. "Moskovskii profaktiv o rabote MOZa," *ZNB* 11–12 (June 1927): 4.

60. L. M. Vasilevskii, *Gigiena zhenskogo truda* (pub. 10,000). Bernstein argues for the normative power of men's bodies; see *The Dictatorship of Sex*, 108.

61. Iu. Lur'e, *Gigiena devochki, devushki, zhenshchiny*, 7, 11. Bernstein found similar descriptions of menstruation; see *The Dictatorship of Sex*, 166.

62. V. E. Dembskaia, *Polovaia gigiena zhenshchiny*, 12 (pub. 10,000).

63. For these ideas in the United States, see Roberta J. Park, "Physiology and Anatomy Are Destiny!? Brains, Bodies and Exercise in Nineteenth Century American Thought," 31–63.

64. Lur'e, *Gigiena devochki, devushki, zhenshchiny*, 11.

65. Vasilevksii, *Gigiena molodoi devushki*, 16.

66. Discomfort with the menstruating body coincided with Russian religious restrictions against menstruating women, who were treated as unclean and capable of destroying the purity of the church. See Eve Levin, *Sex and Society in the World of the Orthodox Slavs, 900–1700*, 169–72. On sexual pollution, see Douglas, *Purity and Danger*, 141–59.

67. Dembskaia, *Polovaia gigiena zhenshchiny*, 13.

68. Antonov, *Pamiatka materi*, 5.

69. V. E. Dembskaia, *Individual'naia gigiena zhenshchiny: Ukhod za zdorov'em i krasotoi*, 23–30. Sander L. Gilman links beauty with health; see *Picturing Health and Illness: Images of Identity and Difference*, 51–66.

70. Vera Ketlinskaia, *Devushka i komsomol*, 62 (pub. 3,000).

71. Ilya Lin, "V chem krasota," *Rabotnitsa* 26 (1927): 15–16; cited in Attwood, *Creating the New Soviet Woman*, 68.

72. Attwood, *Creating the New Soviet Woman*, 71. French health manuals made a similar case; see Stewart, *For Health and Beauty*, 60.

73. *Gigiena i zdorov'e rabochego i ego sem'i*, 21.

74. Semashko, *Nauka o zdorov'e obshchestva*, 19.

75. Zheleznyi, *Kak zhit', chtoby zdorovym byt'?*, 19.

76. Kal'manson and Bekariukov, *Beregi svoe zdorov'e!*, 7; Vasilevskii, *Gigiena pionera*, 25; Zheleznyi, *Kak zhit', chtoby zdorovym byt'?*, 19–20.

77. Semashko, *Iskusstvo odevat'sia*, 19–20.

78. Vasilevskii, *Gigiena pionera*, 26. This connection between personality and clothing informed conversation among costumers. See Nicoletta Misler, "The Science of Dressing

from the Industrial Workshop: The Russian Academy of Artistic Science and Costume—A Summary," in *Revolutionary Costume: Soviet Clothing and Textiles of the 1920s*, ed. Lidya Zaletova et al., 47.

79. Semashko, *Iskusstvo odevat'sia*, 21.

80. Vasilevskii, *Gigiena pionera*, 19; "How Are We Going to Dress? A Discussion: Expressing Your Opinion at the Right Time," *Komsomol'skaia Pravda*, 30 June 1928; reprinted in *Revolutionary Costume*, ed. Zaletova et al., 180; Gorsuch, *Youth in Revolutinary Russia*, 125–37.

81. Zheleznyi, *Kak zhit', chtoby zdorovym byt'?*, 22.

82. For the health dangers inherent in fashionable clothes (high heels and skirts), see Vasilevskii, *Gigiena molodoi devushki*, 25–30; S. D. Astrinskii, *Devushka—budushchaia mat'*, 5 (pub. 10,000). Béraud describes contemporary fashions in *The Truth about Moscow*, 20–22. Short skirts and no corsets were universally recommended.

83. Gorsuch, *Youth in Revolutinary Russia*, 19. Jewelry was incompatible with party life; see A. A. Sol'ts, *O partetike*, 14 (pub. 6,000).

84. Vasilevskii, *Gigiena molodoi devushki*, 34.

85. Chernyshevskii, *What Is to Be Done?*, 281, 358, 376.

86. Vasilevskii, *Gigiena propagandista*, 21; Lebina, *Rabochaia molodezh' Leningrada*, 145–46. French reformers linked syphilis, alcoholism, and tuberculosis. See Barnes, *The Making of a Social Disease*, 138; Vonzblein, *Put' k zdorov'iu*, 7; Sigal, *Vrednaia privychka (Kuren'e tabaka)*, 5–10 (pub. 20,000).

87. I. V. Sazhin, *Pravda o kurenii*, 12–16 (pub. 10,000).

88. Barushkin, *Pochemu vreden tabak?*, 7.

89. A small, direct poster argued similarly "Ni dlia kogo ne mozhet byt' voprosa—Zdorov'iu vred prinosit papirosa!" (Sov. Kavkaz, n.d.), Russian State Library collection. Another series of six posters entitled "Quitting smoking" (n.d.; Russian State Library collection) showed how people learned to smoke (on the street corner), the poison nicotine (death holding a bottle), tobacco killing a frog and a horse, a rendering of non-smoker's lungs (flowers) versus a smoker's lungs (pipes), and the dangers of smoking after twenty years (strained nerves, coughing, sickness). The series ended with a call to remember the workers endangered by tobacco production.

90. Sigal, *Vrednaia privychka*, 16; Sazhin, *Pravda o kurenii*, 19; see also "V obedennyi pereryv," *ZNB* 22 (1926): 7.

91. B. S. Sigal, *I. Sud nad pionerom kurivshim i II. Sud nad neriashlivym pionerom: Dve instsenirovki*, 7–10, 45; idem, *Vrednaia privychka*, 14.

92. Sazhin, *Pravda o kurenii*, 19, 22. He reported of a woman who had given birth to seven healthy children but then went to work in a cigarette factory and had seven miscarriages. Another woman had six miscarriages while at the factory but gave birth to two healthy children after leaving.

93. Proctor, *The Nazi War on Cancer*, 173–83. For more on smoking in Russia, see Andrei Valer'evich Shapovalov, *Ocherki istorii i kul'tury potrebleniia tabaka v Sibiri: XVII—pervaia polovina XX vv.*; Igor Bogdanov, *Dym otechestva, ili kratkaia istoriia tabakokureniia*; and Tricia Starks, "Red Star/Black Lungs: Anti-Tobacco Campaigns in Twentieth-Century Russia."

94. The first studies linking lung cancer and smoking emerged in the late 1920s. The rise was attributed at the time to a number of other issues, including the influenza

pandemic, malnutrition, fallout from chemical weapons, as well as problems unique to urban life, such as automobiles and dust; see Proctor, *The Nazi War on Cancer,* 187–89.

95. Sazhin, *Pravda o kurenii,* 18; Sigal, *Vrednaia privychka,* 12.

96. Gromakova, "Pora pereiti ot slova k delu," *ZNB* 10–11 (1926): 23.

97. Kal'manson and Bekariukov, *Beregi svoe zdorov'e!,* 18.

98. N. Bukharin, "Molodezh' dolzhna stroit' svoi byt po-novomu!," in *Azbuka komsomol'tsa,* ed. Slepkov, 78.

99. Sazhin, *Pravda o kurenii,* 25–27.

100. Semashko, *Puti sovetskoi fizkul'tury,* 31; see also N. A. Semashko, *Nezabyvaemyi obraz,* 15. Sigal also referred to this anecdote in *Vrednaia privychka,* 16.

101. In a Mospoligraph factory workers began an antismoking circle in 1925 in cooperation with the *narkodispanser* (narcotics dispensary), with twenty-five workers giving up smoking for six months. See "Polgoda ne kuriat," *ZNB* 14–15 (1926): 24.

102. In the letter "A Bad Example" the writer complained of the health cell room at Presnenskii soviet, which was always filled with smoke and crowded, which made it a difficult place to breathe. The writer stated that members needed to stick to their own rules; see Paz, "Durnoi primer," *ZNB* 22 (1926): 12.

103. While conceding that smoking was dangerous, Vasilevskii insisted that drinking was even more detrimental to a young woman's health; see *Gigiena molodoi devushki,* 30. For early Russian temperance activities, see Patricia Herlihy, *The Alcoholic Empire: Vodka and Politics in Late Imperial Russia,* 3–35; see also Stephen White, *Russia Goes Dry: Alcohol, State and Society,* 17–19. For Canada, see McCuaig, *The Weariness, the Fever, and the Fret,* 11. For Germany, see Proctor, *The Nazi War on Cancer,* 142.

104. Semashko, *Okhrana zdorov'ia rabochikh,* 44.

105. Semashko, *Sotsial'nye bolezni,* 13.

106. Solomon, "Social Hygiene and Soviet Public Health," in *Health and Society in Revolutionary Russia,* ed. Solomon and Hutchinson, 188–89.

107. Alcoholics were consistently depicted as helpless, weak, and lethal to families. See L. N. Bitte, "Bor'ba s gor'koi," *ZNB* 17–18 (1925): 5–6; see also the agitational trial by Vasilevskaia and Vasilevskii, *Sud nad samogonshchikami,* 27. Dangers to the family were depicted in the 1923 poster "Iad samagona otravliaet zdorov'e trudiashikhsia" (pub. 10,000), Russian State Library collection.

108. L. N. Bitte, "Bor'ba s gor'koi," 5–6. For alcohol's connection to criminality, see *Prestupnyi mir Moskvy: Sbornik statei,* ed. M. N. Gernet.

109. Kagan, *Put' k obshchestvennoi rabote,* 28.

110. B. S. Sigal, *Alkogolizm i molodezh',* 21–23 (pub., 10,000).

111. TsMAM f. 1474, op. 3, d. 2, l. 11; Vasilevskii, *Gigiena pionera,* 29. For KOTiB activities, see Kovgonkin, "Obshchestvennaia bor'ba s narkotizmom," *ZNB* 4–5 (March 1927): 15. See also Sol'ts, *O partetike,* 18–20.

112. "Vse na bor'bu s p'ianstvom" (n.d.; Russian State Library collection) featured a pile of bottles next to a pile of products. Other pictures contrasted the good family with the unhappy one.

113. Semashko, *Okhrana zdorov'ia rabochikh,* 44.

114. This included drinking on the job as well as blue Mondays; see Koenker, *Republic of Labor,* 189–91.

115. Sigal, *Trud i zdorov'e rabochei molodezhi,* 42. Transchel describes "blue Mondays" and other drink-related work problems; see *Under the Influence,* 26–27.

116. Johnson, *Peasant and Proletarain,* 82.

117. In the lower left the viewer was reminded of another victim of religious revelry, namely, the "innocent trees" that sacrificed their lives for these celebrations.

118. White, *Russia Goes Dry,* 23–24. For Komsomol anti-alcohol propaganda in the 1920s, see Gorsuch, *Youth in Revolutinary Russia,* 67–69.

119. The term "hooligan" covered a variety of crimes that disrupted society at various levels. The Soviets undertook campaigns to root out hooliganism in the 1920s. For the meanings of hooliganism for Russian culture in the prerevolutionary period and the 1920s, see Joan Neuberger, *Hooliganism: Crime, Culture, and Power in St. Petersburg, 1900–1914.* For an account of the mock trial, see Avlov, *Sud nad khuliganami.*

120. Kagan, *Put' k obshchestvennoi rabote,* 28.

121. Platonov was sentenced to three years of isolated confinement by the court; see B.S., "Sud nad sifilitikom," *Gigiena i zdorov'e rabochei sem'i* 7 (15 December 1923): 14.

122. For prostitution as a social hygiene problem, see L. M. Vasilevskii, *Prostitutsiia i rabochaia molodezh'* (pub. 10,000).

123. Akkerman, *Sud nad prostitutkoi i svodnitsei,* 38. For more on the character of the madam in literature and agitational trials, see Julie A. Cassiday and Leyla Rouhi, "From Nevskii Prospekt to Zoia's Apartment: Trials of the Russian Procuress," 413–31.

124. Sigal, *Venericheskie bolezni,* 3.

125. Naiman treats this subject at length; see *Sex in Public,* 15–17, 27–44. The scandalous collection *Pis'ma iz uteriannogo portfelia: O poshlosti v bytu,* edited by L. Lebedev and L. Rubinshtein, reprinted "found" letters that detailed crude, sexual exploits of young men who seemingly lacked all moral feeling.

126. Bernstein, *The Dictatorship of Sex,* 130–34; Banting, Kelly, and Riordan, "Sexuality," in *Russian Cultural Studies,* ed. Kelly and Shepherd, 314–16.

127. Attacks against homosexuality were taken up by the state in the late 1920s; see Banting, Kelly, and Riordan, "Sexuality," in *Russian Cultural Studies,* ed. Kelly and Shepherd, 319–20. For a more extensive discussion, see Healey, *Homosexual Desire in Revolutionary Russia.*

128. S. D. Astrinksii, *Beremennost' i venericheskie bolezni,* 30; Akkerman, *Sud nad prostitutkoi,* 191, 193.

129. Kelly, *Refining Russia,* 270; Naiman, *Sex in Public,* 120–21, 137–38; B. S. Sigal, *Polovoi vopros,* 32–39. Bernstein, *The Dictatorship of Sex,* 89–91.

130. V. Ketlinskaia and Vlad. Slepkov, *Zhizn' bez kontrolia (Polovaia zhizn' i sem'ia rabochei molodezhi)* (pub. 10,000). See also A. B. Zalkind, *Polovoi vopros v usloviiakh sovetskoi obshchestvennosti: Sbornik statei.* Jessica Smith details Professor Zalkind's attempt to "industrialize" sex; see *Woman in Russia,* 129. Zalkind came under fire from Semashko for too closely relating sexual advice to political comment. A psychiatrist by training, Zalkind attempted to show that menstruation was tied to the communist periodization of history rather than biology; see Bernstein, *The Dictatorship of Sex,* 28–30. For more on sexuality, see Gorsuch,

Youth in Revolutinary Russia, 14; Sigal, *Polovoi vopros,* 27; Vasilevskii, *Gigiena pionera,* 23–24, 27; Banting, Kelly, and Riordan, "Sexuality," in *Russian Cultural Studies,* ed. Kelly and Shepherd, 323–25. Foreign writers also focussed on sex in the young. For Swedish warnings against childhood masturbation, see Jonas Frykman, "Clean and Proper: Body and Soul through Peasant and Bourgeois Eyes," in *Culture Builders,* ed. Frykman and Lofgren, 240.

131. M. Kaplun, "Vstupaia v brak, osvedomliaites' o zdorov'e drug druga," *ZNB* 2 (1926): 9.

132. Demidovich, *Stat'ia 155.*

133. Sigal, *Venericheskie bolezni,* 25.

134. Bernstein, *The Dictatorship of Sex,* 96–99.

135. Sigal, *Polovoi vopros,* 47. Astrinskii warned that casual sex always ended in sexual disease; see *Devushka—budushchaia mat',* 18. Bernstein argues that in posters only prostitutes engaged in non-procreative sex and that positive, sexually active women were always presented with children; see *The Dictatorship of Sex,* 121.

136. Vasilevskii, *Gigiena molodoi devushki,* 11. Bernstein finds that women who gave birth were depicted as healthier of body and mind; see *The Dictatorship of Sex,* 171.

137. Stewart, *For Health and Beauty,* 106, 117.

138. Horn, *Social Bodies,* 10.

139. Z. O. Mitsnik and A. N. Antonov, *Mat' i rebenok,* 1. Naiman describes a similar trend in Soviet fiction to identify women solely with their biological function as mothers; see *Sex in Public,* 38.

140. Astrinskii, *Devushka—budushchaia mat',* 20. Women were further advised that first pregnancies often ended with a resumption of bleeding within two to three months, and if this occurred they should go to the doctor (21).

141. Antonov, *Pamiatka materi,* 3–4. For similar statements on abortion, see S. D. Astrinskii's long list in *Abort i preduprezhdenie beremennosti,* 12–25; see also Ketlinskaia, *Devushka i komsomol,* 65.

142. Mary Shaeffer Conroy reports that between 1924 and 1929 there were over seven thousand addicts in major cities in Russia but argues that the number was probably far higher. Cocaine and morphine were the two predominant drugs; see "Abuse of Drugs Other Than Alcohol and Tobacco in the Soviet Union," 450–53.

143. S. M. Samet, "K novomu bytu," *ZNB* 6 (March 1927): 13.

144. Frances L. Bernstein, "Prostitutes and Proletarians: The Soviet Labor Clinic as Revolutionary Laboratory," in *The Human Tradition in Modern Russia,* ed. Husband, 115–16, 119–20, 122–23.

145. For an exposition of O. Freilikh's film, see Attwood and Kelly's article "Programs for Identity," in *Constructing Russian Culture,* ed. Kelly and Shepherd, 278–79.

146. GARF f. A-482, op. 1, d. 552, l. 13. In 1928 seven women vied for every available space in the new facility; see Bernstein, "Prostitutes and Proletarians," in *The Human Tradition in Modern Russia,* ed. Husband, 117.

147. Kelly, *Refining Russia,* 264; David L. Hoffmann, "Bodies of Knowledge: Physical Culture and the New Soviet Man," in *Language and Revolution,* ed. Halfin, 269–86; Nye, *Crime, Madness, and Politics in Modern France,* 319–29.

148. The Vseobuch (Central Board of Universal Military Training) was formed in

1918 to improve the health of potential military recruits; see Attwood and Kelly, "Programs for Identity," in *Constructing Russian Culture*, ed. Kelly and Shepherd, 267.

149. Semashko, *Puti sovetskoi fizkul'tury*, 29–30.

150. Ibid., 32.

151. Porter, *Health, Civilization, and the State*, 55.

152. GARF f. A-482, op. 1, d. 156, l. 48. GARF f. 5451, op. 10, d. 502, l. 1. See also Sukharev, *Rabochii, beregi svoe zdorov'e*, 22.

153. Riordan, "The Rise, Fall and Rebirth of Sporting Women," 185–86.

154. James Riordan, *Sport in Soviet Society: Development of Sport and Physical Education in Russia and the USSR*, 32–33; Henry W. Morton, *Soviet Sport: Mirror of Soviet Society*, 160.

155. P. F. Lesgaft set up physical education courses around Russia, with schools also taking up the cause. See McReynolds, *Russia at Play*, 87–95, 107–8; Riordan, "The Rise, Fall and Rebirth of Sporting Women," 187–93. Koenker notes the increased interest among printers' papers in competitive sports over physical culture in the 1920s; see *Republic of Labor*, 187.

156. McReynolds et al., "The Objective Eye," in *Constructing Russian Culture*, ed. Kelly and Shepherd, 75–78; Riordan, *Sport in Soviet Society*, 73.

157. Semashko, *Puti sovetskoi fizkul'tury*, 24–25.

158. GARF f. A-482, op. 1, d. 156, l. 49.

159. Riordan, "The Rise, Fall and Rebirth of Sporting Women," 186–87, 190–91. For a detailed discussion of various Soviet psychologists' theories of gender difference, see Attwood, *The New Soviet Man and Woman*, 60–85.

160. Veronika Gorinevskaia, *Fizicheskaia kul'tura rabotnitsy*, 7 (pub. 6,000).

161. In the chapter "Nature Unveiling before Science" Jordanova demonstrates that dissection was eroticized in the West and that gendered portrayals underscored women's subjugation; see *Sexual Visions*, 87–110; see also Stewart, *For Health and Beauty*, 15. The explicit nature of this poster contrasts markedly with those found in French manuals, where such visuals did not appear.

162. Other sources advised women to do nothing at all during their menstrual period except rest; see Gorinevskaia, *Fizicheskaia kul'tura rabotnitsy*, 45.

163. In her book *Russia at Play* McReynolds argues that pictures of embracing semi-nude wrestlers before the revolution "suggests that the homosexual identity was being co-opted by an evolving heterosexual masculinity" (148). For homosexuality in the 1920s, see Healey, *Homosexual Desire in Revolutionary Russia;* for the body, see John E. Bowlt, "Body Beautiful: The Artistic Search for the Perfect Physique," in *Laboratory of Dreams*, ed. Bowlt and Matich, 37–58.

164. Karen Petrone explores these themes in the 1930s in the context of physculture parades; see *Life Has Become More Joyous, Comrades: Celebrations in the Time of Stalin*, 12, 30–34, 35–39. John F. Kasson theorizes at length on the meaning of the nude—specifically muscular male representations at the turn of the century in the United States—in *Houdini, Tarzan, and the Perfect Man: The White Male Body and the Challenge of Modernity in America*, 21–76.

165. The photo is featured in MOZ, *Doma otdykha*, 185; similar athletic displays appear throughout the book.

166. N. Lebina, *Rabochaia molodezh' Leningrada*, 157; Bernstein, *The Dictatorship of Sex*, 151–58.

167. Semashko, *Okhrana zdorov'ia rabochikh,* 44.

168. Vasilevskii, *Gigiena pionera,* 30. Advice to U.S. youth during the same period similarly emphasized a morning bowel movement as a healthy habit; see Burnham, *How Superstition Won and Science Lost,* 60. According to Kelly, most advice literature to children avoided the topic of bowel movements; see "Shaping the 'Future Race,'" in *Everyday Life in Early Soviet Russia,* ed. Kiaer and Naiman, 261.

169. Semashko, *Puti sovetskoi fizkul'tury,* 56. Semashko did put limits on the ability of the mind to change the body. For example, in 1925 Semashko vigorously challenged theorists who argued that female menstruation was a product of the market economy since it was more "natural" for animals to be in heat for more limited times of the year; see Naiman, *Sex in Public,* 3, 142–43.

170. I. Gel'man, *Polovaia zhizn' sovremennoi molodezhi,* 40–44. For a more thorough discussion of this topic, see Gorsuch, *Youth in Revolutinary Russia,* 108.

171. Dembskaia, *Polovaia gigiena zhenshchiny.* This also appeared in Enlightenment concepts elsewhere; see Stewart, *For Health and Beauty,* 32.

172. Gorsuch, *Youth in Revolutinary Russia,* 114–15. Bernstein examines the "dictatorship" of the glandular system in depth; see *The Dictatorship of Sex,* 56, 41–72.

173. Bernstein, *The Dictatorship of Sex,* 41–72. Naiman points to the numerous works of A. V. Nemilov, which went through multiple printings throughout the 1920s, as proof of the popularity of this brand of biological determinism in the scientific discourse of the revolutionary period; see *Sex in Public,* 191–96. For French arguments of a similar cast, see Stewart, *For Health and Beauty,* 23–27, 92–95.

174. Pierre Bourdieu, *Distinction: A Social Critique of the Judgment of Taste.* Hau argues that the German "life reform movement" became a way for lower-middle-class aspirants to show their hoped for middle-class status while simultaneously demonstrating their distinction from the lower class; see *The Cult of Health and Beauty in Germany,* 5. Nudity, with its consequent shedding of class markers, became the ultimate leveler; 176.

175. Lebina, *Povsednevnaia zhizn' sovetskogo goroda,* 205.

176. Gorsuch, *Youth in Revolutinary Russia,* 88–89; Stites, *Revolutionary Dreams,* 117.

177. Semashko, *Iskusstvo odevat'sia,* 19.

178. McCormick, *The Hammer and the Scythe,* 18.

179. Peterson, "Dirty Women," in *Russia, Women, Culture,* ed. Goscilo and Holmgren, 189.

180. Healey, *Homosexual Desire in Revolutionary Russia,* 142–45; Bernstein, *The Dictatorship of Sex,* 71.

181. K. I. Bukov et al., eds. *Ocherki istorii Moskovskoi organizatsii VLKSM,* 183.

182. Lebina, *Povsednevnaia zhizn' sovetskogo goroda,* 209–11.

183. S. A. Gurevich, *Obzor zhilishchno-kommunal'nogo dela v Moskve i deiatel'nosti Moskovskoi zhilishchno-kommunal'noi inspektsii i sektsii kommunal'noi sanitarii v 1922 g,* 47 (pub. 3,000).

184. Chase, *Workers, Society and the Soviet State,* 187.

185. Anon., "Kak byt' chistymi bez bani," *Gigiena i zdorov'e rabochei sem'i* 3 (1923): 14.

186. Gruber posits this scenario as occurring in Vienna; see *Red Vienna,* 154. Undoubtedly it also held true for overcrowded Moscow.

187. Alchohol was important to masculine culture across classes; see Rebecca Friedman, "From Boys to Men: Manhood in the Nicholaevan University," in *Russian Masculinities*

in History and Culture, ed. Clements, Friedman, and Healey, 33–50; see also, in the same volume, Christine Worobec, "Masculinity in Late-Imperial Russian Peasant Society," 76–93.

188. On the collision of worker concepts of alcohol use and official precepts, see Kate Transchel, "Liquid Assets: Vodka and Drinking in Early Soviet Factories," in *The Human Tradition in Modern Russia,* ed. Husband, 129–41; see also Phillips, *Bolsheviks and the Bottle,* 21, 43, 143, 31, 35.

189. N. N. Petrov, *Chto nado znat' o rake,* 6 (pub. 10,000).

190. Mikh. Maslov, "Bor'ba s ustalost'iu," *Kul'tura i zhizn'* 4 (1922): 34.

191. Semashko, *Puti sovetskoi fizkul'tury,* 32–33. See also Clark, "The 'New Man's' Body," in *Art of the Soviets,* ed. Brown and Taylor, 47. Theorists inspired by Taylor searched for one unified theory that would make everything work. Soviet faith in the regimen was a similar quest for the single method to achieve utopia. For more on the theme, see Martha Banta, *Taylored Lives: Narrative Productions in the Age of Taylor, Veblen; and Ford,* ix.

192. Susan Sontag, *Illness as Metaphor and AIDS and Its Metaphors.*

193. By extension, Gorsuch argues that the success of social engineering was a test of NEP. If youth could become new even as NEP continued, then it was not nearly as threatening a policy as many feared; see *Youth in Revolutinary Russia,* 2–3.

Conclusion

1. Douglas discusses the dangers of the past; see, *Purity and Danger,* 95. Focusing on Andrei Platonov, Mikhail Zoshchenko, and Lev Kassil', in *Constructing the Stalinist Body: Fictional Representations of Corporeality in the Stalinist 1930s* Keith A. Livers situates the "new preoccupation with borders in the 1930s" (10). What was happening in the 1930s, however, may have reflected an intensification of the boundary construction begun in the 1920s.

2. Weiner notes how class and ethnicity both served as categories for later purges; see *Making Sense of War,* 207.

3. Molotov noted the problems of the "cruel discipline" needed by the state but carried out through people who are problematic ("potomu chto net gotovykh, chisten'kikh takikh, ochishchennykh ot vsekh grekhov liudei"). Feliks Ivanovich Chuev and V. M. Molotov, *Sto sorok besed s Molotovym: Iz dnevnika F. Chueva,* 391; quoted in Weiner, *Making Sense of War,* 36.

4. Davis, *Economic Problems,* 85.

5. Vinogradov, Ashurkov, and Kurashov, "Osnovnye tempy razvitiia sovetskogo zdravookhraneniia," in *Okhrana narodnogo zdorov'ia v SSSR,* ed. Kovrigin, 60–61. In English, Davis gives a dramatic account of the intersection of politics, economy, and class in the downfall of Semashko, "Economics of Soviet Public Health," *Health and Society in Revolutionary Russia,* ed. Solomon and Hutchinson, 153–55.

6. For Obukh, see Davis, *Economic Problems,* 58–64. Davis also notes the dismissal of M. Ginzburg, K. Konovalov, V. Goriushin, and G. Dreisin. M. F. Vladimirskii took over as head of Narkomzdrav; see Davis, "Economics of Soviet Public Health," in *Health and Society in Revolutionary Russia,* ed. Solomon and Hutchinson, 156.

7. Semashko, "Politika v dele zdravookhraneniia," in *Desiat' let oktiabria i sovetskaia meditsina,* ed. Semashko, 11–12. Moscow's death rate fell throughout the 1920s as the birth rate rose; see Colton, *Moscow,* 157.

8. Conroy, *The Soviet Pharmaceutical Business,* 132–38; Semashko, "Politika v dele zdravookhraneniia," 12; Weissman, "Origins of Soviet Health Administration," 116; Davis, "Economics of Soviet Public Health," in *Health and Society in Revolutionary Russia,* ed. Solomon and Hutchinson, 146–48.

9. Ewing, *The Science and Politics of Soviet Insurance Medicine,* 69–83.

10. Solomon, "Social Hygiene and Soviet Public Health," *Health and Society in Revolutionary Russia,* ed. Solomon and Hutchinson, 191–93; Davis, "Economics of Soviet Public Health," *Health and Society in Revolutionary Russia,* 153–55.

11. Hoffmann, *Stalinist Values,* 4.

12. This reflected an attempt to bring hygiene into debates on the course of the revolution and involved the use of the term "thermidore." Hoffmann argues that the cultural campaigns of Stalinism fulfilled certain strands of revolutionary utopian thought; see in *Stalinist Values,* 1–14. He supports this argument in a lively essay in *Kritika* 5 (fall 2004), 651–733. Essential to any such evaluation is a look at how the people viewed health provisions and revolutionary promise. Undoubtedly many saw this turn in health care as the fulfillment of the revolution. As Kotkin remarks in *Magnetic Mountain,* "To the vast majority of those who lived it, and even to most of its enemies, Stalinism, far from being a partial retreat let alone a throwback to the Russian past, remained forward-looking and progressive throughout" (6). In *Intimate Enemies* Halfin argues that discussions of the revolution must "turn to the investigation of how historical figures interpreted their historical present and located themselves along the temporal continuum ranging from capitalism to Communism" (2). In *Making Sense of War* Weiner moves into the postwar period, seeing there "the undiminished impetus for revolutionary transformation" (17).

13. According to Hyde, by 1934 75.1 percent of doctors were female; see *The Soviet Health Service,* 98. To meet the needs of workers, new health stations were set up in factories. Rural services were also expanded but still lagged behind urban provisions; see Kaser, *Health Care in the Soviet Union and Eastern Europe,* 40–41.

14. Michaels, *Curative Powers,* 73–102.

15. John Scott provided a personal, chilling account of the effects on medicine and dentistry at the ground level of industrialization in Magnitogorsk; see *Behind the Urals: An American Worker in Russia's City of Steel,* 20–21, 44, 128–30.

16. Hoffmann, *Peasant Metropolis,* 1; Bliznakov, "Soviet Housing," in *Russian Housing in the Modern Age,* ed. Brumfield and Ruble, 107; Khromov and Sveshnikov, *Zdravookhranenie Leningrada,* 39.

17. Davis, *Economic Problems,* 35–41, 85; see also his essay "Economics of Soviet Public Health," in *Health and Society in Revolutionary Russia,* ed. Solomon and Hutchinson, 160–61.

18. Patterson, "Typhus and Its Control in Russia," 85–86.

19. Sir James Purves-Stewart, *A Physician's Tour in Soviet Russia,* 55, 168.

20. Hoffmann, *Stalinist Values,* 40. In 1930 Leningrad launched a campaign calling for the "sanitary minimum" in the city. See Botvinnik, "Kratkaia istoriia razvitiia obshchestvennykh nachal v zdravookhranenii Leningrada," in *Obshchestvennye nachala v sovetskom zdravookhranenii,* ed. Freidmin, 46–47. Hoffmann, *Stalinist Values,* 3; Kelly, *Refining Russia,* 278–96.

21. Having admitted a patient into care in 1973 in Irkutsk, an American doctor wryly commented on the rituals of dust elimination at the hospital: "According to the Soviets,

these measures minimize the dirt that one brings in from the outside. I think they stir up more dust than they stop." William A. Knaus, *Inside Russian Medicine*, 21.

22. By the 1970s, dispensaries numbered nearly 4,000. Over 35,000 health care institutions—hospitals, maternity homes, and dispensaries—catered to the needs of the population. Kaser reports Ministry of Health statistics for over 3,700 dispensaries treating tuberculosis, venereal and dermatological diseases, cancer, and psychiatric disorders; *Health Care in the Soviet Union and Eastern Europe*, 59. See also Ryan, *Organization of Soviet Medical Care*, 82.

23. Hoffmann, *Stalinist Values*, 18–22.

24. Petrone explores the embodiment of Soviet ideology in festival culture, including explorations of physical culture parades; see *Life Has Become More Joyous, Comrades*, 12, 30–34.

25. Hoffmann, *Peasant Metropolis*, 168.

26. Hoffmann, *Stalinist Values*, 22.

27. By the 1960s the House of Leisure extended to over six hundred homes, reaching approximately five million people every year. Over eight million people found therapeutic relaxation in the sanatoriums. See V. V. Poltovanov, "Rest Homes," 18; cited in Hyde, *The Soviet Health Service*, 73, 78.

28. Rebecca Balmas Neary, "Mothering Socialist Society: The Wife-Activists' Movement and the Soviet Culture of Daily Life, 1934–1941," 397.

29. According to Cavanaugh, the message was that "to sanitize was to Sovietize," but often messages were divorced from the reality of implementation or, worse, were "often coercive or humiliating"; "Backwardness and Biology," 214–17. See also Michaels, *Curative Powers*, 46–70. Hirsch notes that by the late 1920s the categorization of people by the state had advanced sufficiently to "step up the transformative agenda" against groups deemed inferior; *Empire of Nations*, 102.

30. In the 1930s one Eskimo noted the positive changes in his life, citing the bathhouse, doctors, clean dishes, European clothes, and even his underwear as evidence. See Yuri Slezkine, *Arctic Mirrors: Russia and the Small Peoples of the North*, 288, 296.

31. As Slezkine remarks in *Arctic Mirrors* of the campaign, "Violence was much less effective if one's task was to make people brush their teeth, use underwear, read books, and boil the meat they ate" (231). On Asia, see Michaels, *Curative Powers*, 46–70; for her evidence on reception, see 103–26.

32. Cavanaugh, "Backwardness and Biology," 218.

33. Hoffmann, *Stalinist Values*, 114, and his "Mothers in the Motherland: Stalinist Pronatalism in Its Pan-European Context."

34. Ransel details not only the problems of the countryside but also the acceleration in the provision of care in the 1930s, especially after 1936; see *Village Mothers*, 65–71.

35. Hoffmann, *Stalinist Values*, 93–97, 110–11. As late as the 1970s, Soviet men rejected coitus interruptus as a means of birth control based on the belief that "if it is practiced frequently it leads to mental illness." Knaus, *Inside Russian Medicine*, 199. The lifting of the abortion ban in the 1950s led to an overreliance on the procedure. Knaus reports an average of six abortions in a woman's reproductive lifetime by the late Soviet period, making the number of abortions performed in the Soviet Union in 1980 ten times greater than the number performed in the United States; 201. Fitzpatrick discusses the ban in

Everyday Stalinism: Ordinary Life in Extraordinary Times: Soviet Russia in the 1930s, 152–55. Greta Bucher's interview with "Tanya" recounts a particularly awful experience at a women's clinic in the 1950s that so frightened the subject that she decided to have no more children; see "'Free and Worth Every Kopeck': Soviet Medicine and Women in Postwar Russia," in *The Human Tradition in Modern Russia*, ed. Husband, 180–81.

36. Hyde, *The Soviet Health Service*, 99. According to Kaser, by 1974 22,000 stations for maternal and child care were operating across the Soviet Union; *Health Care in the Soviet Union and Eastern Europe*, 82. Nearly 700 maternity homes cared for mothers and their children. See Michael Ryan, *The Organization of Soviet Medical Care*, 82.

37. See, e.g., the personal interview and commentary recorded by Bucher in "'Free and Worth Every Kopeck': Soviet Medicine and Women in Postwar Russia," in *The Human Tradition in Modern Russia*, ed. Husband, 175–79.

38. Boym, *Common Places*, 5–11. See also Vera Dunham, *In Stalin's Time: Middle Class Values in Soviet Fiction*; and Hoffmann, *Stalinist Values*, 123–24.

39. Hoffmann, *Stalinist Values*, 71–73, 180–82.

40. Hyde, *The Soviet Health Service*, 103. As a result of a shift in priorities, decreased wages, and declining training, medicine as a profession fell in prestige. This was compounded by the feminization of the profession. By the 1970s women constituted about 70 percent of doctors; see Mark G. Field, "American and Soviet Medical Manpower: Growth and Evolution, 1910–1970," 455–73. For a more extensive discussion of the problems of Soviet medicine in the 1950s, see Field, *Doctor and Patient in Soviet Russia*.

41. Anon., "Narodnoe khoziaistvo SSSR v 1956 g."; quoted in *Zdravookhranenie v SSSR: Statisticheskii spravochnik*, ed. G. F. Konstantinov, 14.

42. Mark Mirsky, *Promoting Public Health: The Story of Soviet Medical Science*, 96.

43. Porter, *Health, Civilization, and the State*, 196–277.

44. William C. Cockerham, *Health and Social Change in Russia and Eastern Europe*, 9. See also Vladimir Shkolnikov, France Mesle, and Jacques Vallin, "Health Crisis in Russia. I. Recent Trends in Life Expectancy and Causes of Death from 1970 to 1993," 123–54; Murray Feshbach and Alfred Friendly, Jr., *Ecocide in the USSR: Health and Nature Under Siege*.

45. Carlson, *An Unhealthy Decade: A Sociological Study of the State of Public Health in Russia, 1990–1999*, 5–8. See also D. D. Venediktov, *Zdravookhranenie Rossii: Krizis i puti preodoleniia*, 65–71.

46. For details on medical provisions, see 157–79; 205–27; for changes in lifestyle, see 91–130, 181–203.

47. Mark G. Field, "The Health and Demographic Crisis in Post-Soviet Russia: A Two-Phase Development," in *Russia's Torn Safety Nets: Health and Welfare during the Transition*, ed. Mark G. Field and Judyth L. Twigg, 16–17, 28. The greatest decline in life expectancy occurred among middle-aged, urban males employed in manual occupations in the most developed regions of the former Soviet Union. See William C. Cockerham, "The Social Determinants of the Decline of Life Expectancy in Russia and Eastern Europe: A Lifestyle Explanation," 119.

48. New diseases, such as AIDS, have spread with alarming rapidity and old ones, such as tuberculosis and cholera, have reemerged. Because of drug shortages, infected people are only getting partial treatment, leading to the specter of drug-resistant strains

of tuberculosis; see David E. Powell, "The Problem of AIDS," in *Russia's Torn Safety Nets*, ed. Field and Twigg, 123–51; see also Field, "The Health and Demographic Crisis," in *Russia's Torn Safety Nets*, 35. Venediktov examines the depopulation problem by region; see *Zdravookhranenie Rossii*, 17–24. He also discusses natal health; see 24–26. See also Field, "The Health and Demographic Crisis," in *Russia's Torn Safety Nets*, 11–14. Most women choose to have no children at all and use rhythm, withdrawal, and ultimately abortion as their primary methods of birth control. See Elena Pervysheva and Laurie Liskin, "Attitudes Toward Family Planning in Russia: Research Results from Moscow and Ivanovo," in *Medical Issues and Health Care Reform in Russia*, ed. Vicki L. Hesli and Margaret H. Mills, 179–83.

49. Diane M. Duffy, "An Assessment of Health Policy Reform in Russia," in *Medical Issues and Health Care Reform in Russia*, ed. Hesli and Mills, 25. Cockerham argues convincingly that policy and stress are not the largest factors contributing to mortality but rather lifestyle choices, which have contributed to the increasingly poor health in the East; see "The Social Determinants of the Decline of Life Expectancy in Russia and Eastern Europe," 122.

50. Cockerham, "The Social Determinants of the Decline of Life Expectancy in Russia and Eastern Europe," 124. He appropriates the concepts of Bourdieu as the basis for his analysis.

51. This data set is from epidemiologists working on the declining health of the former Soviet Union; see Martin Bobak et al., "Socioeconomic Factors, Perceived Control and Self-Reported Health in Russia: A Cross-Sectional Survey," 269–79. Cockerham explores this concept in an article coauthored with M. Christine Snead and Derek F. DeWaal entitled "Health Lifestyles in Russia and the Socialist Heritage," 42–55.

52. Cockerham, "The Social Determinants of the Decline of Life Expectancy in Russia and Eastern Europe," 117–30. See also Murray Feshbach, *Russia's Health and Demographic Crisis: Policy Implications and Consequences.*

BIBLIOGRAPHY

Periodicals and Journals

Ezhenedel'nik Moszdravotdela

Gigiena i zdorov'e

Gigiena i zdorov'e rabochei i krest'ianskoi sem'i

Iskusstvo i promyshlennost'

Izvestiia Narkomzdrava

Klub

Komsomol'skaia Pravda

Kul'turnyi front

Kommunal'noe khoziaistvo

Kommunisticheskii trud

Okhrana materinstva i mladenchestva

Pravda

Rabochii klub

Rabotnitsa

Rupor

Sanitarnoe prosveshchenie

Voprosy zdravookhranenia

Za novyi byt

Zdorov'e

Zhurnal Moskovskogo kommunal'nogo khoziaistva

Primary Sources

Agitsud nad prestupnikami. Voronezh: Voronezhskaia kommuna, 1923.

Akkerman, A. I. *Sud nad prostitutkoi i svodnitsei: Delo grazhd. Evdokimovoi po obvineniiu v soznatel'nom zarazhenii sifilisom i grazhd. Sviridovoi v svodnichestve i soobshchnichestve.* Moscow: Narkomzdrav, 1924.

Andreev, Boris. *Sud nad negramotnym.* Leningrad: Gubono, 1924.

———. *Sud nad starym bytom: Stsenarii dlia rabochikh klubov ko dniu rabotnitsy 8-go Marta (s metodicheskimi ukazaniiami).* Moscow: Doloi negramotnost', 1926.

———. *Tretii front: Stseny iz sovremennogo rabochego byta v trekh deistviiakh.* Moscow: Gosizdat, 1927.

Antonov, A. N. *Kak uberech' rebenka ot Angliiskoi bolezni.* Leningrad: Priboi, 1926.

———. *Ot chego byvaiut letnie ponosy i kak uberech ot nikh rebenka.* Leningrad: Priboi, n.d.

———. *Pamiatka materi.* Leningrad: Priboi, 1925.

———. *Sanitarno-prosvetitel'naia rabota po okhrane materinstva i mladenchestva.* Leningrad: Prakticheskaia meditsina, 1925.

Arkhipov, P. G., D. N. Lukashevich, and I. V. Sazhin, eds. *Sputnik lektora: Konspekty lektzii po anatomii i fiziologii cheloveka.* Petrograd: Petrogradskoe okruzhnoe voenno-sanitarnoe upravlenie, 1922.

Ashikhmin, A. A. *Bolezn' i byt: Bor'ba s sotsial'nymi bolezniami.* Moscow: Gosizdat, 1927.

———. *Sotsial'nye bolezni i zhilishche.* Leningrad: Komissiia sanitarnykh predstaviteleia, 1928.

———. *Tuberkulez i zhilishche.* Leningrad: Sanprosvet Leningradskogo gubzdravotdela, 1925.

———. *Vozdukh nashikh zhilishch.* Leningrad: Leningradskogo gubispolkoma, 1926.

Astrinskii, S. D. *Abort i preduprezhdenie beremennosti.* Moscow: Molodaia gvardiia, 1927.

———. *Beremennost' i venericheskie bolezni.* Moscow: OMM, 1928.

———. *Devushka—budushchaia mat'.* Leningrad: Molodaia gvardiia, 1926.

Avlov, Gr. *Sud nad khuliganami.* Moscow: Doloi negramotnost', 1927.

Barushkin, I. M. *Pochemu vreden tabak?* Moscow: Gosizdat, 1926.

Bellamy, Edward. *Looking Backward: 2000–1887.* Boston: Ticknor, 1888.

Béraud, Henri. *The Truth About Moscow: As Seen by a French Visitor.* Translated by John Pelie. London: Faber and Gwyer, 1926.

Bibanova, E. G. *Kak gotovit' iz rebenka v vozraste do 3-kh let budushchego stroitelia novoi zhizni.* Moscow: Moskovskii rabochii, 1927.

Bogdanov, Alexander. *Red Star: The First Bolshevik Utopia.* Edited by Loren R. Graham and Richard Stites. Translated by Charles Rougle. Bloomington: Indiana University Press, 1984.

Bogomolov, A. K. *Dostizheniia sovetskoi meditsiny.* Moscow: MOZ, 1925.

Bosse, G. *Chelovek—zavod.* N.p.: Proletarii, 1925.

Bravaia, R. M. *Okhrana materinstva i mladenchestva na zapade i v SSSR: Istoricheskii ocherk.* Moscow: Gosmedizdat, 1929.

British Trade Union Delegation. *Russia Today: The Official Report of the British Trade Union Delegation.* New York: International Publishers, 1925.

Bukharin, N., and E. Preobrazhensky. *The ABC of Communism: A Popular Explanation of the Program of the Communist Party of Russia.* Ann Arbor: University of Michigan Press, 1966.

Chernyshevskii, Nikolai. *What Is to Be Done?* Translated by Michael R. Katz. Ithaca, N.Y.: Cornell University Press, 1989.

D. R. *Sud nad domashnei khoziaikoi.* Moscow: Gosizdat, 1927.

Danilevich, A. F. *Rabochee vremia i otdykh.* Moscow: Trud i kniga, 1924.

Dembskaia, V. E. *Individual'naia gigiena zhenshchiny: Ukhod za zdorov'em i krasotoi.* Leningrad: Prakticheskaia meditsina, 1927.

———. *Polovaia gigiena zhenshchiny.* Leningrad: Leningradskaia Pravda, 1928.

Demidovich, E. B. *Stat'ia 155 ugolovnogo kodeksa RSFSR: Sud nad gr. Kiselevym po obvineniiu v zarazhenii tripperom.* Moscow: Narkomzdrav, 1925.

Dewey, John. *Impressions of Soviet Russia and the Revolutionary World: Mexico—China—Turkey.* New York: New Republic, 1929.
Dorokhov, P. *Vspleski: Rasskazy "Novaia Moskva."* Moscow: n.p., 1925.
Dreiser, Theodore. *Dreiser Looks at Russia.* New York: Horace Liveright, 1928.
Dubianskaia, M. P. *Borites' s mukhami, klopami, komarami, vshami: Domashnie nasekomye—nashi vragi.* 2nd ed. Leningrad: Gosudarstvennaia tipografiia im. tov. Zinov'eva, 1926.
———. *Gigiena zhilishch: Ob otoplenii pechami.* Leningrad: Leningradskaia pravda, 1927.
Dzhumaliev, N. *V. I. Lenin i okhrana zdorov'ia trudiashchikhsia.* Kyrgyzstan: Frunze, 1969.
Dzinbikovskaia, A., et al., comp. *Konchilos' schast'e: Sanitarnyi lubok v 2-kh kartinakh.* Petrograd: Politotdel 10-i strelkovoi divizii, 1923.
Fainshmidt, I. I., N. S. Morozovskii, and L. D. Ul'ianov. *Sotsial'no-gigienicheskie usloviia i tuberkulez v Ukrainskom sele.* Kharkov: Nauchnaia mysl', 1928.
Fülüp-Miller, René. *The Mind and Face of Bolshevism: An Examination of Cultural Life in Soviet Russia.* 1926. Translated by F. S. Flint and D. F. Tait. Reprint, New York: Harper & Row, 1965.
Gantt, W. Horsley. *Russian Medicine.* New York: Paul B. Hoeber, 1937.
Gastev, A. *Iunost', idi!* Moscow: VTsSPS, 1923.
———. *Kak nado rabotat': Prakticheskoe vvedenie v nauku organizatsii truda.* Moscow: Ekonomika, 1966.
Geizer, I. *Ozdorovlenie truda i byta: Itogi deiatel'nosti MOZ za period c 1/x—1924 po 1/yii—1925 g.* Moscow: MOZ, 1925.
Gel'man, I. *Polovaia zhizn' sovremennoi molodezhi.* Moscow: Gosizdat, 1923.
———. *Trud, utomlenie i otdykh.* Moscow: VTsSPS, 1925.
Gernet, M. N., ed. *Prestupnyi mir Moskvy: Sbornik statei.* Moscow: Pravo i zhizn', 1924.
Gigiena i zdorov'e rabochego i ego sem'i. Stalingrad: Stalingradskoe izdatel'stvo, 1925.
Ginzburg, B. S. *Okhrana materinstva i mladenchestva (Kratkoe rukovodstvo dlia lektora).* Moscow: OMM Narkomzdrav, 1924.
———. *Populiarnye besedy po okhrane materinstva i mladenchestva (v pomoshch' izbachu): Prilozhenie k khudozhestvennoi vystavke-lubku po okhrane materinstva i mladenchestva.* Moscow: OMM Narkomzdrav, 1925.
———. *Sud nad mater'iu, podkinuvshei svoego rebenka: Delo gr. Tikhonovoi po obvineniiu ee: 1/v prestupno-nebrezhnom otnoshenii k svoemu rebenku povlekshem za soboi riad tiazhelykh zabolevanii; 2/v ostavlenii rebenka na proizvol sud'by: Instsenirovka.* Moscow: Zemlia i fabrika, 1924.
———. *Sud nad vrachom meduchastka.* Moscow: OMM Narkomzdrav, 1925.
Gladkov, F. S. *Cement.* Translated by A. S. Arthur and C. Ashleigh. Evanston, Ill.: Northwestern University Press, 1994.
Gol'dfail', L. Gl., and I. D. Iakhin. *Kurorty, sanatorii i doma otdykha SSSR, 1928.* Moscow: Gosizdat, 1928.
Gorinevskaia, Veronika. *Fizicheskaia kul'tura rabotnitsy.* Moscow: Trud i kniga, 1925.
Gurevich, S. A. *Obzor zhilishchno-kommunal'nogo dela v Moskve i deiatel'nosti Moskovskoi zhilishchno-kommunal'noi inspektsii i sektsii kommunal'noi sanitarii v 1922 g.* Moscow: Sanitornoi chasti MOZ, 1923.
Haines, Anna J. *Health Work in Soviet Russia.* New York: Vanguard Press, 1928.
Halle, Fannina W. *Woman in Soviet Russia.* New York: Viking Press, 1933.

Harper, Samuel Northrup. *Civic Training in Soviet Russia.* Chicago: University of Chicago Press, 1929.

Harrison, Marguerite E. *Marooned in Moscow: The Story of an American Woman Imprisoned in Russia.* New York: George H. Doran, 1921.

Hird, John Wynne. *Under Czar and Soviet: My Thirty Years in Russia.* London: Hurst & Blackett, 1932.

Iordanskii, N. N. *Sanitarno-gigienicheskaia rabota shkoly.* Moscow: Moskovskoe aktsionernoe izdatel'skoe obshchestvo, 1926.

Ivanov, E. M. *40 let deiatel'nosti Moskovskoi sanitarnoi organizatsii, 1883–1923.* Moscow: MOZ, 1925.

Kabo, E. O. *Ocherki rabochego byta: Opyt monograficheskogo issledovaniia.* Moscow: VTsSPS, 1928.

Kagan, A. G. *Rabochaia molodezh' na otdykhe.* Leningrad: Priboi, n.d

Kagan, Liza. *Put' k obshchestvennoi rabote.* Moscow: Gosizdat, 1926.

———. *Rabota gorodskoi iacheiki VLKSM sredi devushek.* Moscow: Molodaia gvardiia, 1927.

Kalashnikov, V. P. *Pamiatka: Domovym sanpredstaviteliam (o gigiene zhilishch).* Leningrad: Leningradskaia pravda, 1927.

Kal'manson, S., and D. Bekariukov. *Beregi svoe zdorov'e! Sanitarnaia pamiatka dlia rabochikh podrostkov.* Leningrad: Molodaia gvardiia, 1925.

Karlgren, Anton. *Bolshevist Russia.* London: George Allen & Unwin, 1929.

Kats, Ia. Iu. *Mediko-sanitarnaia organizatsiia Moskvy i Moskovskoi gub. i novaia ekonomicheskaia politika.* Moscow: MOZ, 1922.

———. *Sistema i metody dispanserizatsii.* Moscow: MOZ, 1925.

———, ed. *Trud i zdorov'e rabochikh.* Moscow: MOZ, 1926.

Katsenel'son, I. S. *Sovety materiam.* Leningrad: Tipografiia pravda, 1927.

Ketlinskaia, Vera. *Devushka i komsomol.* Leningrad: Priboi, 1927.

Ketlinskaia, Vera, and Vlad. Slepkov, *Zhizn' bez kontrolia (Polovaia zhizn' i sem'ia rabochei molodezhi).* Moscow: Molodaia Gvardiia, 1929.

Khlopin, V. G. *Osnovy gigieny.* Moscow: Narkomzdrav, 1921.

Kholodkovskii, Vl. *Moskovskie parki kul'tury i otdykha.* Moscow: Moskovskii rabochii, 1955.

Khrustalev, A. A. *Znakhar' i doktor.* Moscow: Krasnaia nov', 1923.

Kingsbury, Susan M., and Mildred Fairchild. *Factory, Family, and Woman in the Soviet Union.* New York: G. P. Putnam's Sons, 1935.

Knaus, William A. *Inside Russian Medicine: An American Doctor's First-Hand Report.* New York: Everest House, 1981.

Kollontai, A. *Love of Worker Bees.* Translated by Cathy Porter. London: Virago, 1977.

Kradman, D. A. *Fizkul'tura kak chast' kul'turno-prosvetitel'noi raboty.* Leningrad: Knizhnyi Sektor Gubono, 1924.

Langova, N. I., comp. *Vystavka "Okhrana materinstva i mladenchestva."* Moscow: OMM, 1927.

Lawton, Lancelot. *The Russian Revolution, 1917–1926.* London: Macmillan, 1927.

Lebedev, L., and L. Rubinshtein, eds. *Pis'ma iz uteriannogo portfelia: O poshlosti v bytu.* Moscow: Molodaia gvardiia, 1928.

Lebedeva, G. I., ed. *Znakharsha: Skaz.* Moscow: Novaia derevnia, 1924.

Lebedeva, V. P., and G. N. Speranskii, eds. *Kniga materi (Kak vyrastit' zdorovogo i krepkogo rebenka i sokhranit' svoe zdorov'e).* Moscow, 1926.

Leizerov, M. *Chto ty mozhesh' delat' v klube.* Moscow: Gubok, 1926.

———. *Krasnye ugolki.* Moscow: Trud i kniga, 1925.
———. *O rabochem klube.* Moscow: Doloi negramotnost', 1927.
Lenin, V. I. *Collected Works.* Moscow: Progress Publishers, 1960–70.
———. *Polnoe sobranie sochinenii.* Moscow: Gosizdat, 1962.
Leningradskii meditsinskii zhurnal. *Putevoditel' po muzeiu zdravookhraneniia Leningradskogo obzdravotdela.* Leningrad: Leningradskii meditsinskii zhurnal, 1928.
Lissitzky, El. *Russia: An Architecture for World Revolution.* 1930. Translated by Erich Dluhosch. Reprint, Cambridge, Mass.: MIT Press, 1970.
Lur'e, Iu. *Gigiena devochki, devushki, zhenshchiny.* 2nd ed. Moscow: OMM, 1927.
Marts, V. G., ed. *Igry i razvlecheniia: Sbornik statei.* Moscow: TsKRKSM, 1922.
Mayakovsky, Vladimir. *The Complete Plays of Vladimir Mayakovsky.* Translated by Guy Daniels. New York: Washington Square Press, 1968.
McCormick, Anne O'Hare. *The Hammer and the Scythe: Communist Russia Enters the Second Decade.* New York: Alfred A. Knopf, 1929.
McWilliams, R. F., and Margaret McWilliams. *Russia in Nineteen Twenty-Six.* London: J. M. Dent & Sons, 1927.
Melenevskaia. *Okhrana materinstva i mladenchestva: "Obshchestvennoe vospitanie v rannem vozraste."* Moscow: Kul't-ob"edinenie goskino, 1924.
Mendel'son, A. L. *Gipnoz i vnushenie.* Leningrad: Leningradskaia pravda, 1927.
———. *Ob ukreplenii pamiati.* Leningrad: Leningradskaia pravda, 1926.
———. *Vospitanie voli.* Leningrad: Leningradskaia pravda, 1928.
Mil'chakov, Al. *Komsomol v bor'be za kul'turnyi byt.* Moscow: Molodaia gvardiia, 1927.
Miliutin, N. A. *Sotsgorod.* 1930. Reprint, Cambridge, Mass.: MIT Press, 1974.
Mitropol'skii, N. K. *Doloi babok! Doloi oshibki i sueveriia pri rozhdenii i vospitanii detei.* Leningrad: Gosudarstvennaia tipographia im. tov. Zinov'eva, 1926.
Mitsnik, Z. O., and A. N. Antonov. *Mat' i rebenok.* Leningrad: Priboi, 1925.
Mol'kov, A. *Gosudarstvennyi institut sotsial'noi gigieny Narkomzdrava, 1919–1924.* Moscow: Gosudarstvennyi institut sotsial'noi gigieny, 1924.
———. *Materialy dlia besed o podderzhanii chistoty v zhilishche.* Moscow: Gosizdat, 1921.
———, ed. *Sanitarnoe prosveshchenie: V shkole i cherez shkolu.* Moscow: Gosizdat, 1923.
———, comp. *Zdorovoe zhilishche: Programma populiarnoi lektsii.* Moscow: Narkomzdrav, n.d.
Moskovskii komitet nedeli Okhrany materi i mladentsa, ed. *Okhrana materi i mladentsa v Moskve i Moskovskoi gubernii: Illiustrirovannyi sbornik.* Moscow: Moskovskii komitet po provedeniiu nedeli OMM, 1923.
Moskovskii otdel zdravookhranenia. *Doma otdykha: Sbornik statei i materialov (1920–1923 gg.).* Moscow: Gosizdat, n.d.
———. *Kratkii obzor sostoianiia zdravookhraneniia v Moskve i guberniakh.* Moscow: MOZ, 1926.
———. *Materialy o deiatel'nosti lechebno-profilakticheskikh uchrezhdenii MOZa za 1926/7 goda po dannym statisticheskogo otdeleniia MOZa.* Moscow: MOZ, 1928.
———. *Ozdorovlenie truda i revoliutsiia byta: Sbornik trudov instituta MOZa po izucheniiu professional'nykh boleznei.* Moscow: MOZ, 1923.
———, ed. *Piat' let raboty dietstolovykh.* Moscow: MOZ, 1928.
———. *Spravochnik dispanserizirovannykh predpriiatii g. Moskvy na 1-e Oktiabria 1926 g.* Moscow: MOZ, 1927.

———. *Zdravookhranenie v Moskve i Moskovskoi gubernii.* Moscow: MOZ, 1928.

Moskovskii pododtdel okhrany materi i mladentsa, ed. *Mat' i ditia: Sbornik dlia materi.* Moscow: MOZ, 1928.

Moskovskii sovet. *Material k dokladu otdela zdravookhraneniia na plenume Moskovskogo soveta RK i KD 27 Oktiabria 1925 g.* Moscow: Mossovet, 1925.

Moskovskii Sovet RK i KD, Sektsiia domov otdykha MOZ. *Doma otdykha: Sbornik statei i materialov (1920–1923 gg.).* Moscow: Gosizdat, n.d.

Muramevich. *Kak zhivet i rabotaet chelovecheskoe telo.* N.p.: n.p., n.d.

Narodnyi komissariat zdravookhranenia. *Kurorty SSSR: Spravochnik.* Petrograd: Krasnyi pechatnik, n.d.

Nemchenko, L., ed. *Social Insurance in the Soviet Union.* Moscow: Voprossy truda, 1928.

Ne myt'em tak katan'em: Komediia v trekh aktakh piati kartinakh. Moscow: Glavpolitprosvet TsK VLKSM, 1926.

Newsholme, Sir Arthur, and John Adams Kingsbury. *Red Medicine: Socialized Health in Soviet Russia.* Garden City, N.Y.: Doubleday, Doran & Co., 1933.

Nogina, O. P. *Mother and Child Care in the USSR.* Moscow: Foreign Languages Publishing House, 1950.

———. *Organizatsiia i rabota iaslei: Rukovodstvo dlia zaveduiushchikh iasliami i meditsinskogo personala iaslei i iaslei-sadov.* Moscow: Medgiz, 1961.

———. *Tridtsat' let okhrany materi i rebenka v SSSR.* Moscow: Ministerstvo zdravookhraneniia SSSR institut sanitarnogo prosveshcheniia, 1947.

Nogina, O. P., and S. O. Dulitskii, eds. *Okhrana materinstva i mladenchestva: Sbornik statei.* Moscow: MOZ, 1929.

Oborin, A. *O rabote profsoiuzov v gorode i v derevne.* Moscow: Gosizdat, 1926.

Obukh, V. A., ed., and A. K. Bogomolov, comp. *Zdravookhranenie v Moskve (Dispanserizatsiia rabochego naseleniia).* Moscow: MOZ, 1926.

Petrov, B. D., ed. *S. P. Solov'ev: Izbrannye proizvedeniia.* Moscow: Meditsinskoi literatury, 1956.

Petrov, N. N. *Chto nado znat' o rake.* Leningrad: Leningradskaia pravda, n.d.

Pletnev, V. F. *Rabochii klub: Printsipy i metody raboty.* 2nd ed. Moscow: Vserossiiskii proletkul't, 1925.

Purves-Stewart, Sir James. *A Physician's Tour in Soviet Russia.* London: George Allen & Unwin, 1933.

Rebel'skii, I. V. *Instsenirovannye sudy (Kak ikh organizovyvat').* Moscow: Trud i kniga, 1926.

Rodil'nitsa i ee rebenok. Zima: Sovetskaia tipografiia, 1923.

Roman, R., and Veprinskii. *Rabochii, idi v klub! Materialy dlia zhivoi gazety.* Moscow: G. F. Mirimanov, 1925.

Rosenberg, William G., ed. *Bolshevik Visions: First Phase of the Cultural Revolution in Soviet Russia.* 2 vols. Ann Arbor: University of Michigan Press, 1990.

Rubanovskii, Il'ia. *Za knigu ili v pivnuiu?* Moscow: Molodaia gvardiia, 1928.

Sadov, A. A. *Zaraznye bolezni i byt.* Leningrad: Leningradskaia pravda, n.d.

Sakhnovskaia, A. A. *Chesotka i bor'ba s neiu.* Leningrad: Leningradskaia pravda, 1926.

Sanitarnoe prosveshchenie v rabochem klube (Tsikl lektsii-dokladov i illiustrativnykh vecherov). Moscow: Doloi negramotnost', 1925.

Sazhin, I. V. *Pravda o kurenii.* Leningrad: Leningradskaia pravda, n.d.

Scott, John. *Behind the Urals: An American Worker in Russia's City of Steel.* Edited by Stephen Kotkin. Bloomington: Indiana University Press, 1989.
Semashko, N. A. *Chto takoe kurort i kak na nikh lechit'sia.* Moscow: Gosizdat, 1924.
———. *Health Protection in the U.S.S.R.* London: Victor Gollancz, 1934.
———. *Iskusstvo odevat'sia.* Moscow: Gosizdat, 1927.
———. *Kak otdykhat' letom.* Moscow: Gosizdat, 1926.
———. *Nauka o zdorov'e obshchestva (sotsial'naia gigiena).* 2nd ed. Moscow: Narkomzdrav, 1926.
———. *Nezabyvaemyi obraz.* 2nd ed. Moscow: Politizdat, 1968.
———. *Okhrana zdorov'ia rabochikh i rabotnits krest'ian i krest'ianok za desiat' let.* Moscow: Narkomzdrav RSFSR, 1927.
———. *Osnovy sovetskoi meditsiny.* Moscow: Narkomzdrav, 1919.
———. *O svetlom i temnom v rabochem bytu.* Moscow: Gosizdat, 1928.
———. *Puti sovetskoi fizkul'tury.* Moscow: Vysshii sovet fizicheskoi kul'tury, 1926.
———. *Sotsial'nye bolezni.* Moscow: Moskovskii gosudarstvennyi universitet, 1926.
———. *Sotsial'nye prichiny bolezni.* Moscow: Moskovskii gosudarstvennyi universitet, 1926.
———. *Vvedenie v sotsial'nuiu gigienu.* Moscow: Rabotnik prosveshcheniia, 1927.
———, ed. *Desiat' let oktiabria i sovetskaia meditsina.* Moscow: Narkomzdrav RSFSR, 1927.
Shtrum, I. *Sovetskaia vlast' i sanitarnoe prosveshchenie.* Kharkov: UKRPUR, 1921.
Sigal, B. S. *Alkogolizm i molodezh'.* Moscow: Molodaia gvardiia, 1925.
———. *Kak vyrastit' zdorovogo rebenka.* Moscow: Molodaia gvardiia, 1927.
———. *Polovoi vopros.* Moscow: Molodaia gvardiia, 1925.
———. *Sud nad mater'iu, vinovnoi v plokhom ukhode za det'mi, povlekshem za soboi smert' rebenka.* Leningrad: Gosudarstvennaia tip. im. tov. Zinov'eva, 1926.
———. *Sud nad mater'iu vinovnoi v rasprostranenii skarlatiny.* Moscow: Zhizn' i znanie, 1925.
———. *I. Sud nad pionerom kurivshim i II. Sud nad neriashlivym pionerom: Dve instsenirovki.* Moscow: Zhizn' i znanie, 1927.
———. *Trud i zdorov'e rabochei molodezhi.* Leningrad: Molodaia gvardiia, 1925.
———. *Venericheskie bolezni.* Moscow: Molodaia gvardiia, 1926.
———. *Vrednaia privychka (Kuren'e tabaka).* Moscow: Gosmedizdat, 1929.
Slepkov, A., ed. *Azbuka komsomol'tsa.* Moscow: Novaia Moskva, 1926.
Smidrovich, S. *Rabotnitsa i novyi byt.* Moscow: Gosizdat, 1927.
Smith, Jessica. *Woman in Soviet Russia.* New York: Vanguard Press, 1928.
Sol'ts, A. A. *O partetike.* Moscow: Kommunisticheskii universitet, 1925.
Spandar'ian, O. *Pochemu Varia otdala svoikh detei v pionery.* Moscow: Gosizdat, 1926.
Sputnik po okhrane materinstva i mladenchestva. Moscow: OMM, 1921.
Strashun, I. D. *Bor'ba za zdorov'e—bor'ba s religiei.* Moscow: Bezbozhnik, 1925.
Strashun, I. D., and A. O. Edel'shtein, eds. *Sanitarnoe prosveshchenie.* Moscow: Narkomzdrav, 1925.
Strong, Anna Louise. *The First Time in History: Two Years in Russia's New Life (August, 1921 to December, 1923).* New York: Boni & Liveright, 1924.
Subbotin, Leonid. *Zhakhar'-obmanshchik i babkina loshad': Komediia v 3 deistviiakh.* Moscow: Novaia derevniia, 1925.
Sud nad domashchnei khoziakoi. Moscow: Gosizdat, 1927.
Sukharev, V. *Rabochii, beregi svoe zdorov'e: K ozdorovleniiu rabochei sem'i.* Moscow: Gosizdat, 1926.

Trotsky, Leon. *The Military Writings of Leon Trotsky.* New York: New Park Publications, 1979–81.
———. *My Life: An Attempt at an Autobiography.* New York: Charles Scribner's Sons, 1930.
———. *Problems of Everyday Life: And Other Writings on Culture and Science.* New York: Monad Press, 1973.
Tsentral'noe statisticheskoe upravlenie, Narodnoe khoziaistvo soiuza SSR v tsifrakh. Moscow: MKKh, 1925.
Vainshtein, A. *Doma otdykha i sanatorii dlia zastrakhovannykh.* Moscow: Voprosy truda, 1925.
Vasilevskaia, L. A., and L. M. Vasilevskii. *Sud nad akusherkoi Lopukhinoi, sovershivshei operatsiiu aborta, sledstviem chego iavilas' smert' zhenshchiny, i instsenirovannyi pokazatel'nyi sud.* N.p.: Oktiabr', 1923.
———. *Sud nad samogonshchikami, delo Karpova Tikhona i ego zheny Agaf'i po obvineniiu v izgotovlenii i tainoi torgovle samogonkoi.* N.p.: Oktiabr', 1923.
Vasilevskii, L. M. *Gigiena molodoi devushki.* Moscow: Novaia Moskva, 1926.
———. *Gigiena pionera.* 2nd ed. Moscow: Novaia Moskva, 1925.
———. *Gigiena propagandista (Agitatora, lektora, prepodavatelia).* Moscow: Molodaia gvardiia, 1924.
———. *Gigiena zhenskogo truda.* Leningrad: Leningradskogo gubernskogo soveta professional'nykh soiuzov, 1925.
———. *Prostitutsiia i rabochaia molodezh'.* Moscow: Novaia Moskva, 1924.
Veselov, M. O. *15-let: Bor'ba za pogolovnuiu gramotnost' v Moskovskoi oblasti.* Moscow: Gosizdat, 1932.
Vonzblein, Iu. N. *Put' k zdorov'iu.* Leningrad: Leningradskaia pravda, 1926.
Vsia Moskva 1928. Moscow: Moskovskii rabochii, 1928.
Wells, H. G. *Russia in the Shadows.* New York: George H. Doran Co., 1921.
Wicksteed, Alexander. *Life under the Soviets.* London: John Lane, 1928.
———. *My Russian Neighbors: Recollections of Ten Years in Soviet Moscow.* New York: McGraw-Hill, 1934.
Wiedenfeld, Kurt. *The Remaking of Russia.* London: Labour Publishing, 1924.
Winter, Ella. *Red Virtue.* London: Victor Gollahncz, 1933.
Zaitsev, Vl. *Trud i byt rabochikh podrostkov.* Moscow: Voprosy truda, 1926.
Zalkind, A. B. *Polovoi vopros v usloviiakh sovetskoi obshchestvennosti: Sbornik statei.* Leningrad: Gosizdat, 1926.
Za novyi byt v nashei smene: Prezidium konferentsii zdraviacheek shkol Baumanskogo raiona. Moscow: MOZ i MONO, 1926.
Zenkovsky, Serge A., ed. *Medieval Russia's Epics, Chronicles, and Tales.* 1963. Reprint, New York: Penguin Books, 1974.
Zetkin, Klara. *Reminiscences of Lenin.* London: Modern Books Ltd., 1929.
Zheleznyi, A. *Kak zhit', chtoby zdorovym byt'?* Moscow: Novaia Moskva, 1925.
Zhitomirskii, V., and A. Ostrovskii. *Sem' zaraz ub'em zaraz: Sanitarnyi lubok v 2-kh kartinakh.* Moscow: Zhizn' i znanie, 1926.

Secondary Sources

Accampo, Elinor A., Rachel G. Fuchs, and Mary Lynn Stewart, eds. *Gender and the Politics of Social Reform in France, 1870–1914.* Baltimore, Md.: Johns Hopkins University Press, 1995.

Alexander, John T. *Bubonic Plague in Early Modern Russia: Public Health and Urban Disaster.* Baltimore, Md.: Johns Hopkins University Press, 1980.

———. "Medical Developments in Petrine Russia." *Canadian-American Slavic Studies* 8, no. 2 (1974).

Alexopoulos, Golfo. *Stalin's Outcasts: Aliens, Citizens, and the Soviet State, 1926–1936.* Ithaca, N.Y.: Cornell University Press, 2003.

Amato, Joseph A. *Dust: A History of the Small and the Invisible.* Berkeley: University of California Press, 2000.

Anemone, Anthony. "The Monsters of Peter the Great: The Culture of the St. Petersburg Kunstkamera in the Eighteenth Century." *Slavic and East European Journal* 44 (winter 2000).

Armstrong, David. *The Political Anatomy of the Body.* Cambridge: Cambridge University Press, 1983.

Ashurkov, E. D., et al., eds., *N. A. Semashko: Izbrannye zdravookhraneniia.* Moscow: Meditsinskaia literatura, 1954.

Attwood, Lynne. *Creating the New Soviet Woman: Women's Magazines as Engineers of Female Identity, 1922–53.* New York: St. Martin's Press, 1999.

Baehr, Stephen Lessing. *The Paradise Myth in Eighteenth-Century Russia: Utopian Patterns in Early Secular Russian Literature and Culture.* Stanford, Calif.: Stanford University Press, 1991.

Bailes, Kendall E. "Alexei Gastev and the Soviet Controversy over Taylorism, 1918–24." *Soviet Studies* 29 (July 1977).

Baker, Keith Michael. *Condorcet: From Natural Philosophy to Social Mathematics.* Chicago: University of Chicago Press, 1982.

Ball, Alan M. *Imagining America: Influence and Images in Twentieth-Century Russia.* Lanham, Md.: Rowman & Littlefield, 2003.

———. *Russia's Last Capitalists: The Nepmen, 1921–1929.* Berkeley: University of California Press, 1987.

Banta, Martha. *Taylored Lives: Narrative Productions in the Age of Taylor, Veblen, and Ford.* Chicago: University of Chicago Press, 1993.

Barnes, David S. *The Making of a Social Disease: Tuberculosis in Nineteenth-Century France.* Berkeley: University of California Press, 1995.

Barsukov, M. I., ed. *Annaly istorii meditsiny: Sbornik trudov.* Moscow: Gosizdat, 1963.

———, ed. *Ocherki istoriografii sovetskogo zdravookhraneniia.* Moscow: Meditsina, 1965.

———. *The Organization of Hygiene and Sanitation Services in the USSR.* Washington, D.C.: U.S. Department of Commerce, 1968.

Bates, Barbara. *Bargaining for Life: A Social History of Tuberculosis, 1876–1938.* Philadelphia: University of Pennsylvania Press, 1992.

Beer, Daniel. "The Medicalization of Religious Deviance in the Russian Orthodox Church, 1880–1905." *Kritika* 5 (summer 2004).

Bernstein, Frances. *The Dictatorship of Sex: Lifestyle Advice for the Soviet Masses.* De Kalb: Northern Illinois University Press, 2007.

———. "Envisioning Health in Revolutionary Russia: The Politics of Gender in Sexual-Enlightenment Posters of the 1920s." *Russian Review* 57 (April 1998).

Bobak, Martin, et al. "Socioeconomic Factors, Perceived Control and Self-Reported Health in Russia: A Cross-Sectional Survey." *Social Science and Medicine* 47 (July 1998).

Bock, Gisela, and Pat Thane, eds. *Maternity and Gender Policy: Women and the Rise of the European Welfare States, 1880s–1950s.* London: Routledge, 1991.

Bogdanov, Igor. *Dym otechestva, ili kratkaia istoriia tabakokureniia.* Moscow: Novoe literaturnoe obozrenie, 2007.

Bonnell, Victoria E. *Iconography of Power: Soviet Political Posters under Lenin and Stalin.* Berkeley: University of California Press, 1997.

———. *Roots of Rebellion: Workers' Politics and Organizations in St. Petersburg and Moscow, 1900–1914.* Berkeley: University of California Press, 1983.

———, ed. *The Russian Worker: Life and Labor under the Tsarist Regime.* Berkeley: University of California Press, 1983.

Borrero, Mauricio. *Hungry Moscow: Scarcity and Urban Society in the Russian Civil War, 1917–1921.* New York: Peter Lang, 2003.

Bourdieu, Pierre. *Distinction: A Social Critique of the Judgment of Taste.* Cambridge, Mass.: Harvard University Press, 1984.

Bowlt, John E., and Olga Matich, eds. *Laboratory of Dreams: The Russian Avant-Garde and Cultural Experiment.* Stanford, Calif.: Stanford University Press, 1996.

Boym, Svetlana. *Common Places: Mythologies of Everyday Life in Russia.* Cambridge, Mass.: Harvard University Press, 1994.

Bradley, Joseph. *Muzhik and Muscovite: Urbanization in Late Imperial Russia.* Berkeley: University of California Press, 1985.

———. "'Once You've Eaten Khitrov Soup You'll Never Leave!' Slum Renovation in Late Imperial Russia." *Russian History* 11, no. 1 (1984).

Brooks, Jeffrey. *Thank You, Comrade Stalin! Soviet Public Culture from Revolution to Cold War.* Princeton, N.J.: Princeton University Press, 2000.

Brown, Mathew Cullerne, and Brandon Taylor, eds. *Art of the Soviets: Painting, Sculpture and Architecture in a One-Party State, 1917–1992.* Manchester, Eng.: Manchester University Press, 1993.

Brumfield, William C., ed. *Reshaping Russian Architecture: Western Technology, Utopian Dreams.* Cambridge: Woodrow Wilson International Center for Scholars and Cambridge University Press, 1990.

Brumfield, William C., and Blair A. Ruble, eds. *Russian Housing in the Modern Age: Design and Social History.* Cambridge: Cambridge University Press, 1993.

Buchli, Victor. *An Archaeology of Socialism.* Oxford: Berg, 1999.

Bukov, K. I., et al., eds. *Ocherki istorii Moskovskoi organizatsii VLKSM.* Moscow: Moskovskii rabochii, 1976.

Burnham, John C. *How Superstition Won and Science Lost: Popularizing Science and Health in the United States.* New Brunswick, N.J.: Rutgers University Press, 1987.

Carlson, Per. *An Unhealthy Decade: A Sociological Study of the State of Public Health in Russia, 1990–1999.* Stockholm: Almqvist & Wiksell, 2000.

Cassedy, James H. *American Medicine and Statistical Thinking, 1800–1860.* Cambridge, Mass.: Harvard University Press, 1984.

Cassiday, Julie A. *The Enemy on Trial: Early Soviet Courts on Stage and Screen.* De Kalb: Northern Illinois University Press, 2000.

———. "Flash Floods, Bedbugs and Saunas: Social Hygiene in Maiakovskii's Theatrical Satires of the 1920s." *Slavic and East European Review* 76, no. 4 (1998).

Cassiday, Julie A., and Leyla Rouhi. "From Nevskii Prospekt to Zoia's Apartment: Trials of the Russian Procuress." *Russian Review* 58 (July 1990).

Cavanaugh, Cassandra. "Backwardness and Biology: Medicine and Power in Russian and Soviet Central Asia, 1868–1934." Ph.D. diss., Columbia University, 2001.

Chase, William J. *Workers, Society and the Soviet State: Labor and Life in Moscow, 1918–1929.* Urbana: University of Illinois Press, 1987.

Chatterjee, Choi. *Celebrating Women: Gender, Festival Culture, and Bolshevik Ideology, 1910–1939.* Pittsburgh, Pa.: University of Pittsburgh Press, 2002.

Clark, Charles E. *Uprooting Otherness: The Literacy Campaign in NEP-Era Russia.* Selinsgrove, Pa.: Susquehanna University Press, 2000.

Clark, Katerina. *Petersburg, Crucible of Cultural Revolution.* Cambridge, Mass.: Harvard University Press, 1995.

———. *The Soviet Novel: History as Ritual.* 1981. Reprint, Bloomington: Indiana University Press, 2000.

Clements, Barbara Evans. *Bolshevik Feminist: The Life of Aleksandra Kollontai.* Bloomington: Indiana University Press, 1979.

Clements, Barbara Evans, Rebecca Friedman, and Dan Healey, eds. *Russian Masculinities in History and Culture.* New York: Palgrave, 2002.

Clowes, Edith W., Samuel D. Kassow, and James L. West, eds. *Between Tsar and People: Educated Society and the Quest for Public Identity in Late Imperial Russia.* Princeton, N.J.: Princeton University Press, 1991.

Cockerham, William C. *Health and Social Change in Russia and Eastern Europe.* New York: Routledge, 1999.

———. "The Social Determinants of the Decline of Life Expectancy in Russia and Eastern Europe: A Lifestyle Explanation." *Journal of Health and Social Behavior* 38 (June 1997).

Cockerham, William C., M. Christine Snead, and Derek F. Dewaal. "Health Lifestyles in Russia and the Socialist Heritage." *Journal of Health and Social Behavior* 43 (March 2002).

Colton, Timothy J. *Moscow: Governing the Socialist Metropolis.* Cambridge, Mass.: Harvard University Press, Belknap Press, 1995.

Conroy, Mary Shaeffer. "Abuse of Drugs Other Than Alcohol and Tobacco in the Soviet Union." *Soviet Studies* 42 (July 1990).

———. "Health Care in Prisons, Labour and Concentration Camps in Early Soviet Russia, 1918–1921." *Europe-Asia Studies* 52, no. 7 (2000).

———. *The Soviet Pharmaceutical Business during Its First Two Decades, 1917–1937.* New York: Peter Lang, 2006.

Coopersmith, Jonathan. *The Electrification of Russia, 1880–1926.* Ithaca, N.Y.: Cornell University Press, 1992.

Cowan, Ruth Schwartz. *More Work for Mother: The Ironies of Household Technology from the Open Hearth to the Microwave.* New York: Basic Books, 1983.

David, Michael Zdenek. "The White Plague in the Red Capital: Tuberculosis and Its Control in Moscow, 1900–1941." Ph.D. diss., University of Chicago, forthcoming.

Davis, Christopher M. *Economic Problems of the RSFSR Health System, 1921–1930.* Birmingham, Eng.: University Centre for Russian and East European Studies, 1978.

Deák, František. "'Blue Blouse' (1923–1928)." *Drama Review* 17 (March 1973).

Denbeste-Barnett, Michelle D. "Earnestly Working to Improve Russia's Future, 1867–1905." Ph.D. diss., Southern Illinois University, Carbondale, 1997.

Dernitsyn, T. M., et al., eds. *Profsoiuzy Moskvy: Ocherki istorii.* Moscow: Profizdat, 1975.

Diagilev, V. A. *Istoriia Moskvy.* 6 vols. Moscow: Pervaia akademii nauk SSSR, 1957.

Dodge, Norton T. *Women in the Soviet Economy.* Baltimore, Md.: Johns Hopkins University Press, 1966.

Douglas, Mary. *Purity and Danger: An Analysis of Concepts of Pollution and Taboo.* 1966. Reprint, London: Routledge, 2002.

Dubos, René. *Mirage of Health: Utopias, Progress, and Biological Change.* 1959. Reprint, New York: Harper Colophon Books, 1979.

Duffy, John. *The Sanitarians: A History of American Public Health.* Urbana: University of Illinois Press, 1990.

Dunham, Vera. *In Stalin's Time: Middle-Class Values in Soviet Fiction.* Cambridge: Cambridge University Press, 1976.

Elias, Norbert. *The Civilizing Process: Sociogenetic and Psychogenetic Investigations.* 1939. Reprint, Oxford: Blackwell Publishers, 2000.

Eliav-Feldon, Miriam. *Realistic Utopias: The Ideal Imaginary Societies of the Renaissance, 1516–1630.* Oxford: Clarendon Press, 1982.

Emmons, Terence, and Wayne S. Vucinich, eds. *The Zemstvo in Russia: An Experiment in Local Self-Government.* Cambridge: Cambridge University Press, 1982.

Engelstein, Laura. *The Keys to Happiness: Sex and the Search for Modernity in Fin-de-Siècle Russia.* Ithaca, N.Y.: Cornell University Press, 1992.

Erlich, Alexander. *The Soviet Industrialization Debate, 1924–1928.* Cambridge, Mass.: Harvard University Press, 1960.

Feldberg, Georgina D. *Disease and Class: Tuberculosis and the Shaping of Modern North American Society.* New Brunswick, N.J.: Rutgers University Press, 1995.

Feshbach, Murray, and Alfred Friendly Jr. *Ecocide in the USSR: Health and Nature Under Siege.* New York: Basic Books, 1992.

———. *Russia's Health and Demographic Crisis: Policy Implications and Consequences.* Washington, D.C.: Chemical and Biological Arms Control Institute, 2003.

Field, Mark G. "American and Soviet Medical Manpower: Growth and Evolution, 1910–1970." *International Journal of Health Services* 5, no. 3 (1975).

———. *Doctor and Patient in Soviet Russia.* Cambridge, Mass.: Harvard University Press, 1957.

———. *Soviet Socialized Medicine.* New York: Free Press, 1967.

Field, Mark G., and Judyth L. Twigg, eds. *Russia's Torn Safety Nets: Health and Social Welfare during the Transition.* New York: St. Martin's Press, 2000.

Figes, Orlando, and Boris Kolonitskii. *Interpreting the Russian Revolution: The Language and Symbols of 1917.* New Haven, Conn.: Yale University Press, 1999.

Finer, S. *The Life and Times of Edwin Chadwick.* London: Methuen, 1970.
Fitzpatrick, Sheila. *The Commissariat of Enlightenment: Soviet Organization of Education and the Arts under Lunacharsky, October 1917–1921.* Cambridge: Cambridge University Press, 1970.
———. *The Cultural Front: Power and Culture in Revolutionary Russia.* Ithaca, N.Y.: Cornell University Press, 1992.
———. *Everyday Stalinism: Ordinary Life in Extraordinary Times: Soviet Russia in the 1930s.* Oxford: Oxford University Press, 1999.
———. *The Russian Revolution.* Oxford: Oxford University Press, 2001.
Fitzpatrick, Sheila, Alexander Rabinowitch, and Richard Stites, eds. *Russia in the Era of NEP: Explorations in Soviet Society and Culture.* Bloomington: Indiana University Press, 1985.
Foucault, Michel. *The Birth of the Clinic: An Archaeology of Medical Perception.* 1973. Reprint, New York: Vintage Books, 1994.
———. *Discipline and Punish: The Birth of the Prison.* 1977. Reprint, New York: Vintage Books, 1995.
———. *The History of Sexuality: An Introduction.* 1978. Reprint, New York: Vintage Books, 1990.
Frank, Stephen P. *Crime, Cultural Conflict, and Justice in Rural Russia, 1856–1914.* Berkeley: University of California Press, 1999.
Freidmin, S. Ia., ed. *Obshchestvennye nachala v sovetskom zdravookhranenii.* Leningrad: Meditsina, 1966.
Frieden, Nancy Mandelker. *Russian Physicians in an Era of Reform and Revolution, 1856–1905.* Princeton, N.J.: Princeton University Press, 1981.
Frierson, Cathy A. *Peasant Icons: Representations of Rural People in Late Nineteenth-Century Russia.* New York: Oxford University Press, 1993.
Frykman, Jonas, and Orvar Lofgren, eds. *Culture Builders: A Historical Anthropology of Middle-Class Life.* New Brunswick, N.J.: Rutgers University Press, 1987.
Gauldie, Enid. *Cruel Habitations: A History of Working-Class Housing, 1780–1918.* London: Ruskin House, 1974.
Geoghegan, Vincent. *Utopianism and Marxism.* London: Methuen, 1987.
Gerovitch, Slava. "Love-Hate for Man-Machine Metaphors in Soviet Physiology: From Pavlov to Physiological Cybernetics." *Science in Context* 15 (2002).
Gilman, Sander L. *Picturing Health and Illness: Images of Identity and Difference.* Baltimore, Md.: Johns Hopkins University Press, 1995.
———. *Smoke: A Global History of Smoking.* London: Reaktion, 2004.
Glants, Musya, and Joyce Toomre, eds. *Food in Russian History and Culture.* Bloomington: Indiana University Press, 1997.
Gleason, Abbott, Peter Kenez, and Richard Stites, eds. *Bolshevik Culture: Experiment and Order in the Russian Revolution.* Bloomington: Indiana University Press, 1985.
Goering, Laura. "'Russian Nervousness': Neurasthenia and National Identity in Nineteenth-Century Russia." *Medical History* 47 (January 2003).
Goldman, Wendy. *Women, the State and Revolution: Soviet Family Policy and Social Life, 1917–1936.* Cambridge: Cambridge University Press, 1993.
Gorham, Michael S. *Speaking in Soviet Tongues: Language, Culture and the Politics of Voice in Revolutionary Russia.* De Kalb: Northern Illinois University Press, 2003.

Gorsuch, Anne E. *Youth in Revolutionary Russia: Enthusiasts, Bohemians, Delinquents.* Bloomington: Indiana University Press, 2000.

Goscilo, Helena, and Beth Holmgren, eds. *Russia, Women, Culture.* Bloomington: Indiana University Press, 1996.

Goubert, Jean-Pierre. *The Conquest of Water: The Advent of Health in the Industrial Age.* Cambridge: Polity Press, 1989.

Graham, Loren R. *Science and Philosophy in the Soviet Union.* New York: Alfred A. Knopf, 1972.

———. *Science in Russia and the Soviet Union: A Short History.* New York: Cambridge University Press, 1993.

Grossman, Ia. L., ed. *Sanitarno-prosvetitel'naia rabota v sanatoriiakh i domakh otdykha (metodicheskie materialy).* Moscow: Gosizdat, 1964.

Gruber, Helmut. *Red Vienna: Working-Class Culture, 1919–1934.* New York: Oxford University Press, 1991.

Gutkin, A. Ia., and Z. G. Frenkel, eds. *Zdravookhranenie v sovetskoi Rossii za X let (1917–1927).* Leningrad: Prakticheskaia meditsina, 1927.

Hachten, Elizabeth Andrews. "Science in the Service of Society: Bacteriology, Medicine, and Hygiene in Russia, 1855–1907." Ph.D. diss., University of Wisconsin–Madison, 1991.

Hagen, Mark von. *Soldiers in the Proletarian Dictatorship: The Red Army and the Soviet Socialist State, 1917–1930.* Ithaca, N.Y.: Cornell University Press, 1990.

Haigh, Basil. "Design for a Medical Service: Peter the Great's Admiralty Regulations (1722)." *Medical History* 19 (1975).

Haimson, Leopold H. *The Russian Marxists and the Origins of Bolshevism.* Boston: Beacon Press, 1955.

Halfin, Igal. *Intimate Enemies: Demonizing the Bolshevik Opposition, 1918–1928.* Pittsburgh, Pa.: University of Pittsburgh Press, 2007.

———, ed. *Language and Revolution: Making Modern Political Identities.* London: Frank Cass, 2002.

Hanson, Stephen E. *Time and Revolution: Marxism and the Design of Soviet Institutions.* Chapel Hill: University of North Carolina Press, 1997.

Hatch, John. "The Politics of Mass Culture: Workers, Communists, and the Proletkul't in the Development of Workers' Clubs, 1921–1925." *Russian History* 13, nos. 2–3 (1986).

———. "Hangouts and Hangovers: State, Class and Culture in Moscow's Workers' Club Movement, 1925–1928." *Russian Review* 53 (January 1994).

Hau, Michael. *The Cult of Health and Beauty in Germany: A Social History, 1890–1930.* Chicago: University of Chicago Press, 2003.

Healey, Dan. *Homosexual Desire in Revolutionary Russia: The Regulation of Sexual and Gender Dissent.* Chicago: University of Chicago Press, 2002.

Hellbeck, Jochen. "Working, Struggling, Becoming: Stalin-Era Autobiographical Texts." *Russian Review* 60 (July 2001).

Hellebust, Rolf. "Aleksei Gastev and the Metallization of the Revolutionary Body." *Slavic Review* 56 (autumn 1997).

———. *Flesh to Metal: Soviet Literature and the Alchemy of Revolution.* Ithaca, N.Y.: Cornell University Press, 2003.

Herlihy, Patricia. *The Alcoholic Empire: Vodka and Politics in Late Imperial Russia.* Oxford: Oxford University Press, 2002.

Hertzler, Joyce Oramel. *The History of Utopian Thought.* New York: Cooper Square Publishers, 1965.

Hesli, Vicki L., and Margaret H. Mills, eds. *Medical Issues and Health Care Reform in Russia.* Lewiston, N.Y.: Edwin Mellen Press, 1999.

Hirsch, Francine. *Empire of Nations: Ethnographic Knowledge and the Making of the Soviet Union.* Ithaca, N.Y.: Cornell University Press, 2005.

Hoffmann, David L. "Mothers in the Motherland: Stalinist Pronatalism in Its Pan-European Context." *Journal of Social History* 34 (fall 2000).

———. *Peasant Metropolis: Social Identities in Moscow, 1929–1941.* Ithaca, N.Y.: Cornell University Press, 1994.

———. *Stalinist Values: The Cultural Norms of Soviet Modernity, 1917–1941.* Ithaca, N.Y.: Cornell University Press, 2003.

Hoffmann, David L., and Yanni Kotsonis, eds. *Russian Modernity: Politics, Knowledge, Practices.* New York: St. Martin's Press, 2000.

Hoffmann, David L., et al. "Ex Tempore: Stalinism and the 'Great Retreat.'" *Kritika* 5 (fall 2004).

Holquist, Peter. "'Information Is the Alpha and Omega of Our Work': Bolshevik Surveillance in Its Pan-European Context." *Journal of Modern History* 69 (September 1997).

———. *Making War, Forging Revolution: Russia's Continuum of Crisis, 1914–1921.* Cambridge, Mass.: Harvard University Press, 2002.

———. "Violent Russia, Deadly Marxism? Russia in the Epoch of Violence, 1905–21." *Kritika* 4 (summer 2003).

Horn, David G. *Social Bodies: Science, Reproduction, and Italian Modernity.* Princeton, N.J.: Princeton University Press, 1994.

Houtaud, Alphonse d', and Mark G. Field. *Cultural Images of Health: A Neglected Dimension.* Commack, N.Y.: Nova Science Publishers, 1995.

Hoy, Suellen. *Chasing Dirt: The American Pursuit of Cleanliness.* New York: Oxford University Press, 1995.

Hughes, Lindsey. *Russia in the Age of Peter the Great.* New Haven, Conn.: Yale University Press, 1998.

Husband, William B., ed., *The Human Tradition in Modern Russia.* Wilmington, Del.: Scholarly Resources, 2000.

Hutchinson, John F. *Politics and Public Health in Revolutionary Russia, 1890–1918.* Baltimore, Md.: Johns Hopkins University Press, 1990.

Hyde, Gordon. *The Soviet Health Service: A Historical and Comparative Study.* London: Lawrence & Wishart, 1974.

Iarovinskii, M. Ia. *Zdravookhranenie Moskvy, 1581–2000, gg.* Moscow: Meditsina, 1988.

Institut organizatsii zdravookhraneniia i istorii meditsiny im. N. A. Semashko. *Leninskie idei ob okhrane zdorov'ia naroda.* Moscow: Medgiz, 1961.

Johansson, Kurt. *Aleksej Gastev: Proletarian Bard of the Machine Age.* Stockholm: Minab/Gotab, 1983.

Johnson, Robert Eugene. *Peasant and Proletarian: The Working Class of Moscow in the Late Nineteenth Century.* New Brunswick, N.J.: Rutgers University Press, 1979.

Jordanova, Ludmilla. *Sexual Visions: Images of Gender in Science and Medicine between the Eighteenth and Twentieth Centuries.* New York: Harvester Wheatsheaf, 1989.

Kamminga, Harmke, and Andrew Cunningham, eds. *The Science and Culture of Nutrition, 1840–1940.* Amsterdam: Rodopi, 1995.

Kanevskii, L. O., E. I. Lotova, and Kh. I. Idel'chik, eds. *Osnovnye cherty razvitiia meditsiny v Rossii v period kapitalizma, 1861–1917.* Moscow: Medgiz, 1956.

Kaser, Michael. *Health Care in the Soviet Union and Eastern Europe.* Boulder, Colo.: Westview Press, 1976.

Kasson, John F. *Civilizing the Machine: Technology and Republican Values in America, 1776–1900.* New York: Grossman Publishers, 1976.

———. *Houdini, Tarzan, and the Perfect Man: The White Male Body and the Challenge of Modernity in America.* New York: Hill & Wang, 2001.

———. *Rudeness and Civility: Manners in Nineteenth-Century Urban America.* New York: Hill & Wang, 1990.

Kelly, Catriona. *Refining Russia: Advice Literature, Polite Culture, and Gender from Catherine to Yeltsin.* Oxford: Oxford University Press, 2001.

———. *Utopias: Russian Modernist Texts, 1905–1940.* London: Penguin Books, 1999.

Kelly, Catriona, and David Shepherd, eds. *Constructing Russian Culture in the Age of Revolution, 1881–1940.* Oxford: Oxford University Press, 1998.

———. *Russian Cultural Studies: An Introduction.* Oxford: Oxford University Press, 1998.

Kharkhordin, Oleg. *The Collective and the Individual in Russia: A Study of Practices.* Berkeley: University of California Press, 1999.

Khromov, B. M., and A. V. Sveshnikov. *Zdravookhranenie Leningrada: Kratkii istoricheskii ocherk.* Leningrad: Lenizdat, 1969.

Kiaer, Christina, and Eric Naiman, eds. *Everyday Life in Early Soviet Russia: Taking the Revolution Inside.* Bloomington: Indiana University Press, 2006.

Kieckhefer, Richard. *Magic in the Middle Ages.* New York: Cambridge University Press, 1989.

Koenker, Diane. "Men against Women on the Shop Floor in Early Soviet Russia: Gender and Class in the Socialist Workplace." *American Historical Review* 100 (December 1995).

———. *Moscow Workers and the 1917 Revolution.* Princeton, N.J.: Princeton University Press, 1981.

———. *Republic of Labor: Russian Printers and Soviet Socialism, 1918–1930.* Ithaca, N.Y.: Cornell University Press, 2005.

Koenker, Diane, William G. Rosenberg, and Ronald Grigor Suny, eds. *Party, State and Society in the Russian Civil War: Explorations in Social History.* Bloomington: Indiana University Press, 1989.

Konstantinov, G. F. *Zdravookhranenie v SSSR (Statisticheskii spravochnik).* Moscow: Medgiz, 1957.

Kopp, Anatole. *Town and Revolution: Soviet Architecture and City Planning, 1917–1935.* New York: George Braziller, 1970.

Kopp, James J. "Cosimo Noto's *The Ideal City* (1903): New Orleans as Medical Utopia." *Utopian Studies* 1, no. 2 (1990).

Kotkin, Stephen. *Magnetic Mountain: Stalinism as a Civilization.* Berkeley: University of California Press, 1995.

Koven, Seth, and Sonya Michel, eds. *Mothers of a New World: Maternalist Politics and the Origins of Welfare States.* London: Routledge, 1983.

Kovrigin, M. D., ed. *Okhrana narodnogo zdorov'ia v SSSR.* Moscow: Meditsinskaia literatura, 1957.

Kowalsky, Sharon. "Making Crime Soviet: Women, Deviance, and the Development of Criminology in Early Soviet Russia." Ph.D. diss., University of North Carolina, Chapel Hill, 2004.

Kozlov, I. I., ed. *Zdravnitsy profsoiuzov SSSR: Kurorty, sanatorii, pansionaty i doma otdykha.* Moscow: Profizdat, 1973.

Krementsov, Nikolai. *The Cure: The Story of Cancer and Politics from the Annals of the Cold War.* Chicago: University of Chicago Press, 2002.

Kumanev, V. A. *Sotsializm i vsenarodnaia gramotnost': Likvidatsiia massovoi negramotnosti v SSSR.* Moscow: Nauka, 1967.

Ladd-Taylor, M. *Mother-Work: Women, Children, Welfare and the State, 1890–1930.* Urbana: University of Illinois Press, 1994.

———. *Raising a Baby the Government Way: Mothers' Letters to the Children's Bureau, 1915–1932.* New Brunswick, N.J.: Rutgers University Press, 1986.

Leavitt, Judith Walzer. *Brought to Bed: Childbearing in America, 1750–1950.* New York: Oxford University Press, 1986.

Leavitt, Sarah A. *From Catharine Beecher to Martha Stewart: A Cultural History of Domestic Advice.* Chapel Hill: University of North Carolina Press, 2002.

Lebina, N. B. *Povsednevnaia zhizn' sovetskogo goroda: Normy i anomalii, 1920–1930 gody.* St. Petersburg: Letnii sad, 1999.

———. *Rabochaia molodezh' Leningrada: Trud i sotsial'nyi oblik, 1921–1925 gody.* Leningrad: Nauka, 1982.

Levin, Eve. *Sex and Society in the World of the Orthodox Slavs, 900–1700.* Ithaca, N.Y.: Cornell University Press, 1989.

Levinston, Harvey A. *Revolution at the Table: The Transformation of the American Diet.* New York: Oxford University Press, 1988.

Lewis, Jane. *The Politics of Motherhood: Child and Maternal Welfare in England, 1900–1939.* London: Croom Helm, 1980.

Lewis, R. A. *Edwin Chadwick and the Public Health Movement.* London: Longmans & Green, 1952.

Lindenmeyr, Adele. *Poverty Is Not a Vice: Charity, Society, and the State in Imperial Russia.* Princeton, N.J.: Princeton University Press, 1996.

Lindenmeyer, Kriste. *"A Right to Childhood": The U.S. Children's Bureau and Child Welfare, 1912–1946.* Urbana: University of Illinois Press, 1997.

Livers, Keith A. *Constructing the Stalinist Body: Fictional Representations of Corporeality in the Stalinist 1930s.* Lanham, Md.: Lexington Books, 2004.

Mackaman, Douglas Peter. *Leisure Settings: Bourgeois Culture, Medicine, and the Spa in Modern France.* Chicago: University of Chicago Press, 1998.

Madriaga, Isabel de. *Catherine the Great: A Short History.* 1990. Reprint, New Haven, Conn.: Yale University Press, Yale Nota Bene, 2002.

Mally, Lynn. *Culture of the Future: The Proletkult Movement in Revolutionary Russia.* Berkeley: University of California Press, 1990.

———. "Performing the New Woman: The Komsomolka as Actress and Image in Soviet Youth Theater." *Journal of Social History* 30 (fall 1996).

———. *Revolutionary Acts: Amateur Theater in the Soviet State, 1917–1938.* Ithaca, N.Y.: Cornell University Press, 2000.

Manning, Roberta T. *The Crisis of the Old Order in Russia: Government and Gentry.* Princeton, N.J.: Princeton University Press, 1982.

Manuel, Frank E., and Fritzie P. Manuel. *Utopian Thought in the Western World.* Cambridge, Mass.: Harvard University Press, Belknap Press, 1979.

Martin, Dale B. *The Corinthian Body.* New Haven, Conn.: Yale University Press, 1995.

McCuaig, Katherine. *The Weariness, the Fever, and the Fret: The Campaign against Tuberculosis in Canada, 1900–1950.* Montreal: McGill-Queen's University Press, 1999.

McGrew, Roderik E. *Russia and the Cholera, 1823–1832.* Madison: University of Wisconsin Press, 1965.

McGuire, Robert A. *Red Virgin Soil: Soviet Literature in the 1920s.* Princeton, N.J.: Princeton University Press, 1968.

McReynolds, Louise. *Russia at Play: Leisure Activities at the End of the Tsarist Era.* Ithaca, N.Y.: Cornell University Press, 2003.

Michaels, Paula A. *Curative Powers: Medicine and Empire in Stalin's Central Asia.* Pittsburgh, Pa.: University of Pittsburgh Press, 2003.

Mirsky, Mark. *Promoting Public Health: The Story of Soviet Medical Science.* Moscow: Novosti Press Agency, 1972.

Morton, Henry W. *Soviet Sport: Mirror of Soviet Society.* New York: Collier Books, 1963.

Naiman, Eric. *Sex in Public: The Incarnation of Early Soviet Ideology.* Princeton, N.J.: Princeton University Press, 1997.

Neary, Rebecca Balmas. "Mothering Socialist Society: The Wife-Activists' Movement and the Soviet Culture of Daily Life, 1934–1941." *Russian Review* 3 (1999).

Neuberger, Joan. *Hooliganism: Crime, Culture, and Power in St. Petersburg, 1900–1914.* Berkeley: University of California Press, 1993.

Nove, Alec. *An Economic History of the U.S.S.R.* London: Allen Lange, 1969.

Nye, Robert A. *Crime, Madness, and Politics in Modern France: The Medical Concept of National Decline.* Princeton, N.J.: Princeton University Press, 1984.

Oakley, Ann. *The Captured Womb: A History of the Medical Care of Pregnant Women.* Oxford: Basil Blackwell, 1984.

Ott, Katherine. *Fevered Lives: Tuberculosis in American Culture since 1870.* Cambridge, Mass.: Harvard University Press, 1996.

Outram, Dorrinda. *The Body and the French Revolution: Sex, Class and Political Culture.* New Haven, Conn.: Yale University Press, 1989.

Palmer, Phyllis. *Domesticity and Dirt: Housewives and Domestic Servants in the United States, 1920–1945.* Philadelphia, Pa.: Temple University Press, 1989.

Park, Roberta J. "Physiology and Anatomy Are Destiny!? Brains, Bodies and Exercise in Nineteenth-Century American Thought." *Journal of Sport History* 18, no. 1 (spring 1991).

Patenaude, Bertrand M. *The Big Show in Bololand: The American Relief Expedition to Soviet Russia in the Famine of 1921.* Stanford, Calif.: Stanford University Press, 2002.
Patterson, K. David. "Typhus and Its Control in Russia, 1870–1940." *Medical History* 37 (1993).
Pedersen, Susan. *Family, Dependence, and the Origins of the Welfare State: Britain and France, 1914–1945.* Cambridge: Cambridge University Press, 1993.
Peiss, Kathy. *Cheap Amusements: Working Women and Leisure in Turn-of-the-Century New York.* Philadelphia, Pa.: Temple University Press, 1986.
Peris, Daniel. *Storming the Heavens: The Soviet League of the Militant Godless.* Ithaca, N.Y.: Cornell University Press, 1998.
Perrie, Maureen, and Andrei Pavlov. *Ivan the Terrible.* London: Longman, 2003.
Peterson, Alan, and Robin Burton, eds. *Foucault, Health and Medicine.* London: Routledge, 1997.
Petrone, Karen. *Life Has Become More Joyous, Comrades: Celebrations in the Time of Stalin.* Bloomington: Indiana University Press, 2000.
Phillips, Laura L. *Bolsheviks and the Bottle: Drink and Worker Culture in St. Petersburg, 1900–1929.* De Kalb: Northern Illinois University Press, 2000.
Pick, Daniel. *Faces of Degeneration: A European Disorder, c. 1848–c. 1918.* Cambridge: Cambridge University Press, 1989.
Pinnow, Kenneth M. "Violence against the Collective Self and the Problem of Social Integration in Early Bolshevik Russia." *Kritika* 4 (summer 2003).
Porter, Dorothy. *Health, Civilization and the State: A History of Public Health from Ancient to Modern Times.* London: Routledge, 1999.
Porter, Roy. *The Greatest Benefit to Mankind: A Medical History of Humanity.* New York: W. W. Norton, 1997.
Porter, Theodore M. *The Rise of Statistical Thinking, 1820–1900.* Princeton, N.J.: Princeton University Press, 1986.
Potova, E. I. *Bor'ba s infektsionnimi bolezniami v SSSR, 1917–1967.* Moscow: Meditsina, 1967.
Proctor, Robert N. *The Nazi War on Cancer.* Princeton, N.J.: Princeton University Press, 1999.
Rabinbach, Anson. *The Human Motor: Energy, Fatigue, and the Origins of Modernity.* Berkeley: University of California Press, 1990.
Rabinow, Paul. *French Modern: Norms and Forms of the Social Environment.* Chicago: University of Chicago Press, 1989.
Rabinowitch, Alexander. *The Bolsheviks Come to Power.* New York: W. W. Norton, 1976.
———. *Prelude to Revolution: The Petrograd Bolsheviks and the July 1917 Uprising.* Bloomington: Indiana University Press, 1968.
Raeff, M. *The Well-Ordered Police State.* New Haven, Conn.: Yale University Press, 1983.
Ransel, David L., ed. *The Family in Imperial Russia: New Lines of Historical Research.* Urbana: University of Illinois Press, 1978.
———. *Mothers of Misery: Child Abandonment in Russia.* Princeton, N.J.: Princeton University Press, 1988.
———. *Village Mothers: Three Generations of Change in Russia and Tataria.* Bloomington: Indiana University Press, 2000.

Rees, E. A. *State Control in Soviet Russia: The Rise and Fall of the Workers' and Peasants' Inspectorate, 1920–1934.* New York: St. Martin's Press, 1987.

Retish, Aaron. "Creating Peasant Citizens: Rituals of Power, Rituals of Citizenship in Viatka Province, 1917." *Revolutionary Russia* 16 (June 2003).

———. "Peasant Identities in Russia's Turmoil: Status, Gender, and Ethnicity in Viatka Province, 1914–1921." Ph.D. diss., The Ohio State University, 2003.

Riordan, James. "The Rise, Fall and Rebirth of Sporting Women in Russia and the USSR." *Journal of Sport History* 18 (spring 1991).

———. *Sport in Soviet Society: Development of Sport and Physical Education in Russia and the USSR.* Cambridge: Cambridge University Press, 1977.

Rosen, George. *A History of Public Health.* New York: MD Publications, 1958.

Ryan, Michael. *The Organization of Soviet Medical Care.* London: Basil Blackwell & Mott, 1978.

Sadov, A. A. *Zaraznye bolezni i byt.* Leningrad: Leningradskaia pravda, n.d.

Samoilov, V. O. *Istoriia Rossiiskoi meditsiny.* Moscow: Epidavr, 1997.

Schulz, Heinrich E., Paul K. Urban, and Andrew I. Lebed, eds. *Who Was Who in the USSR.* Metuchen, N.J.: Scarecrow Press, 1972.

Service, Robert. *The Bolshevik Party in Revolution: A Study in Organizational Change, 1917–1923.* New York: Barnes & Noble Books, 1979.

Shapovalov, Andrei Valer'evich. *Ocherki istorii i kul'tury potrebleniia tabaka v Sibiri: XVII—pervaia polovina XX vv.* Novosibirsk: Progress-Servis, 2002.

Shkolnikov, Vladimir, France Mesle, and Jacques Vallin. "Health Crisis in Russia. I. Recent Trends in Life Expectancy and Causes of Death from 1970 to 1993." *Population: An English Selection* 8 (1996).

Sieder, Reinhard. "Housing Policy, Social Welfare, and Daily Life in 'Red Vienna,' 1919–34." *Oral History Journal* 13 (1985).

Siegelbaum, Lewis H. "The Shaping of Soviet Workers' Leisure: Workers' Clubs and Palaces of Culture in the 1930s." *International Labor and Working-Class History* 56 (fall 1999).

———. *Soviet State and Society between Revolutions, 1918–1929.* Cambridge: Cambridge University Press, 1992.

Sigerist, Henry. *Medicine and Health in the Soviet Union.* New York: Citadel Press, 1947.

———. *Socialized Medicine in the Soviet Union.* New York: W. W. Norton, 1937.

Skocpol, Theda. *Protecting Soldiers and Mothers: The Political Origins of Social Policy in the United States.* Cambridge, Mass.: Harvard University Press, 1992.

Slezkine, Yuri. *Arctic Mirrors: Russia and the Small Peoples of the North.* Ithaca, N.Y.: Cornell University Press, 1996.

Smart, Carol, ed. *Regulating Womanhood: Historical Essays on Marriage, Motherhood and Sexuality.* London: Routledge, 1992.

Snead, M. Christine, and Derek F. DeWaal. "Health Lifestyles in Russia and the Socialist Heritage." *Journal of Health and Social Behavior* 43 (March 2002).

Solomon, Susan Gross. "David and Goliath in Soviet Public Health: The Rivalry of Social Hygienists and Psychiatrists for Authority Over the *Bytovoi* Alcoholic." *Soviet Studies* 41 (April 1989).

Solomon, Susan Gross, and John F. Hutchinson, eds. *Health and Society in Revolutionary Russia.* Bloomington: Indiana University Press, 1990.

Sontag, Susan. *Illness as Metaphor and AIDS and Its Metaphors.* New York: Anchor Books, 1990.

Soskin, V. L. *Sovetskaia massovaia kul'tura: U istokov (1917–1927 gg.).* Novosibirsk: Novosibirskii gosudarstvennyi universitet, 2001.

Starks, Tricia. "Red Star/Black Lungs: Anti-Tobacco Campaigns in Twentieth-Century Russia." *Journal of the Social History of Alcohol and Drugs* 21, no. 1 (fall 2006).

Steinberg, Mark. *Proletarian Imagination: Self, Modernity, and the Sacred in Russia, 1910–1925.* Ithaca, N.Y.: Cornell University Press, 2002.

Steiner, Evgeny. *Stories for Little Comrades: Revolutionary Artists and the Making of Early Soviet Children's Books.* Seattle: University of Washington Press, 1999.

Steinmetz, George. *Regulating the Social: The Welfare State and Local Politics in Imperial Germany.* Princeton, N.J.: Princeton University Press, 1993.

Stewart, Mary Lynn. *For Health and Beauty: Physical Culture for Frenchwomen, 1880s–1930s.* Baltimore, Md.: Johns Hopkins University Press, 2001.

Stites, Richard. *Revolutionary Dreams: Utopian Vision and Experimental Life in the Russian Revolution.* New York: Oxford University Press, 1989.

———. *Russian Popular Culture: Entertainment and Society since 1900.* Cambridge: Cambridge University Press, 1992.

Stovall, Tyler. *The Rise of the Paris Red Belt.* Berkeley: University of California Press, 1990.

Teller, Michael E. *The Tuberculosis Movement: A Public Health Campaign in the Progressive Era.* New York: Greenwood Press, 1988.

Thurston, Robert W. *Liberal City, Conservative State: Moscow and Russia's Urban Crisis, 1906–1914.* New York: Oxford University Press, 1987.

Tomes, Nancy. *The Gospel of Germs: Men, Women and the Microbe in American Life.* Cambridge, Mass.: Harvard University Press, 1998.

Transchel, Kathy S. *Under the Influence: Working-Class Drinking, Temperance, and Cultural Revolution in Russia, 1895–1932.* Pittsburgh, Pa.: University of Pittsburgh Press, 2006.

Turner, Bryan S. *The Body and Society: Explorations in Social Theory.* Oxford: Basil Blackwell, 1984.

———. *Regulating Bodies: Essays in Medical Sociology.* London: Routledge, 1992.

Tuve, Jeanette E. *The First Russian Women Physicians.* Newtonville, Mass.: Oriental Research Partners, 1984.

Venediktov, D. D. *Zdravookhranenie Rossii: Krizis i puti preodoleniia.* Moscow: Meditsina, 1999.

Vigarello, George. *Concepts of Cleanliness: Changing Attitudes in France Since the Middle Ages.* Cambridge: Cambridge University Press, 1988.

Vucinich, Alexander. *Social Thought in Tsarist Russia: The Quest for a General Science of Society, 1861–1917.* Chicago: University of Chicago Press, 1976.

Waters, Elizabeth. "Child-Care Posters and the Modernization of Motherhood." *Sbornik-Study Group on the Russian Revolution* 13 (1987).

———. "Teaching Mothercraft in Post-Revolutionary Russia." *Australian Slavonic and East European Studies* 1 (July 1987).

Weindling, Paul. *Health, Race and German Politics between National Unification and Nazism, 1870–1945.* Cambridge: Cambridge University Press, 1989.

Weiner, Amir. *Making Sense of War: The Second World War and the Fate of the Bolshevik Revolution.* Princeton, N.J.: Princeton University Press, 2001.

Weiner, Dora. *The Citizen-Patient in Revolutionary and Imperial Paris.* Baltimore, Md.: Johns Hopkins University Press, 1993.
West, Sally. "The Material Promised Land: Advertising's Modern Agenda in Late Imperial Russia." *Russian Review* 57 (July 1998).
White, Stephen. *The Bolshevik Poster.* New Haven, Conn.: Yale University Press, 1988.
———. *Russia Goes Dry: Alcohol, State and Society.* Cambridge: Cambridge University Press, 1996.
———, ed. *New Directions in Soviet History.* Cambridge: Cambridge University Press, 1992.
Wildman, Allan K. *The End of the Russian Imperial Army.* Princeton, N.J.: Princeton University Press, 1980–87.
Williams, Christopher. "Soviet Public Health: A Case Study of Leningrad, 1917–1932." Ph.D. diss., University of Essex, 1989.
Wood, Elizabeth. *The Baba and the Comrade: Gender and Politics in Revolutionary Russia.* Bloomington: Indiana University Press, 1997.
Youngblood, Denise J. *Movies for the Masses: Popular Cinema and Soviet Society in the 1920s.* Cambridge: Cambridge University Press, 1992.
Zaletova, Lidya, et al., eds. *Revolutionary Costume: Soviet Clothing and Textiles of the 1920s.* New York: Rizzoli Publications, 1989.
Zanozin, V. N., and E. A. Adamenko, eds. *Blagotvoritel'nost' i miloserdie: Rubezh XIX–XX vekov.* Saint Petersburg: Liki Rossii, 2000.
Zdorov'e naseleniia i metody ego izucheniia (izbrannye proizvedenia). Moscow: Statistika, 1979.

INDEX